The
GOOD
HEALTH
Handbook

DR PETER MANSFIELD

The
GOOD
HEALTH
Handbook

Help yourself get better

GRAFTON BOOKS
A Division of the Collins Publishing Group

LONDON GLASGOW
TORONTO SYDNEY AUCKLAND

Grafton Books
A Division of the Collins Publishing Group
8 Grafton Street, London W1X 3LA

Published by Grafton Books 1988

British Library Cataloguing in Publication Data

Mansfield, Peter, *1943–*
    The good health handbook.
    1. Man. Health. Self-care – Manuals
    I. Title
    613

ISBN 0–246–13169–1

Printed in Great Britain by
Hartnolls Ltd, Bodmin, Cornwall

Dedicated to the memory of

MAJOR-GENERAL SIR ROBERT McCARRISON, CIE, MD, FRCP
astute observer, painstaking scientist, and clear visionary

through whose writings, neglected by medical opinion for over fifty years,
I among others have begun to realize the relationship
between food and health

Contents

Acknowledgements

This book stems from the learning of many lives, most of them long complete, but generously shared with me by several teachers. My greatest debt is to some I have never met who took the trouble to write their insights down – Drs Max Bircher-Benner, Edward Bach, Henry Lindlahr, Robert McCarrison, Lionel Picton, Are Waerland and George Scott Williamson in particular. Dr John Horder taught me my craft and introduced me to Dr Innes Pearse, who opened most of these authors to me; Drs Barbara and Gordon Latto acquainted me with several of the others, and taught me much besides that they had learned themselves. Dr Michael Balint got me listening to people, and helped me understand them. Tony Neate, Eric and Christine Gregory and through them Colin Bloy, Bruce MacManaway and Muz Murray have widened my horizons by leaps and bounds in the last few years, and helped me to tie up a good many loose ends.

Invaluable information, encouragement and much excellent advice has come from Mary Langman these seventeen years, without which my knowledge of the Pioneer Health Centre would be inaccurate, unbalanced and very incomplete; she probably still has reservations. Meanwhile Celia Monument was taking endless pains, well beyond the reasonable call of secretarial duty, over disorderly piles of manuscript. By producing from these several respectable pamphlets and a small book she prepared me to tackle something bigger. Leslie Kenton then put in some timely encouragement which crystallized the idea that became this book.

But no-one of my temperament can get anywhere without the homely wisdom, sublime tolerance and abiding love of a good woman. Ever since we met, Pamela has kept my cup filled to overflowing – often by pouring from her own. In this way Duncan, Hazel and Geoffrey entered our lives: my excitement at seeing health so vividly at work in them got the book finished.

Peter Mansfield
July 1987

The
GOOD
HEALTH
Handbook

Introduction

WHY DOCTORS DISAPPOINT

There can never before have been a time when so many doctors have been available to people in the Western world, nor been so frequently consulted by them. The mass of media effort devoted to sickness and health indicates the fascination they provide. Yet people frequently nowadays come away from consultations with their doctors vaguely disappointed or openly dissatisfied.

The reasons vary. Often the doctor has simply not heard what the person has said. If he is very overworked he may try to save time by anticipating a common problem, cut short the description and get straight down to the treatment. So long as the doctor opens his mind at least a little way to each new consultation and does not immediately reach for a prescription pad, he will be right most of the time. But when he guesses wrongly the patient will not be pleased, and the treatment will probably be ineffective too.

There are other ways of working. The doctor may listen carefully but classify the story according to how he[1] intends to deal with it. He may for instance decide to call it a 'common cold', for which he is prepared to relieve symptoms only; or 'sino-bronchitis', which justifies antibiotic treatment. This is a reasonably practical and honest way to work, so long as the doctor stays alert for problems that occur rarely. But it frustrates patients who in the past have not been helped by his standard treatment and who want to tackle their problem some other way.

A conventional second opinion can be less satisfactory still. Medical and surgical specialists, by choosing these careers, show much more commitment to medicine and science as systems of thought. They tend to work systematically within a clearly defined part of the body. Though they may have time to listen to the patient's story in more detail, they are more likely to spend this pursuing answers in depth to technical questions that interest them. In consequence specialists usually show less inclination to accept departures from their expectations, not more. And they can always terminate their involvement by declaring that the problem does not lie 'in my department'.

All these methods of working, and their drawbacks, arise from pressure felt by doctors to close cases as soon as they can and work on down the queue. Few family doctors that I know like this situation very much; most would rather get to know their patients individually and learn to respond accurately to

---

[1] I shall use the male pronoun for doctors throughout; feminist readers will soon see that this is very far from being any kind of insult to the female sex.

every subtle nuance in each one's story. They could even set themselves up for this if they chose, by carrying smaller lists of patients and offering each more time.

But they need to realize that choice early in their careers: for with it comes a correspondingly smaller income, and less esteem among their colleagues. Most young doctors enter their calling with enthusiasm and positively welcome a huge workload at first. By the time they have tired of it they are dependent on the high income it earns and set about using that to protect themselves from what they see as excessive demand. Very few have the leisure or mental agility to recognize their true situation, and fewer still the courage to dismantle it. So the image of the overworked doctor, slightly aloof for his own preservation, is fed and maintained from one generation to the next.

This self-defensive apparatus also prevents doctors from discovering many truths for which their training does not prepare them. Few ever see how deftly people frame their complaints in a form the doctor will accept, so as to streamline the process of consultation and obtain the service they want. And they can never know anything of the wide range of problems people no longer bother doctors with, realizing in advance that they are unlikely to be helpful. Consequently, the experience most doctors accumulate during their careers is very partial and peculiar, tending to reinforce any preconceptions and biases they have asserted from the beginning. And the more confidently they maintained those preconceptions, the more firmly are they reinforced by the people choosing to consult them.

Doctors in this position are very unlikely to face new problems with open minds. They will prefer to fit unusual stories firmly into one of the mental pigeon-holes their habits have prepared, editing and shoe-horning as necessary. When the consequences are not what they expect, they tend to blame the patients before questioning their own mental rigidity. The patient usually tires of this situation long before the doctor and goes in search of a different interpretation of their problem. The great growth of complementary and alternative systems of medicine is the principal consequence.

ALTERNATIVES

To use these is not necessarily unwise, but opens up many pitfalls for the unwary. No mechanism yet exists to place people reliably with a form of therapy appropriate to their needs. With a few honourable exceptions, training for the complementary therapies is insufficient to prepare their practitioners for full professional independence. Standards of competence, ethical codes of practice and a unified system of official registration all await construction and acceptance. Even within each alternative discipline two or more schools of thought may co-exist uncomfortably, each with its own training scheme and sometimes more than one professional register. This fosters disorderly political strife rather than common purpose, a situation which no professional group or authority has yet seriously sought to reconcile.

The Working Party on Alternative Medicine, appointed by the British Medical Association's Board of Science and Education, reported conservatively in 1986, as they were bound to do. The whole of medicine is now constructed on the principles of material science, by whose criteria no other system can be justified. It will take broader minds to explore the territory beyond those safe confines, where things seem to happen that science cannot yet explain. Before that can be attempted, all the professions involved will need to learn much greater generosity of mutual regard.

My own experience has separated me from this materialist trend, or I could not have recognized it. I came to medicine sideways, from another university course. I did not like the exclusiveness of medical society, and stayed outside it. While still at medical school I pursued my interest in 'whole' people by opting for general practice, and later combined an extended training for this with four years of research into its basis. During this time my tutor fed and guided my curiosity with great wisdom, and introduced me to the only concept of health that has ever satisfied me. That concept has been the basis of my work ever since, and is the subject of Chapter One.

There followed an exciting and hectic period, during which I had to reinterpret all I had so far learnt. I found myself understanding people's problems differently, and giving different advice. This had a quite unforeseen effect. Those people felt free to treat me as a person myself, unprotected by any professional distance. That took some coping with, but proved well worth while. Not only was I forced under their critical scrutiny to practise as I preached; people began to tell me their experience directly, without massaging it into a form they thought I would accept.

So began a process of experiment and re-evaluation which gave me the different perspectives I now exercise. Along the way my wife and I founded a club for health cultivation, to be supported later by Templegarth Trust, a charity which promotes in various ways what we are learning.

One of the successful experiments made by the Trust was to gather together local practitioners of various therapeutic disciplines so that we could confer together with patients whose problems were particularly difficult and thereby learn to understand and trust one another. The result has been an extraordinarily fruitful growth in the service we are able collectively to offer, a local and temporary solution to the national problem I have been discussing.

USING THIS BOOK

It would be marvellous to extend this approach widely, and allow a creative solution of that problem to emerge. But it would take some time, and require as a motive force the kind of coherent pressure from consumers that we have recently seen working on chemical additives in food.

Meanwhile we shall remain prey to inadequate advice from our medical services, both orthodox and alternative. You deserve whatever help you can get to cope with this. And you may then be able to provide the pressure which will encourage the right kind of permanent change.

That is why I have written this book.

Part One offers a comprehensive and practical alternative outlook on health and disease from which you will see more clearly how to cope with your problems and any unhelpful medical responses to them. My basic proposition is that we live not just in one world but simultaneously in two, superimposed on one another but counterbalanced, like a landscape and its reflection in a lake. The landscape is tangible but meaningless, whereas the reflection is a dream-like vision in the mind's eye, laden with personal significance. I explore their nature and relationship in detail, then show how they clarify the facts of life and disease. This proposition arises for my part from fifteen years of practical experiment and discussion, amongst many thousands of people with a wide variety of needs and interests. And it draws on many centuries of sound healing tradition, embellished sometimes with new insights from this century.

Part Two is designed for reference, when in need of practical alternative ideas in particular situations. It examines a long list of the problems which in my experience most conventionally trained doctors deal with badly, and offers practical ways of tackling them. And I have carefully avoided recommending anything you cannot safely do for yourself or confidently ask of a practitioner qualified as I describe.

None of the recommendations will interfere with orthodox medicines you may wish to go on using, except where I have drawn attention to it. Consequently you are not obliged to confess use of these methods to your doctor or endure any kind of show-down with him. But if they work you can almost certainly find a tactful way of telling him, which is bound in the long run to help him open his mind, however he may react at first. Without this kind of feed-back, your doctor cannot fairly be expected to improve the way he handles your kind of problem.

Whenever in the past many individual consumers have acted coherently on an issue which concerns them all they have accomplished great things. I have a strong hunch that appropriate medical care will prove to be one of those issues.

Note

Cross-references appear in SMALL CAPITALS. Words in *italics* followed by an asterisk are listed in the index where they are explained and/or can be explored through cross-references.

PART ONE

1 *Good Living*

IMPRISONED BY IDEAS

If you ask experienced people which of life's various necessities they value most, good health ranks very high among their answers. But if you then ask what they mean by that you will get only the vaguest of replies. People confuse good health with fitness, beauty or energy, with being average or 'normal' or with a lack of bodily imperfections and illnesses. Some cannot distinguish health from disease at all. Yet when buildings devoted to the treatment of disease can be called Health Centres and our National Health Service devotes itself entirely to the medical identification, treatment and prevention of disease, you can understand their confusion.

Doctors and health service administrators are no better off. For two generations they have been so totally preoccupied with delivering medical care that they rarely have a chance to think about health. A few on the international scene with a bit more time, in 1979 at the World Health Organization's historic Alma Ata meeting led the cry 'Health for All by the Year 2000!' What exactly this means remains only vaguely defined, however. And its practicality is discounted by doctors who can see how inadequately our medical services deal with today's demands, represented by lengthening queues of chronically sick people.

Since society takes its lead from doctors and health authorities, it too stolidly assumes that the only way to make people healthy is to treat their diseases as best we can. Our huge investment in medical care and drugs indicates where we have put our faith. Yet as evidence accumulates of the hopelessness of this approach, people show no signs of questioning or changing it. Instead most conclude pessimistically that health is unattainable, an idealistic goal we can in practice never reach.

That conclusion is by no means inescapable. There is nothing to stop us scrapping it entirely, re-examining the practical realities with fresh minds and drawing from them more useful ideas. There are still, for instance, many people who never see a doctor for years at a time yet remain stubbornly resilient and contented without their help. This kind of tough independence is highly desirable, and appears to be more than a matter of luck. What is it that protects these people from the kind of weakness others show? What keeps all of us free of infection most of the time, despite frequently repeated exposure to germs and viruses that are able at times to make us ill? Surely the answers to questions like these must get us closer to understanding the nature of health.

THE PRIMAL ADAPTIVE SYSTEM

Michel Odent is the first widely-read medical writer in forty years to take these questions seriously. By reconsidering what we know about the way our bodies work, he is able to draw revolutionary conclusions.

Self-defence, he says, is a misleadingly negative view of your immune system, whose primary purpose is to maintain your unique personal integrity or wholeness in very positive ways, regardless of the particular threats to your health that may exist at any given moment. What is more, your immune system is not alone in this function. Fundamental brain and hormonal mechanisms are so inextricably involved that Odent can no longer distinguish them as having separate functions. With immunity they make up your 'primal adaptive system', without which a separate unique life would not be possible.

He is forced to speculate a good deal to bridge gaps in our knowledge which have not yet aroused the curiosity of the major research foundations, and he may be mistaken in some details. But no error in his assembly of the facts can undermine his basic insight from them, which enables us at last to escape from the prison of our present ideas. Odent has re-discovered why, if you look for health in the state of your body, you will never find it. This is because your health is a way of carrying on – a working mechanism or process – and does not relate to your current state at all. If you were to liken life to a journey, your health is represented neither by a shiny new vehicle nor by your destination, but by your general day-to-day approach to travelling.

It turns out Odent is not the first to grasp this. Clear understanding can be found in the writings of the nineteenth-century French biologist Antoine Béchamp, and something of the kind is implied in ideas of a 'natural healing force' which date in various authors back to ancient times. The naturalistic physicians of the early part of this century based their entire practice on it. And the 1940s 'Peckham Experiment' (see pp. 12–13), the only comprehensive attempt doctors and biologists have ever made to identify the nature of human health, not only confirmed the beliefs of those old physicians but laid firm foundations for a modern understanding of the mechanism of health.

All these writings are fascinating studies in themselves, and will prove to have been far ahead of their time. I cannot do them justice here, and have paused only long enough to acknowledge our debt to them. My chief purpose is to set before you what they enable us to understand today.

TWO DIMENSIONS: QUANTITY AND QUALITY

If we work forward from Odent's starting-point, it quickly follows that there is a world of difference between what we do and the way we do it.

Our earliest curiosities as children are to discover what, when and where everything is, and our parents take pleasure in telling us. Under their guidance we grow up in a Western civilization based almost entirely on material science and technology which is totally preoccupied with refining our collective answers to those same basic questions. Our entire culture takes it for granted that knowledge of the quantity of things and their arrangement in space and time is an essential prerequisite of living. So we expect competitors in any kind of race to explore the layout and condition of the course thoroughly first.

But quantity is sterile in itself. At best it only defines a flat, featureless landscape or agenda in which living can take place. It does not live itself: that only begins when quantities start moving to some qualitative purpose. The landscape must deepen, vibrate and take shape in response to quite different fundamental questions – how, why and who?

The making of a baby is a vivid example of this process; it even begins with thickening and moulding of a piece of flat, featureless embryonic tissue! We do not wonder why or how this happens with half the curiosity or intelligence it deserves. That is understandable when we are babies ourselves; our nature is so nearly identical with the life process which is making us that we do not at first realize we are separate from other living things. Until we do, questions like how, why and who we are cannot make sense.

But these questions arise in us all sometime during childhood, and the answers our elders give us are unwilling, evasive and immature by comparison with their responses to our material curiosities. They cannot plead any excuse except the feeble answers and scant encouragement they received in their turn. Our culture does not like reflecting on the enormous quantity of material resources now at our disposal, and considering the qualitative questions that they raise. Most scientists are uncomfortable with quality and prefer to believe that everything comes down to quantity in the end. If this cannot be demonstrated now, they believe it will be one day. Meanwhile opinions, value judgements and arbitrary preference are regarded with suspicion, second-rate substitutes for the hard data they would prefer.

The truth, evident to any artist, is that quality and quantity are quite different and separate dimensions of reality. We even devote half our brain to each, with quite different mental processes operating either side of the thick bundle of connecting nerves which re-unite them. No person can function as a whole without operating synchronously and harmoniously within both at once. But modern Western education is heavily predisposed to train our quantitative faculties, and in most people quality remains grossly underdeveloped and misunderstood.

Consequently we are all too familiar with the kind of material that relates to quantity. All logical, deductive, step-by-step reasoning belongs here, together with all measurements of any kind. People are regarded as essentially the same, with differences between them arising more or less at random for quantitative genetic reasons. Consequently statistical methods can be applied to their behaviour and needs as if they were random variables, reducing our collective aspirations to numbers and rates. Extended into economics, this principle scarcely distinguishes human beings from the

11

machinery with which they work. A host of numerical indicators are related to each other mathematically, likening the behaviour of the entire economy to a predictable mechanism. Correspondingly, in medicine and biology we are utterly preoccupied with exploring the chemical mechanisms operating within parts or systems of the body, assuming it to be no more than an elaborate machine.

When we begin to search all this knowledge for meaning, we enter the realm of quality. This is on the surface a very intimate world, private to each living individual, though as we shall see it also equips individuals to connect sensitively with each other. Everything that occurs within the qualitative realm is completely subjective and incapable of proof to others, yet totally convincing to anyone who actually experiences it. Here belong all deep emotion, instinct, motivation, purpose, creativity, judgement, belief, insight and moral sense. Qualitative understanding – instantaneously complete, clear and apparently inspired – is quite unlike the step-wise quantitative logic we can mobilize deliberately to reason our way through arguments.

In living we each assert, through exercise of the primal adaptive mechanism recognized by Odent, a qualitative identity we receive at conception. This motivates what we do with the raw quantitative material at our disposal, bending it to serve our purpose. The matter of our bodies and their surroundings mean nothing in themselves; they merely provide us with tools, and situations in which to use them. In the end it is only quality which means anything to any of us. Access to it does not depend in any way on material riches, only on the vigour with which we set about the process of living.

This is a very basic distinction to grasp, whose validity I cannot prove to you in any objective way. It may seem sensible to you on the basis of your own experience or you may just be sufficiently perplexed with life to follow through any interesting suggestions. Either way we have to explore the distinction a lot further before we can actually make use of it. To begin with, we need to look a bit more closely at how life in quality actually works.

NEIGHBOURLY RELATIONS: FIELDS OF INFLUENCE

The idea of hosts of individual people vigorously pursuing their independent lives automatically conjures up visions which range from chaos at best to a highly destructive kind of anarchy at worst. Yet on the rare occasions when such an experiment has been made for long enough, that chaos has eventually given birth to a much higher order of harmony than we can otherwise experience.

One of the best-recorded examples took place as the Pioneer Health Centre was getting under way in Peckham in 1936. It was designed as a family leisure club, and it was important that members should find their feet in it naturally without reference to rules and regulations. This was at first very trying to all concerned since children would rush in after school and run madly through the place, wrecking anything in their path; but the director managed to keep his nerve.

He was rewarded after eighteen months with a strikingly cooperative and considerate spirit, which took root even in the wildest breast. Once it pervaded the building, newcomers were automatically infected by it; chaotic behaviour never returned. Nowhere was the change more obvious than in the gymnasium, where dozens of children could now work independently for hours without collision or conflict. They had developed a mutual self-discipline which transcended anything that could have been imposed on them, and much more effectively prevented accidents.

This development should not really surprise us. Nature is after all made up of a great multitude of independent organic beings that manage to work together at many levels – from single cell microbes up to colonies of ants, hives of bees and herds of deer. Even within every bee there are many millions of individual cells, each functioning in most day-to-day respects independently of the cells right next door. Yet these multitudes of separate cells manage to function in wonderful harmony with each other as a whole bee, which is able in turn to manage a sophisticated communal life on very little brain-power. However they do it, we should be able to manage. But how do they?

There are no convincing clues from material biology. We know of chemical and nervous influences which can modify the climate of life for all the cells of the organism or just for some of them. But we have no material explanation for the intimately coordinated growth, movement and relationship of cells in the organism's structure. Why should cells of a certain type, identical under the microscope, behave in one place as part of a finger and in another as part of a leg muscle? How does something as complex as a brain come to differentiate itself from a fold of skin and then commission itself for a completely separate and highly specialized function?

Rupert Sheldrake is making great strides in tackling these questions, and in a particularly interesting way. As an outstanding biological scientist, he has developed his ideas along lines which can be experimentally tested. And he has seriously upset some members of the academic biological establishment by using their own time-honoured methods to produce results which support his own hypotheses yet cannot be explained by theirs!

Sheldrake does not believe we can explain form in nature just by genetic programming, since the genes in each cell are essentially the same. It is asking a lot to suggest that they can be selectively programmed for life to respond as flexibly as they do to unpredictably changing functions and needs. Instead, he suggests the existence of interwoven fields of influence, pervading the whole of the universe, which record all the subtle shades of form and behaviour pattern ever adopted anywhere by individuals of every species and variant of organism. Each individual cell tunes into the fields most appropriate to itself, and these guide its development into the particular form and function it fits best. So a particular germ cell, by responding best to the fields associated with its parents, discovers how to become the particular and unique child of those parents.

You should read more of this idea in Sheldrake's own words, but for the time being note that his *Fields of Formative Causation*, however unfamiliar, are not merely whimsical figments of his fertile imagination. From his studies of various creatures from slime moulds to people he has assembled, and published, respectable scientific evidence in support of their existence.

In one human experiment Sheldrake used picture-puzzles, which are meaningless random patterns until you have 'seen' the image hidden in them. Two newly created puzzles were shown under standard conditions to a panel of students in a Far Eastern university, and each pattern was 'seen' in the time allowed by a similarly small proportion of them. Sheldrake then introduced both puzzles to a large television audience in Britain, but they were deliberately let in on the secret of one of them. The effect of this was to make the solution of one puzzle much better known in Britain than the other. When Sheldrake repeated his original test with a new group of students in a different Eastern university, far more of them 'saw' the better known image, without any direct help from the viewers and students previously involved. The best available explanation is that English viewers had unknowingly strengthened the world-wide field of familiarity with the revealed picture, so that more of the students managed to tune in to it when shown the puzzle.

Fields of influence of this kind form the framework of the quality dimension and are quite incomprehensible as material quantities. They need to be explored, lived by and checked for validity in your personal experience; there is no other way you can prove or believe in them. They are not capable of logical, deductive proof in the quantitative sense: Sheldrake's clever use of scientific method to undermine objections to their acceptance is as far as deduction can take us. Instead, each of us has to see for himself whether they make useful sense. If they do, that is good enough reason for us to go on believing in them.

In fact, nature makes very little sense otherwise. If Sheldrake were not making his claims, we should have to propose something like them for ourselves. But our purpose would be more general than his, and requires a slight shift in the emphasis of the idea.

THE RAINBOW CRAYON

We are already familiar with the idea of Quantitative Space, within which material objects move to make up the hard world we can touch and see. What we need is a medium in which qualitative events can happen, superimposed on quantitative space but run on entirely different lines. Within it, qualities can move in response to *fields of qualitative influence*, including those Sheldrake associates with formative causation.

The term which lends itself most naturally to this realm is *Qualitative Space*. Within it operate the harmonizing influences which enable large and complex communities of organisms to maintain their unity, and without which even the simplest solitary cell would disintegrate in chaos. It does not exist somewhere else, like the 'heaven' and 'hell' depicted in medieval paintings. Instead it overlaps with quantitative space, like a tracing or carbon copy. In fact it can be accurately likened to the colour which gives life to a black-and-white technical drawing.

So exactly does this likeness convey the impression I intend, that I shall employ it as short-hand throughout the remainder of this book. From now on 'colour' will be used to refer to *qualitative space*, and 'mono(chrome)' refers correspondingly to *quantitative space*. We can put the idea to use straight away to form a working idea of health.

From the moment of your conception as a 'mono' egg until you give up trying, your life consists of 'colouring' events – in your own flesh and all around you – with your own personal rainbow crayon. You can think of your health as the skill of your hand behind that crayon. It enables you to *create* – develop and match your personal world to the 'colour' of the greater patterns around you. These patterns are the fields of 'colour' influence, which tell your primal adaptive system and everyone else's how to behave towards one another.

There is nothing selfish or competitive built into this idea, as there tends to be in quantitative notions. A good 'colour' scheme for the whole pattern always suits and satisfies all of its parts just as nicely: healthy growth cannot be at anyone's expense. At every level from the microscopically small to the universally large, 'colour' patterning provides the benign unifying force that has always been at work mending injuries and balancing relationships in nature, whether we have acknowledged it or not.

Biologists have many fertile years of new research ahead of them before ideas like this will find a place in the accepted cannon of scientific truth. But we ordinary mortals do not have to wait that long. Everyone who wishes to can experience and appreciate health directly for themselves.

SIGNS OF LIFE

Whether or not you realize it, your private 'colour' nature works itself out at various levels within you. In the first place it tells your primal adaptive system *who* you are, stamping every fragment of your body with your personal insignia. On the defensive side, that is how you can recognize and deal with intruders so confidently. More positively, however, it governs your instinctive behaviour in accordance with your purposes in life – *why*, or to what end, you do things. We are all more or less flawed, however, and your purposes and nature may be more or less healthy according to your particular imperfections. How are you to know where you stand?

You need to examine *how* you ever do anything. As we have seen, living is not a passive state but a highly active process whereby you read and respond to a constant succession of situations. In doing so you make intelligent use of the material resources available, but these are only the 'mono' traffic of your affairs, and in themselves say nothing about you. How you handle the situations is much more informative. You may not make your identity or purpose very obvious, nor even be conscious of them yourself; but the way you act is readily available for anyone to see, repeatedly demonstrated in all sorts of situations.

If you watch the way other people act, you will quickly realize that each one tends to work along the same lines regardless of the situation. Some assertive characters consistently get results in their favour, but tend to prosper at other people's expense. Their motives are often all too obvious, and none too flattering. Others seem too little inclined to assert themselves, so that they are constantly being taken advantage of. It is much harder to discover the intimate nature of such a person; some are cowards, others just sensitive and unsure of themselves. Those you find it easiest to admire combine the best in both these extremes. They always respect both themselves and others, and act in every situation for the mutual benefit of all.

It is clear that the last of these ways of life is the only creative and harmonious one, and indicates a person who is well worked out. Exactly who they are or why they do things may interest you, but is not your immediate concern. Their actions indicate what matters, that everything about them is wholesome. You would entrust yourself and your interests to the keeping of such a person, and never willingly or knowingly to any other kind.

Your customary pattern of action declares all about your health that others need to know, unconsciously and honestly. When people have had time to discover your action-pattern, they begin to feel they know you. The converse is of course also true. You can read the nature of others, and watch the progress of their growth in how they behave. Once you have learned to read action-pattern, you begin to recognize and work in 'colour'. You are already equipped to do this instinctively, through your ordinary appetites. You do not need to be taught, but you may need to break unfavourable habits your education has superimposed.

The most important is a tendency to think of motivation in negative terms. The science of behaviour has largely been worked out from our responses to painful experiences, and many suppose that our lives are entirely preoccupied with avoiding pain. Of course thirst, tiredness, boredom, hunger and loneliness necessarily make us uneasy, because they threaten our existence and must prompt us to correct them. But a life relieved of all pain is not necessarily happy, and by no means complete. We need the positive motive of a sense of fulfilment powerful enough to mobilize our utmost capabilities.

We experience fulfilment as a profound happiness or ease much more satisfactory than mere lack of discomfort. It occurs not only at those rare high points of accomplishment but whenever our actions are healthy. It is how we know we have grown in 'colour'. And that occurs whenever our action, however small, responds truly to the appropriate field of 'colour' influence.

The pursuit of ease becomes the motive of anyone who has discovered 'colour', because no other gratification comes anywhere near. Since it occurs in response to action, it begins to recur as we establish a 'colourful' action-pattern – one sensitive to all the appropriate fields of 'colour' influence. Ease is therefore the reason we aspire to 'colour' at all. Happiness indicates health reliably, even when its source is not otherwise obvious.

Ease is highly infectious. It works like yeast in the relationships producing it, enticing them faithfully into line with the fields of 'colour' influence. Onlookers can choose to resist it, but once they have yielded to 'colour' influence they too are eased and take up 'painting'. An uneasy grandmother can respond to the 'colourful' life of her daughter's home, and does not need to ask openly about her family's happiness: she simply eases into their 'colour' pattern and experiences it for herself.

It comes down to this. 'Colour' tells you how to live and health is the skill with which you do it, manifested in the wholesomeness of your customary action-pattern. Ease is your tuning signal, motive and reward. Participation is fluent and spontaneous and requires nothing but willingness; 'mono' resources only provide the clay you mould into your 'colour' image. The more you practise, the easier it gets. It is self-sustaining, self-reinforcing and highly infectious.

IN THE THICK OF IT: STRESS

Health is deeply rooted because it needs to be. It is the power by which you cope with the many formidable challenges life presents.

Hans Selye coined the term 'stress' to represent all these challenges, and advanced greatly our understanding of their effects on us in 'mono'. He showed how quantitative and qualitative stresses are the essential agenda of our lives, providing us with opportunities for healthy action to create and maintain order in our affairs despite the stress. While we continue to succeed we remain at ease, positively enjoying the challenges. We even invent games and sports to extend ourselves when we cannot get enough! But our power of coping has its limits, and as we approach them the order of our lives comes under strain.

At first exposure to a single overwhelming stress, you oppose it strongly with an appropriate protective reaction, then relapse into shock while you recover from the effort this has taken. Selye called this the alarm phase, which will recur whenever the same stress challenges you – provided that is seldom.

If instead the stress is repeated regularly within periods of less than three days, your resistance disappears and gives way to a phase of adaptation. This outward acceptance is accomplished by a flood of anti-stress hormones into your blood-stream, which for a time heighten very much your sense of well-being. But as the hours pass this effect wears off, and you are left exhausted by the internal effort it has cost you. So your mood swings through irritability to depression, which slackens to mental fatigue before true ease is eventually restored. A further dose of the same stress at any time during this adaptive cycle produces more hormones, which restore the false well-being and reactivate the cycle.

Adaptation is gearing up your efforts in a distorted pattern designed to roll with the punches of stress rather than oppose them. At first sight this appears healthy, even though it makes you dependent on the stimulus of stress. But ease is gone, because your buoyancy is artificially contrived. You are uneasily preoccupied with plundering your energy reserves to keep the hormones flowing. You cannot at the same time attend so well to outward living; so your life in 'colour' dramatically declines. Yet at any stage you could rest from the stress for long enough to allow ease to return, and so restore your health. The situation is entirely in your hands.

If ease does not return things go on getting worse, because life in 'colour' is no longer sustainable indefinitely. In adapting to stress you are drawing on reserves of energy faster than you can replace them. The false well-being of 'mono' gets briefer and more irritable and the depression more profound and stubborn. Eventually after a period of months or years the reserves are exhausted and you are left feeling unwell most of the time.

This is a profoundly dependent condition from which you will need to be rescued. Unease no longer describes it; you have entered the phase of true *dis-ease*, which is wistfulness for 'colour' no longer vivid. You know things are wrong but cannot now tell what will put them right. Even if you knew, you may no longer possess the energy to work your way back.

Meanwhile order in your life and your body has broken down, to be replaced by *dis-orders* of various kinds, only too recognizable in 'mono'. These will progress if unchecked, rapidly destroying the material reserves that remain. Eventually you can no longer maintain a separate physical identity and it is submerged in death.

SURVIVING, DYING OR LIVING?

Most people now spend the majority of their lives in some form of adaptation or in the exhaustion which follows its neglect. Many babies, faced from birth with well-meaning but brutish handling, enter adaptation there and then; they whimper and cringe their way through life, lacking the confident curiosity to welcome 'colour' and explore its wonders. Their primal adaptive systems are imperfectly commissioned and they will never be capable of truly free existence.

This *maladaptation* is not living at all, but mere survival. People in this unhappy state never discover ease, which is as near to a birth-right as we possess. Their creativity is stifled. Lacking any 'colour' vision, they tend to take sides and feed conflicts with rigidly held opinions. Their security is threatened by any departure from a comfortably familiar routine, however benign the change may be. Freedom from quantitative want is their highest aspiration.

We can descend into survival at any stage in life, by exchanging the uncertainty of creative living for the apparent security of establishment. Many young adults surrender to survival as they settle down to a predictable career and make a routine of family life. Their increasing dependence is masked by their prosperity, until unemployment or misfortune exposes it; by then most are incapable of a creative response.

In survival, simple neglect of 'colour' fades it away. Vivid, whole people blur into vague smudges. Their ability to cope with stress shrinks for lack of exercise, and the uneasiness which warns of dissipation is dulled. So even a sheltered survival eventually declines into exhaustion, unprotected by any reserves of resilience. Disease begins, and disorder inexorably follows. The process of dying has begun.

This can occur at any age, but need not occur at all. Even people who bear terrible 'mono' wounds from coping with overwhelming stress, are able to live in 'colour' with what remains, if they choose. To rally a little health despite your disorders is to be healed, even if death must soon follow in any case. If you can do it in time to recommission your primal adaptive system and harness sufficient energy to restore order throughout your body and its surroundings, you will also be cured.

MEDICINE AND HEALTH

Medicine takes on a very different perspective when seen this way. We can recognize its long-established role in caring for those in the dying phase of 'mono' existence, and note its uncomfortable efforts to prevent this by teaching survival behaviour. It does not appear to understand living, or 'colour', at all. So it seems to be most at home in the very situations which offer least opportunity for doing any good! How could it come to be at such a disadvantage?

The establishment of medicine was led by demand, and as we have seen, this only begins to occur in the exhaustion phase. So doctors have always been faced with people who are already dying, so far as their health is concerned. They have consequently acquired great experience and understanding of all aspects of this condition, and by their occasional successes in restoring people to survival have developed a slight acquaintance with that mode also.

Medical science, impressive as it is, is founded entirely on this experience. It is only comfortable in 'mono' and its principal flaw is built into it as a consequence of this one-dimensional perspective. Since people formerly approached doctors only in extreme need, disorder was by then usually present in 'mono', and the doctor became skilful at tracing this disorder. Consequently he came to believe that the 'mono' disorder was the cause of the patient's disease. In that implicit belief medical scientists fell to classifying and describing all the disorders they encountered, basing on this knowledge the treatment and prognosis offered to every patient.

This is fundamentally misconceived. The disorder is a final consequence in 'mono' of the adaptive process we have called survival, in which uneasy and vain attempts are made to maintain ourselves under stress. It is this maladaptive process, in fading 'colour', that mushrooms into the open awareness of disease, perhaps after many years. Unheeded, it is eventually responsible for the accumulating disorder manifest in 'mono'. When doctors search for a 'mono' disorder and use that to account for the patient's 'colour' disease (his 'symptoms'), they have mislaid a dimension and set the effect over the cause.

This error has its worst results when people consult the doctor before disorder has had time to appear in 'mono'. They are vividly aware of their 'colour' disease and take great pains over their attempts to describe it for the doctor's benefit. He may even be sufficiently impressed to make a diligent, systematic search for a causative disorder which does not show up. But he then stops believing in the disease, because he cannot substantiate it in 'mono'. The patient may be supposed neurotic, his desperate attempts to convince the doctor otherwise only confirming the impression. Stalemate is probable, with the patient left to fend for himself. At best he will be invited to return after an interval, when a real disorder has had a chance to develop.

This advice is absurd, but demonstrates how traditional thinking makes realistic prevention impossible. Searching for early signs of disorder in 'mono' is already far too late. Finding none provides no guarantee they will not appear tomorrow. A boat is afloat right up to the moment when it actually hits the rocks: until then, any examination of her current 'mono' position will reveal nothing wrong. Only if we notice her 'colour' navigation can we begin to realize danger and be in time to prevent it.

Even if medical examination of the body in 'mono' could give reliable assurances about its future, it would not be a healthy approach. Back bearings from 'mono' disorders are not to the taste of healthy people, who are quite properly preoccupied with living in 'colour'. It is unnatural to let action be ruled by fear of possible future 'mono' disasters, and most of those who think this way are not living but surviving. People who repeatedly seek medical assurance that disorders have not yet arisen are too preoccupied with them. We cannot cross the road as skilfully and safely as we might if we too much fear being run over.

We must instead take seriously the unease and disease in 'colour' which mark the beginnings and early progress of trouble, and help people to identify the stresses underlying them. We can usually choose to relieve these or permanently increase our capacity for coping with them in healthy and 'colourful' ways. Then we really have forestalled development, years or decades later, of the degeneration that would otherwise have followed. Which precise disorders might have occurred need not concern us at all.

DOCTORING FOR HEALTH

This calls for quite revolutionary changes in the way doctors think and work. Discovery of preventable disorder should arouse him to dismay – a personal breakthrough into 'colour'. He may then start to listen with respect to the 'colour' of people's complaints.

He will go on to examine in a new way, for quality of function before quantitative state. Distorted action-patterns can then be revealed and traced back to the stresses causing them. The doctor then sets these before their victim, together with an appropriate range of 'colourful' alternative courses of action, as choices for his consideration. His patient can then select his future without didactic prescriptions but fully informed.

To be of any use at all, doctors will in future submit themselves to this process whilst in training as a matter of course. What they have not experienced personally they do not have to offer. To know 'colour' well enough to cultivate it in others, doctors require to be healthy themselves.

In this way we can build up the new body of knowledge and the climate of opinion in which Health Cultivation becomes our main activity. This would not be medical at all, though latter-day general practitioners will be found, alongside health visitors, social workers and teachers, amongst those leading the movement from within. It must be pleasant enough to appeal to people still healthy as an enticing leisure pursuit. It must provide opportunities to discover 'colour' for yourself and get your bearings in it. All the information you need should be available, and all the resources that promote health must be easily at your disposal. This will include access to fresh wholesome food and other opportunities to extend yourself to your full 'colour' potential.

A Health Cultivation Service would strongly underpin family life. This begins with approaches to birthgiving which reinforce wholesome parental instincts and functions and do not undermine them in the name of safety. And it would give young people challenges real enough to search out their uttermost resources of character and build on them. We need to sustain the post-war impetus of men like Kurt Hahn, one of the founders of the Outward Bound movement, who in 1947 declared, 'I refuse to arrange a world war in every generation to rescue the young from a depressing peace'.

Despite all that health cultivation has to offer, medical care on some scale will still be necessary for the indefinite future. Forty years of a comprehensive free medical service have achieved much, and several generations of survivors from pre-health days will continue to need the diagnostic and therapeutic functions in which doctors excel. Furthermore, hostile environmental factors beyond our personal control will go on claiming casualties, even after the backlog of preventable disorder has been cleared.

But your medical needs dwindle as soon as you begin to manage your own 'colour' affairs. To do that you must first get your bearings in the available territory, and plot your present position. The next two chapters provide a full-'colour' map to help you.

2 Under Pressure

Knowing something of your capabilities, you can begin to explore how you use them to cope with disease. This chapter is concerned with the self-limiting kind experienced by all of us in some degree throughout life, in which prompt and complete recovery is the rule. Understanding why will help you manage better any disease whose outcome is less certain.

Before it can make any sense to you we need to consider the two distinct backgrounds from which disease arises. We start by considering the more ancient and natural of them.

DEALING WITH DISRUPTION

To establish our proper place in nature we have always needed to maintain, with all other neighbouring organisms, relationships based on mutual self-interest and respect. Throughout our lives we must each defend our own share of space from encroachment by all the others.

But in health you do not attempt to sterilize your surroundings, hiding behind a *cordon sanitaire*. On the contrary, you trade actively with organisms of all other species as well as your own, and to great mutual benefit. Health conjures these paradoxical needs, for both self-preservation and relationship, into the stable yet resilient natural order we have marvelled at, whose 'colour' you may enjoy whether or not you understand it.

Being alive means acting always to maintain this natural order, among all the organisms involved with you in every situation, and keeping yourself whole in the process. In a perfectly natural world this would be easy and joyful. But the natural order has always been subject to a tidal movement of climatic and population pressures, which favour or disadvantage different species according to the conditions they produce.

We can see this process at work in the creation of a garden. A particular gardener must decide, from a 'colour' vision he wishes to create, what special 'mono' rules of life and death will operate there, additional to the ordinary rules operated within nature as a whole. He determines which plants will form the community of the garden and which he will weed out. Skilfully chosen and applied, these rules can create a very special microcosm of the ordinary world, reflecting a wholesome partnership of human and natural creativity.

While the gardener's effort is sustained, the garden prospers and grows; each season matures it further. But he must continually weed out plants he does not wish to include, and keep animals at bay that he has no desire to feed or house. He is aroused whenever his garden's identity is encroached upon by such intruders, and is only at ease when the threat has been dealt with.

This arousal is the unease we have already associated generally with challenges to the health and integrity of any living thing. It provides the motive for self-preservative action, and its presence is essential to health. Since the garden exists first and foremost because the gardener intends it, his will maintains its 'colour' integrity, his body is its primal adaptive system. As soon as his will weakens, the garden loses its grip on the independence he conceived for it, because he cannot be bothered to maintain it any more. Outside pressures begin to blur its separate identity, which is eventually submerged in its uncultivated surroundings.

Just the same principle applies to the self-preservation of the gardener. Understanding it helps you to comprehend some of the strange and painful things that can happen to you in the pursuit of health.

HOLDING YOUR OWN

In the natural give-and-take of life, your personal experience is just like the garden's. Your essential nature expresses its 'colour' purpose as your will, which informs your primal adaptive system of its function. That remains constantly alert not only to immediate material influences but also to less tangible currents within qualitative space. This enables you to respond intuitively to the 'colour' influences which favour your purposes.

That is how good food, prepared with respect for its 'colourful' vitality, can satisfy you so profoundly when you need it, and leave you indifferent when you do not. As you chew the last mouthful you know that your meal is complete, long before your pedestrian digestive processes could possibly reach that conclusion. The 'colour' of the meal registers directly on your primal adaptive system, a profound impression you only savour with such food. In contrast preserved, processed or counterfeit meals depend on 'mono' tastes, smells and textures – even their sheer bulk – to satisfy you only partially.

The same 'colour' mechanism makes you just as quick to take alarm at threatening influences. Attunement in qualitative space helps you to distinguish what is hostile even before the intruder's 'mono' nature makes this apparent.

Suppose you meet a clump of germs, carried in the air as a particle of dust and urgently in need of a body to colonize. Since they enter in your breath, they will stick first to the lining of some part of the respiratory passage from your nostrils to your lungs and set about penetrating it.

In health you are promptly aroused to mobilize appropriate defences. These can be deployed with amazing precision and subtlety, often overthrowing the threat with scarcely any disruption of your daily life. Or you may become uneasy according to the adversity of your circumstances, the aggressiveness of the germs and the size of their colony. Even so you can continue to function just a little subdued, reserving only the resources required to deal with the threat, so long as these are not overwhelmed.

If they are, you must temporarily abandon your usual activities and concentrate on getting well. You are now frankly *dis*-eased, and may for a while be dependent on help from others. Everything you have is concentrated on the effort of asserting yourself against the germ colony – inflaming your lymph glands and blood circulation to suppurate against it, or form abscesses around it which can migrate and burst harmlessly to the outside, according to the need.

ASSERTING YOURSELF

People very often misunderstand this inflammatory effort. It is certainly the disease, very uncomfortable and sometimes exhausting. Its vigour corresponds to the outrage you feel at being so heavily encroached upon. You would be less diseased if you cared less about surviving, but then you might not be sufficiently aroused to succeed.

Disease is not the problem, as people usually suppose. On the contrary, it is part of the solution! Symptoms are welcome evidence of a self-preservative response. They even tell you which part is threatened so you can choose to place your reinforcements there.

This insight should prompt you to rethink the remedies you use at home. Most restore comfort by suppressing symptoms and so may also frustrate their healing purpose. This approach can easily complicate or delay recovery. It certainly puts at risk your progress towards health.

You need therefore to choose your remedies for their 'colour' implications, which is where Part Two will help you. But the main features of a good cure can be put briefly. It works alongside symptoms instead of opposing them. It takes you right through the middle of the problem, face to face with it. This way you not only solve it properly, but you may grow as well.

A cure helps you discover how the original symptoms came about. That is a lesson about yourself which may very much enrich the 'colour' of your life. Many survivors bless the misfortune of their heart attack for discovering how to live. But many others do not survive. Why wait for so deadly a clue as that? Learn instead the meaning of any disease you encounter and take the trouble to act on it. You are then much less likely ever to require the drastic correction imposed by catastrophic illness.

While cure is possible quite often, even after years of chronic illness, it can be very hard to bear for it not only calls for fundamental changes in long-established habits but may provoke for a time even worse symptoms than you ever had before. Evidently the healing effort represented by your past symptoms was insufficient or you would have got better instead of declining gradually. Once you have made the changes which will let you succeed, the effort will increase – and so will the symptoms. But you will probably turn the corner towards recovery within a few weeks, when your symptoms will dwindle permanently. This 'healing crisis' never exceeds your ability to cope, but often taxes it extremely. Coming through that kind of challenge burnishes your self-esteem.

Spectacular symptoms may be a source of pride in less threatening circumstances too. A vigorous, appropriate response to challenge is a sign of good health, not of bad. Children who sicken briskly with the frequent ailments they collect at school, usually sparkle most of the time in between. When compared with the commonplace alternative – continual vague symptoms, poor thriving and limping unhappiness – this is much to be preferred.

To ail little, if at all, is obviously better still. More would succeed were the tide of fortune within nature the only kind of disruption you had to face. It has instead been overlaid with powerful unnatural forces.

DEAD THREATS

The industrial and technological trends of recent centuries have increased explosively the range and amount of physical and chemical pollutants to which you are exposed. Many of these are novelties of our time, which no organism has ever experienced before. Unlike the natural ebb and flow of fortune for which your self-preservative faculties evolved, these new threats menace every part of nature along with us.

The simplest are chemical contaminations of your surroundings and lines of supply. Pollution of the air and water almost everywhere, and of the soil in which your food is grown, is now a serious concern even for investors in the practices which cause it. They are not exempt from the symptoms of irritability and allergy which are affecting more and more people, particularly the young.

Damage and neglect of the health of the soil has other consequences of a higher order. The plants and animals we cultivate for food cease to be healthy themselves and therefore lose some of their value for us. The 'mono' consequences of this include contamination with pesticides and additives and lack or imbalance of nutrients. But we can now demonstrate experimentally that 'colour' is affected too. Evidence is accumulating that unhealthy food, however satisfactory its 'mono' analysis, cannot sustain your 'colour' vitality nearly so well as healthy food.

Industrialization of agriculture, food processing and distribution have taken this devitalization several steps further. Few people now eat sufficient food that is fresh enough to be still alive. Even healthy food loses 'colour' when cooked and saved or preserved in unnatural ways. When foods are invented or counterfeited with chemical ingredients, matters get rapidly worse; not even 'mono' nutrients are safe then.

Modern food production has another insidious consequence. It reduces the range of items available, regardless of quality. At one time most foods were only available for limited seasons, in great variety and from richly diverse

25

regional methods of culture and processing. Now we have transcontinentally standardized production of fewer varieties, many of which are available throughout the year. Continuous dependence on a narrow range of foodstuffs, many of them adulterated with artificial preservatives, is hard for us to tolerate.

You respond with the only defences you have, evolved to cope with living things at every possible port of entry. When you breathe in these challenging substances in overwhelming quantities, you react in your nose and lungs with mucus, sneezing or congestion; sometimes coughing and wheezing. When they are swallowed you hurry them out again by vomiting or diarrhoea, or else endure the griping soreness and inefficiency of unsettled intestines and digestion. If in spite of this you are forced to absorb them, disturbed body processes fight back with energy borrowed from daily living, so that you tire more easily. Disturbances of metabolism register in headaches, reduced tolerance and buoyancy, and the host of other ways people can feel unwell. Even getting rid of the cause of these symptoms may intoxicate and damage your kidneys, liver, lungs and skin – the organs most directly involved in excretion.

LOW SOCIETY

All these factors tend to derange your body maintenance, making you more susceptible to stresses of every kind. You may tolerate hard work less well or be far less tenacious in pursuit of difficult intentions. You resist infection more feebly and break down more quickly under any kind of pressure.

There is no shortage of that. Much work is 'colourless' drudgery, fulfilling nothing except a 'mono' wage. We are cramped too close together in our cities and easily get in one another's way. We then blame our neighbours for unhappiness they suffer as much as we do. And if we make the effort to break out of difficult circumstances, our surroundings respond so sluggishly that we are more likely to give up than succeed.

So we are seldom eased of the effort required just to survive. Cultivation of quality in our lives becomes a luxury many feel unable to afford, even if they still believe in it. This particularly affects how we bring up our children, who risk developing less depth of personal 'colour' with which to face more 'mono' difficulties than ever before.

There are three unhealthy ways they can respond. They may withdraw into the timid, hopeless inertia that awaits anyone who cannot replace long-term joblessness with a purpose of his or her own. Their frustration may erupt as violently destructive vandalism, venting their need for wholesome personal adventure on its most immediate obstacle. At best they may abandon others to their fate and scramble ruthlessly for competitive advantage. Many quite ordinary people take pride in this as the apparent prerequisite of business success. But war and theft feed from the same soil. The seeds of crime and civic virtue sprout uncomfortably close.

Virtue of any kind thrives best on opportunity, which far too few of us have. Even people worn out by the effort of survival can draw wholesome strength from any chance to live as free beings. They have only to dare, and most children still do. Parents just need the courage to let them. Creating sufficient real opportunities is a job for society at large, and well within our present scope. Perfect nourishment at every level of being, from a luxuriant and responsive environment offering a rich variety of 'colourful' and adventurous activity, only awaits our willing investment.

3 *In Decline*

We have assumed so far that the vast healing power available to us is always successful in overthrowing disruption and restoring us to a full life, if we are determined that it will.

In youth this is nearly always true. But at some stage in every life vitality declines. We all know it must eventually expire in death, the one future common to all living things. When and how that vitality ebbs away is the main subject of this chapter.

MATURITY

In developed countries the expectation of life has been increasing steadily for at least a century. But this has changed very little the age when our elders can expect to die, which has been remarkably stable for much longer. The striking difference is that almost everyone can now expect to achieve maturity.

This does not occur at any particular age, but few reach their peak before forty, just giving time to digest the experience of parenthood and recover from the more exhausting exertions of that phase. To discover the fallacies in your received wisdom, exposed as you rear a family of your own, overwhelmingly repays any incipient decline in physical vigour that may by then have begun.

From then on your 'colour' is revealed to others in your face, corroborating the action-pattern they discover as they get to know you better. You display the trophies of hard lessons and the penalties imposed for those unlearnt. Yet the 'colour' of your talents and experiences is never more completely at your disposal and command, to exercise however you may choose.

If by this stage you have found a creative purpose, life still offers endless possibilities; by applying yourself efficiently you can easily maintain the momentum of your 'colour' painting. This exercise sustains your primal adaptive system in prime condition, so that you can continue to uphold yourself strongly at every level. You respect yourself along with others, and easily affirm your own opinions without offending theirs. You can handle your emotions wholesomely, aware which need urgent expression and which can safely await the right opportunity. And you can see the point of maintaining your body, as a fit vehicle for any activity your 'colour' aspirations may prompt.

This is not a check-list you hold in 'mono', to review mentally at prudent intervals. It is integral with health, part of your 'colour' hologram. Your faculties are spontaneously upheld, at every level of subtlety, so long as your sense of purpose is strong.

This is therefore the foremost requirement for health in the second half of life. Time and again we see the most unlikely candidates defy bodily weaknesses into a ripe old age, inspired by their preoccupations. The number of musicians still in harness in their eighties is particularly remarkable, and demonstrates the special power of music to express meaning and facilitate life. But music is not unique in this respect. I know two very youthful yoga teachers, and a couple researching together the origins of childhood handicap, all busier than ever in their seventies. I first learned about health from an enthusiastic author, already eighty-six. My own former doctor was still springing about the glorious garden he shared with his devoted wife shortly before his death at ninety-two.

None of these are particularly fit, in the mechanical or metabolic sense. Several are overweight and pear-shaped. Some have physical weaknesses, such as an arthritic hip. Though each cares passionately for the quality of what they eat, their diets vary widely. But they are all exceptional enthusiasts, bent on a purpose large enough to absorb them totally. Not one is preoccupied with self-maintenance, yet all are remarkably successful at it. Every one, without being childish, possesses a child-like sense of fun. Though they may tire more easily than younger people, they do not tire of life.

These people are at ease in their old age. They have continued to grow throughout their lives and are exploring wholes large enough to excite them still. Their 'mono' equipment, though worn, has been animated by 'colour' adventure.

AGEING

Meanwhile an inexorable tide has nevertheless been creeping out, retarded by health but not abolished. The power available for 'mono' living begins to ebb somewhere in your thirties, however prudently you draw on it. The attrition your body easily withstands in youth preoccupies more effort as you age.

We know something now of the 'mono' mechanisms that are at work. Even where no obvious external injury occurs, remorseless damage by free radicals – violent splinters of chemical glass – wears away at the pristine perfection of your molecular infrastructure. But the ultimate 'colour' meaning of this decline remains obscure. Why should you cease to heal this kind of damage as well as in youth just because you are older? Evidently the cyclical rhythms of decay and rebirth in nature at large are paramount. Immortality is simply against the rules.

By careful attention to all your needs you can appreciably extend the time this process takes. On the other hand, self-abuse tends to hasten it. Consequently after forty, 'mono' ageing is no longer so closely related to years as to the attrition resulting from the balance of these physical processes. The age others guess you to be from your bodily appearance is a fairly reliable guide to this 'mono' decline. Eventually we shall learn how to forecast the outlook of our bodies from practised judgements of that kind, supported by relevant measurements.

In health you age overall, in balance; no one part wears out before the others. Your 'colour' signature retains its full rainbow spectrum, though its energy may eventually wane. But decades of uneasy survival unbalance that and pave the way for diseased decline into disarray.

DEGENERATION

Now that most people in the developed world reach physical maturity, degenerative bodily disorders have become a major preoccupation. One or other will affect most of us adults contemporary with this book. They are neither natural nor inevitable, though their foundations in our own lives are firmly laid by now and require major revisions of lifestyle to uproot them. But increasing proportions of each succeeding generation can hope to avoid that insidious decline from living into survival which undermines your primal adaptive system, permits disease and makes progressive disorder possible.

The form it takes depends on your inherent nature, as affected by adverse environmental influences over which you have no personal control, and by the individual action-pattern by which you have chosen to live. These superimpose a specific disruptive effect on your 'rainbow' signature, weakening some 'colours' and frustrating the flow of energy in others. The disturbed rainbow that results, with some dim bands and others unnaturally bright, sets the unhealthy pattern of body maintenance which shows eventually in an accumulating series of 'mono' mistakes.

Well-directed technological research will one day enable us to discriminate the 'colour' disturbance patterns that forebode particular disorders, establishing a new era of predictive or 'colour' medicine. But we can already speculate about some of the connections.

One class of disorders appear to result from accumulations in the body of irritant substances, whether consumed as contaminants or residual from diseased metabolism. Many have been present at low levels in our environment for millions of years, but some of them are entirely new. The overall mass of chemicals in circulation has increased hugely in the industrial age, and has inevitably penetrated our bodies, proving easier to absorb than to excrete. Lead and other metals, pesticides and fluorides from agriculture, chlorinated hydrocarbons from treated water supplies, and airborne solvents, hydrocarbons and aerosol propellants, are all capable of dissolving in your tissues and accumulating there.

Some of them appear to select particularly vulnerable sites and upset their function immediately. Others seem to be dumped in any tissue away from the main metabolic stream, awaiting an opportunity for excretion which never comes. Eventually these deposits reach an intolerable size and provoke a healing response.

Though designed for dealing with wounds and other traditional challenges, inflammation is the stock response best suited to this comparatively new situation. We recognize the consequent swelling, heat, redness and pain as rheumatism of some kind if it occurs in muscles or ligaments; as neurological degeneration if the brain and nerves are affected; or as eczema, bronchitis or asthma, liver or kidney disease if poisons we are trying to excrete have damaged the organs involved.

Not all chronic disorders arise in this way, however. Much arterial degeneration, culminating in catastrophes such as heart attacks and strokes, come about through imperfect healing of the many small wounds in the lining skin of these blood vessels, which must pulsate vigorously at least 100,000 times daily throughout life. No machine could accomplish as much, and we depend on continuous replacement of the lining cells, and prompt repair when they are torn. Insufficient supplies of the fatty acids essential to the structure of these cells not only weakens them so that they tear more easily, but also hinders replacement and repair. When these essential fatty acids are in short supply the different kind of fat used to store energy is usually over-represented, gets more time to form deposits in blood vessel wounds that are healing too slowly, and thickens the eventual scars. So arteries age faster and fail sooner for the life-long lashings of animal fat, sugar and white bread that batter them every time a consenting Westerner eats.

CANCER

Cancer is the most problematic degeneration pattern for the scientist and yet the easiest for us to understand. When your health is sufficiently under-mined, at any level and for whatever reason, your primal adaptive system weakens and your body becomes less coherent. In these circumstances your tissues can mutiny and get away with it.

Malignant growths behave the same wherever they occur. A bodily tumour is just like a disorderly group of immature or unsophisticated people, reject-ing self-disciplined membership of some larger social group. If that society is watchful and wise, enjoying the full support and cooperation of all its other members, developments of this kind are spotted early and promptly settled. If however the society is uncertain of its purposes, its members disaffected or poorly supported, revolt is easily engendered and its early signs will pass unnoticed. Rapid growth and uncontrolled spread of the rebellion is then much more likely than in more unified circumstances.

The occurrence of cancer is a direct reflection of the failure of health, disordering life downwards from the level where the failure occurs. So a bodily cancer may sometimes arise not in that person but from the unhealthy relationships of a hostile community life. Malignant social behaviour arises in a precisely corresponding manner, within an unwholesome culture. 'Cancerous' social trends such as vandalism and violent crime, religious, racial and industrial strife will increase in step with bodily cancers, because they originate at different levels in the same social diseases.

Apparently rational people may react to cancer quite unreasonably, especially those professionally concerned with it. This uncharacteristic behaviour is not so perplexing as it may seem. More directly than any other, this disorder exposes illusions we nourish in ourselves, bringing us up against fundamental things. If we are not prepared to face them as mature adults, they assume nightmarish proportions in childish minds. Organizations, individuals and whole cultures may go to extraordinary lengths to evade or ignore the truths most uncomfortable to them.

The awful knowledge cancer arouses in the minds of most of us is how vulnerable our bodies are. Cancer seems able to destroy, at will and at any age, the bodies of even the strongest and most powerful people.

DYING

Most people take death to be the end of everything, and suppose dying to be an entirely undesirable prelude to it. They can think of nothing to be said for either, and hold both in dread. Considering we are sure eventually to face at least one of these processes, we pay them far too little positive attention.

Death happens in one of five ways, of which suicide is inherently the ugliest and most aggressive. It would be anathema to any creature with a shred of health left in it, because it requires that an otherwise viable life shall wilfully determine to destroy itself. That contortion calls for something near the opposite of health, in which one knows that however bad things may be now one can always simply wait on unexpected new events to change them. We are often called upon to accept our fortune, seldom to determine it.

Yet I have met a few apparently sound-minded people who earned my respect rather than any contradiction, and were soberly determined on suicide. If it is to be prevented other than by force, the brink of self-destruction is not the place to start. And there are many others who wish to die whose health prevents them making any fatal move. The largest number do not even go that far, but are sufficiently desperate for help to make a gesture.

Death by accident, however tragic and unpredictable, does not usually occur by pure chance. Some people's action-patterns are more accident-prone than others. And when an accident happens, however improbable, it often seems in retrospect to have been an inevitable consequence of extraordinary circumstances that in turn could not have been prevented. Perhaps sometimes an ostensibly untimely death makes more wholesome sense than we suppose, though this is small comfort to shocked and grieving relatives unless they can believe in the survival of our essential 'colour' beyond 'mono' extinction.

The next most straightforward reason for death is the premature failure of some vital part of your body – often arterial disease of the heart (coronary disease) or some other organ. Despite their suddenness these are predictable causes of death and should be preventable. We have noted already (Chapter

One) that this depends on adopting a sufficiently long-term perspective and on the introduction of methods for analysing the stresses affecting children and young adults. A reliable system of predictive medicine is perfectly feasible, once we give its development the priority it warrants.

These deaths are unambiguously premature: they kill people's bodies before in 'colour' they are ready to expire. Whatever unwholesome action-pattern may have set up the 'mono' breakdown, the 'colour' signature of the victim is often still quite vital when he dies. The death is unbalanced and wasteful, making it hard to console those who mourn him. Yet it is merciful, since it rarely involves the victim in prolonged suffering or anticipation.

Cancer, though essentially of this kind, is exceptional. It often does diminish the sufferer by inches during the weeks or months leading up to death. Pain and other symptoms may be severe and distressing. Medical treatment sometimes adds to these difficulties, at least in the short run. On the other hand it uniquely challenges the victim and his family to face mortality squarely, and gives them time to sort out their approach to it. Sometimes the victim discovers tremendous reservoirs of will and recovers his health for an indefinite period – effectively cured.

Perhaps even more remarkable is the extraordinary peace with which people in this position can face death, if that proves inevitable and imminent after all. The explanation is not so immediately obvious, though it derives from considerations already dealt with in the previous chapter.

Whenever any wild creature succumbs to an adverse tide of fortune, its decline is marked by infestation with predatory insects and microbes which in health it could keep in a harmless minor relationship. Once it is dead, these creatures take over its corpse and begin to recycle it through their own bodies. We take advantage of this process to make compost efficiently and inoffensively from kitchen and garden refuse, with which to fertilize the growth of next year's crops.

At this level, within a large enough natural context, one creature's death or another's good fortune always makes sense. This does not reduce the unfortunate individual's distress if it clings to 'mono' survival despite the odds against it. But most creatures faced with inevitable decline are able to accept the situation, and acquire great ease and dignity from this. They have, in effect, abandoned their personal interest in favour of a larger one appropriate to the wider natural order of which their spent whole is just one part. In these circumstances the personal dis-ease of death is exchanged for the ease of real and conscious participation in a larger being, whose life may not previously have been apparent to the dying one.

We betray the 'colourless' plumage of Western culture by failing to understand this and act from it. Dignified acceptance of the inevitable, anticipating with curiosity what experience it may lead to, ennobles all concerned. Bringing such full-'colour' realism to bear on otherwise unpalatable 'mono' circumstances is healing in the truest sense. It greatly eases pain and distress and connects everyone with the resources necessary to cope with them. It is the realistic and legitimate objective of care in all situations of this kind, where 'colour' remains when 'mono' resources are exhausted.

More often, at present, the opposite pertains. People of any age may descend into the 'colourless' survival described in Chapter One, all true living done. Their gradual 'mono' decline and death may take decades, and involve many protracted physical disorders not in themselves lethal. Homes for the elderly are multiplying fast to cater for the huge population of ageing people in this category. It is rapidly becoming the prevalent way of death.

Though not inherently undignified, this kind of gradual decrepitation is in practice often demeaning unless sufficient love and manpower is invested in caring for it. But such gradual wastage is highly undesirable in any case, and may well prove to be generally preventable. If so, good lifelong nourishment with fresh live food, and a cultural climate which encourages real vitality at every step, will prove essential to that objective.

Simultaneous expiry of the 'colour' will to live and the 'mono' resources for it is the desirable substitute for this living death. It is the most natural end available to mankind, and the perfect consummation of a life well lived. At present it occurs rarely but, however commonplace it may become, will always be a privilege to witness. It carries that great peace which crowns any wholesome death, transforming the survivors' grief into a tasteful celebration. It is often foreseen, and may be consciously invited. Some dying this way apparently see beyond their death as through a very thin veil, and approaching the end are able to speak with clear and prophetic wisdom.

Intimacy with them is rarely lost in death by those they love, and is sometimes greater afterwards than it could be in life – a discovery which may take the surviving companion unawares. And it is not rare for a distressed mourner to encounter the deceased as a voice, a vivid dream or a ghostly vision. This happened on a massive scale during the Second World War, when a number of officers in the armed services became involved in the intense traffic of spiritual messages to parents from fallen young men anxious to reassure them as to their happiness in the afterlife.

One of these officers was Air Chief Marshal Lord Dowding, Commander-in-Chief of Royal Air Force Fighter Command during the Battle of Britain, who wrote two fascinating books about his experiences. Another was Major Bruce MacManaway, who went on to become a widely respected contemporary proponent and practitioner of healing by 'colour' influence.[1] Two less fanciful or impressionable people would be hard to find, and they resolutely affirmed their experience at no small risk to their reputations. Perhaps they would encounter less incredulity now.

There is much for us to learn about living from the nature of death and what may follow it. Many cultures ostensibly more primitive than ours not only cope easily with mortality but seem also to possess a grace in living that we cannot match. The two are as indissolubly connected as opposite sides of the same coin. If our 'mono' lives are only a brief temporal interlude in a timeless

---

[1] Ambiguous, but both my sense and the healing use of coloured light happen to apply.

'colour' consciousness, then the truths about living and dying are one and the same, held within a unified field of qualitative influence. The culture that ignores these fields has not only forgotten how to die. We can no longer remember that we once knew how to live.

4 *Getting Better*

Up to now we have been concerned with understanding the basis of health and disease in a more appropriate way than we are used to, so that you have no need to distinguish all the separate disorders to which humankind is prone. Instead you can see the links between them and the life processes whose breakdown allows them to begin. You have discovered the prior importance of dis-ease, which gives you years of opportunity to prevent most degenerative disorders if you are prepared to take it seriously from the beginning. And you have begun to realize what healing power there is in the ordinary forces of daily living, once you choose to get out of their way and let them operate.

The main purpose of this book is to equip you practically for that choice. There is in any case no other way to convince yourself that what I say is true. To explore the realities of life you must set about living, and most people nowadays have some unsolved problem which can be used as a starting-point. So Part Two is designed to guide your first steps back to health, starting wherever you now find yourself. Simply look up the topic which most arouses your interest, and follow the references from there.

The arrangement of Part Two means that a number of practical approaches which are applicable to many topics are repeated. Those which fit neatly into the format, such as BOOKS, DIETS and SUPPLEMENTS, have been turned into topics themselves. But it is impossible to give a sensible account of all the available therapies in this way, because they overlap so richly. Also, since any one therapy may not be available near you, it is more important to know which alternatives are similar than to understand the differences between them.

This chapter is therefore devoted to an account of therapies in general. It is not a catalogue but a personal reflection on my experience in using and cooperating with them. Quite apart from my temperamental preference for dealing with them in this way, there is as yet no full consensus of their relative merits on which I can draw. On subjects this controversial, it is only safe to tell you what I know personally to be the case. This leaves some therapies at a disadvantage, since I happen never to have had the opportunity of cooperating with them in practice and will not presume knowledge I do not possess. On the other hand, my fundamental proposition – the proper distinction between quality and quantity – has much to offer in explaining the various therapies and drawing them together, which may lend credibility to several therapies where that is lacking up to now. No doubt others will hasten to correct me, which should encourage this important debate to develop along fruitful lines. Such an outcome would amply justify what follows.

HOLISM

Throughout the development of all the therapies now offered as alternative or complementary to Western medicine, their proponents have struggled to express what exactly distinguishes them from the conventional option. Holism, the philosophy that underlies holistic medicine, is the concept at the heart of this issue, and we have to know what we mean by it.

We have only to study the origin of the word to realize what it stands for in principle. It shares its roots with 'hale', 'whole', 'healthy' and 'holy', all of which imply that completeness, roundness and perfection which is beautiful to witness and to share. 'Mono' thought and language cannot do the concept justice. I have resorted to 'coloured' prose in my struggle to convey it and wish I commanded other arts to help me.

Of the two essential principles discussed in Chapter One, I am perfectly convinced. Wholeness in not a matter of structure but of action, and it originates not in quantitative matter but in qualitative influence. That influence is expressed directly in grace of movement, by which we get those glimpses of quality that give our own lives meaning. Furthermore, it is habitual wholesomeness of movement which generates wholeness of form – whether in sculpted stone, living flesh or human relationships.

This exposes a flaw in the behaviour of many complementary therapists who like to consider themselves holistic. It is not sufficient to believe that the whole person is greater than the sum of his parts, nor even to treat each person as a whole – every healing tradition asserts this, including Western medicine. Holism is as holism does. Any therapist whose behaviour tends to build up his patient's integrity, and reconcile his whole person to the realities of his life, can justly claim to be holistic. Any who in practice does not behave this way is not holistic, whatever he may claim.

There are therefore no holistic therapies, only holistic therapists. Any doctor worth his salt is holistic in his behaviour, however rigid or compartmentalized his training may have been. I know of no alternative healing traditions which in themselves set out to antagonize or confront the established therapies; on the contrary, their rhetoric and teaching declares the essential unity of all healing methods, if it refers to the subject at all. But there are in every school of thought individuals whose behaviour is divisive, whose practice is egocentric, self-centred or doctrinaire, or whose patients are made dependent and vulnerable. Therapists of this kind tend to uphold their own discipline at the expense of others, and are chiefly responsible for the deplorable tendency for therapies to split away from one another and multiply – just as specialisms within medicine are so roundly criticized for doing!

In spite of this difficulty, you cannot automatically condemn every healing faction just for asserting a separate identity. People are unique, and some are uniquely able. Any who discover in themselves powerful healing gifts that cannot be fully contained within an existing tradition are fully justified in establishing a minority of one. If they are also gifted teachers, they may go on to inspire others by their example and so found a new healing tradition. It is the mediocre effort of a less inspired disciple that usually perverts this perfectly healthy process.

So how are you to distinguish the good from the mediocre? You cannot rely on 'mono' qualifications or diplomas, which vary enormously in scope and substance. Registration with a professional body is in principle more hopeful, as this should be constituted of accomplished practitioners within the tradition, their collective judgement of 'mono' competence and 'colour' professionalism worth something. Unfortunately there are some rival bodies even in this field, and their inability to reconcile their differences is bound to undermine your confidence in each of them to some extent.

You should be very wary of anyone who advertises his or her services regularly in newspapers or magazines. To declare your arrival in a neighbourhood is reasonable enough, and some professional training schools place such an advertisement on behalf of their graduates when they commence in practice. But a continual need to advertise implies failure to establish an attractive reputation, and indicates if anything a mediocre or suspect practitioner.

Ultimately it is a good local reputation you should look for. Any truly holistic therapist earns the esteem of his clients by setting up reasonable expectations and then fulfilling them. The passage of time will confirm rather than undermine an honest reputation, which is then likely to reach your ears from several independent sources. If these include some that you have personal reason to trust, you can be reasonably confident in approaching that therapist. Almost invariably he or she will possess a worthwhile qualification and be willing to discuss its meaning with you. In any case you can expect an explanation of what he has to offer you, once you have given him the opportunity to assess your case.

That process involves time and expense however, and it is well worth your while choosing the therapy in advance as carefully as you select the therapist. Most will offer you something, and a good practitioner of a less appropriate therapy may serve you better than a novice in something more suitable. But good therapists may be available to you in several disciplines, one or two of which may suit your needs especially well. What follows is intended to help you set off in the most promising direction.

It is still possible both to recognize the kinship that exists between separately identified approaches to therapy and to identify nine main schools of thought to which they all relate. New therapies will doubtless keep on coming, and some will eventually fall out of currency; but each of these schools of thought has by now established an impressive record of historical permanence. I shall therefore pay my respects to each in turn.

Paramount among them, in Western tradition at least, stand two overlapping disciplines which can be traced back through many centuries. They are distinguished from each other chiefly by their degree of establishment, since their philosophies largely coincide. They are identified most closely nowadays with Naturopathy and Holistic Medicine.

NATURALISTIC MEDICINE

A natural philosophy of some kind has strongly underpinned all systems of healing since well before Hippocrates, at least until the nineteenth century. For most of that time the proper philosophy has been disputed by various contending schools of thought, each of which has organized itself as defender of the truth as they saw it. As often as not, the dispute has not been so much over the content of the truth as how it should be preserved and taught. There has always been tension between those healers that have qualified through 'mono' scholarship and long 'colour' apprenticeship within a clearly defined professional tradition and hierarchy and those who emerged informally by reputation through practising their natural 'colour' talents and insights. The former has usually resembled a priesthood or religious order, and the medieval church was indeed an important healing institution. Whenever in history this institutional tendency has been strong, unofficial healers have been the butt of its hostility. Some of the fury vented on witches originated in this way, however it may have been rationalized. That the gift of healing should arise spontaneously in uncultured people has never pleased those who care too much for rank and institutional establishment or are too complacent in possession of it.

This conflict is always sharpest during periods of transition, because it is pressure from the informal sector that imposes change upon an establishment that is out of touch. To begin with they ignore that pressure, believing it will eventually go away. When it refuses to they turn to ridicule, criticizing it for failing to meet the very criteria of excellence which are in dispute. When all else fails heads roll, and new figures emerge in the establishment who co-opt the proposed changes – and usually claim to have upheld them all along!

The established medical tradition was reasonably holistic until late last century, mainly for lack of temptation to be otherwise. Many of the texts and handbooks written by doctors of that time still seem quite radical; Biltz's *The Natural Method of Healing* (two volumes, published in 1898) and Lindlahr's *Natural Therapeutics* (four volumes published around 1925, but republished in an edition by Jocelyn Proby in 1975) are outstanding examples.

Among the unofficial naturopaths of that period, Sebastian Kneipp is far the best remembered. He was parish priest in the Bavarian village of Bad Wörishofen, where throughout the second half of the last century he exerted his gift for healing on the principal resource of the place, its cold spring water. Kneipp's account of hydrotherapy – *My Water Cure* – appeared in the 1880s and was immensely popular. It became the practice of many new spa clinics throughout Europe and is still taught at Wörishofen to thousands of student therapists, medical and non-medical.

Many doctors in continental Europe incorporated these natural methods into their practice, and many reputable clinics are still run along these lines. The most famous and accomplished of these doctors was Dr Max Bircher-Benner, whose teachings survive in the world famous Zürich clinic that bears his name. Probably the best nutritional scientist and clinician the world has so far produced, Bircher-Benner recognized and taught the importance of 'colour' throughout the first forty years of the present century. The cures he accomplished with raw food diets, hydrotherapy, air bathing and sun bathing were quite remarkable and by no means confined to his own patients.

In 1937 Dr Dorothy Hare of the Royal Free Hospital in London studied with Dr Bircher-Benner to discover how a cure had been achieved in the previous year for a case she had considered hopeless and sent to Zürich as a last resort. On her return she applied the Zürich methods to twelve severely handicapped sufferers from rheumatoid arthritis that occupied her wards. Their progress was recorded on film and detailed in *Proceedings of the Royal Society of Medicine*, Volume XXX. Within weeks, seven walked out of the hospital carrying their own suitcases; only two proved to be beyond help.

With spectacular results like this, why did the spa tradition of natural treatment die out so ignominiously in Britain? Doctors cannot claim to have been innocent of its benefits – they simply chose to ignore them. Somewhere in the unwritten history of twentieth-century medicine there must be several murky chapters. Most obviously, chemistry began to emerge during the same period, and became the centre of a sharp division amongst practitioners which grumbled on throughout the first half of this century. Those without a deeply rooted commitment to naturalistic philosophy were quick to follow where the chemists led, though to begin with they had little enough to offer. The lobby against naturalism must have been strong to dissuade doctors from demonstrations such as Hare's. But the discovery of spectacular pharmaceuticals like penicillin decided matters, and in mid-century the medical establishment adopted the chemical or allopathic complexion it has retained ever since.

Naturopathy survived informally, even in Britain, but almost entirely without the help of doctors. Drs Gordon and Barbara Latto are towering exceptions who almost alone have practised naturalistic medicine throughout the fifty years of its eclipse. But several schools of naturopathy have continued to train non-medically qualified practitioners throughout the period. Their emphasis on biologically correct nutrition has saved them from becoming involved with chemistry, though most naturopaths nowadays deal in individual nutrient supplements in a way their elders would not have approved. Besides this they employ exercise, bathing in air, sun and water, and breathing techniques to promote metabolism, excretion and whole-person function. All their treatments are eminently sensible and safe, but they require personal effort and daily repetition over a period of months. Given these the results can be dramatically rewarding. How else could they have survived in the private sector alongside a hostile, free, state-sponsored medical service?

It was four decades before doctors again took techniques such as these seriously, when some of them began to realize the limitations and long-term effects of unnatural chemical medication. True to precedent this debt of influence has not been appreciated, and is unlikely ever to be acknowledged.

Instead, the large minority of the British medical profession which has recently separated itself to form the British Holistic Medical Association is currently recasting naturopathic techniques into their own idiom. If present trends continue, we can expect this new outlook eventually to supersede the allopathic tradition with a full range of naturalistic values and convey to these the mantle of establishment. The allopathic tradition is never likely to vanish entirely, having added some legitimate and useful remedies to the common stock. But however hard its devotees may struggle to retain the paramount position they have enjoyed since 1940, it is bound eventually to slip from their grasp.

Holistic medicine has yet to earn that central position in professional affairs. Even among those doctors already practising it, few appreciate their debt to any naturopathic tradition, believing instead they have invented it in modern times. Nevertheless, if you wish to consult a registered medical practitioner who acknowledges holistic principles at least to some extent, you can turn to members of the BHMA with some confidence. They may not yet have worked out their new role but they have at least abandoned the old.

THE COMPLEMENTARY THERAPIES

The healing traditions which have begun to penetrate the telephone directories in rich diversity constitute between them the seven clans I have arranged around holism and naturopathy in the diagram on the following page. Although several of these are comprehensive traditions in their own right, capable of tackling all forms of disease and offering a more satisfactory explanation for it than most doctors can, none is ever likely to oust the medical profession from the centre of the stage. Whatever their merits, the best they can reasonably hope for in the foreseeable future is freedom both to continue teaching and practising their own tradition and to inform, enlighten and complement the established profession through a relationship of mutual respect.

ALLOPATHIC MEDICINE

Allopathy was a term introduced by Hahnemann, the founder of homoeopathy, to characterize the prevailing medical tradition and distinguish it from his brainchild. Allopathy employs 'mono' treatments that neutralize or oppose the manifestations of a disease, whereas homoeopathy uses 'colour' remedies prepared from substances that would reproduce those manifestations. This distinction implicitly criticizes the basis of the allopathic system for making no attempt to uproot the causal processes that underlie disease. Over a century later this criticism is being strongly taken up by many who have never heard of Hahnemann.

Yet allopathic medicine still has its proper place. It remains the most satisfactory treatment for the diseases of glandular deficiency such as

KINSHIP AMONG THERAPIES

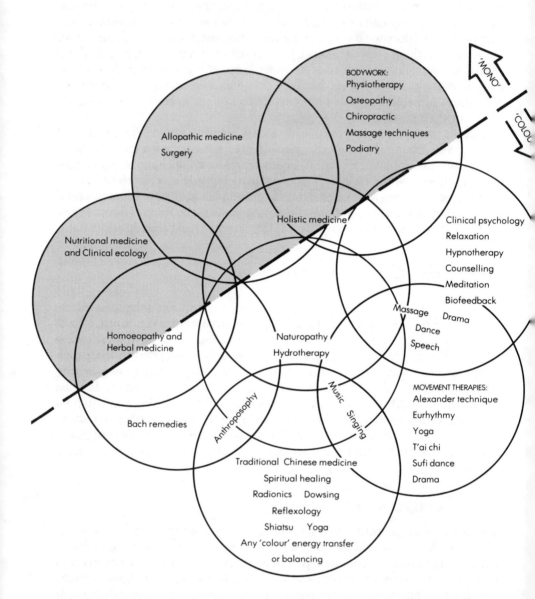

diabetes once these are irreversibly established. It offers effective suppression of the diseases of intolerance and exhaustion, such as asthma and depression, unless and until their cause can be discovered and dealt with. And it offers acceptable means for postponing failure of heart, lungs or kidneys where any of these has become inevitable. Any of its other remedies may reasonably be employed in short-term crises, but indefinite reliance on them is unwise since the balance of benefits and adverse effects will eventually turn out unfavourably. In most of the situations where these drugs are now used continuously for years, some other remedial approach is in the long run likely to be safer and more useful.

Surgery is the most spectacular and glamorous development associated with medicine, made possible by the development of effective chemical anaesthetics. It has a strong simplistic appeal for ordinary people, who find it much easier than medicine to understand. Many would like to think that, if only sufficient resources could be made available, spare-part surgery would quickly supersede all other methods in dealing with degenerate hearts, lungs, livers, joints and limbs.

This prospect is absurd and naïve, but few surgeons can be relied upon to say so. It is obviously stupid to dissipate health heedlessly for five decades and then devote huge resources to mending the consequences. Even birth defects are not exempt from this. The health of both parents at the time of conception determines nearly all the common malformations that can affect babies. To leave this to chance and call in the surgeon when luck deserts you is as senseless as mopping up spillage from a blocked sink without turning off the tap! Yet that is how things stand officially in Britain, at the time of writing.

Nevertheless surgery will always have a place, alongside adequate preventative measures, in dealing with those few cases that defy prevention. It never stands alone, relying always on the general healing capabilities of the patient to take advantage of the surgeon's skill. The public must not be aroused to expectations technology cannot fulfil, however good this makes the surgeons feel.

NUTRITIONAL AND ECOLOGICAL MEDICINE

Two main trends have remained within the general professional and disciplinary framework of medicine, yet embarked on radically new techniques of diagnosis and treatment. *Nutritional Medicine**1 recognizes the importance of correct diet to health, but has tended to medicalize the subject by comparison with the naturopathic approach. Laboratory tests of your nutrient levels and toxic load therefore have an important place, and prescriptions of nutritional supplements are given in place of drugs.

Closely akin but slightly more specialized is *Clinical ecology,** which pays special attention to the environmental causes of disease such as allergy and chemical intolerance, and employs a provocation/neutralization principle to

1 Words in italics followed by an asterisk appear in the Index where they are explained and/or can be explored through cross-references.

identify irritants and prepare vaccines to neutralize them. It can be shown that if one dilution of a dissolved substance provokes in you an irritable response, there will be a more dilute strength of the solution which exactly neutralizes this effect. Identification of the substances that affect a particular person, and their neutralizing dilutions, enables the clinical ecologist to offer protective treatment. In the long run, however, he too depends on proper nutrition and appropriate supplements to restore the patient's immunity to normal, when neutralizing vaccines should cease to be necessary.

BODYWORK

The value of *physiotherapy** has been recognized by doctors for many years already, and a minority now realize how greatly manipulative techniques extend its range of usefulness. Even so, departments of physiotherapy in National Health Service hospitals are overworked and understaffed, which forces them to depend on non-specific methods of treatment which can be supervised less closely. Little is done to meet the acute needs of patients outside hospital, and access to what there is often comes too late to be of much use. This has created a demand for private physiotherapy, which many practitioners elect to fill once their experience is sufficient. Chartered Physiotherapists in private practice tend on the whole to be enterprising people, and usually make a point of adding manipulative techniques to their basic skills to extend their range. This brings them into a position broadly comparable with osteopaths.

*Osteopathy** separated from allopathic medicine over a century ago by asserting the value of skeletal manipulation in restoring bodily functions of all kinds at a time when allopathy was still chiefly fascinated with the diagnosis of structural pathology. It was the first healing tradition to arise in Western culture recognizing how 'mono' manipulations and massage can bring about 'colour' changes. Osteopaths have successfully treated such conditions as asthma and nervous tension which do not obviously relate to muscular or skeletal malfunction. *Chiropractic** is a more specialized manipulative technique which concentrates on the spine.

Since then various people have explored these possibilities further, developing *Therapeutic Massage,** *Alexander Technique,** *Keller work,** *Rolfing** and others, all of which are more or less closely allied. *Podiatry** is rather distinct, a mechanical approach to correction of your walking rhythm and posture which promises eventually to reduce osteoarthritis drastically. In Britain it has been taught as a post-grade diploma to chiropodists, who in the main practise it privately.

*Yoga** is one of the few disciplines that defies limitation to just one school. It is a very old tradition, in which the manipulation of 'colour' through posture and movement predominates over its 'mono' benefits on suppleness. Nevertheless many more people are able to take advantage of group yoga tuition for practice at home than could ever afford or have access to personal bodywork.

HYPNOTHERAPY AND PSYCHOLOGY

The last of the complementary therapies with which the medical establishment has formally established professional working relationships covers the whole area of mental functioning. Conventional psychiatry has come to rely heavily on drug treatment that is highly inappropriate for most sane people with emotional or mental problems, and merely suppresses their effects. Clinical psychology is usually a much more useful approach, since it seeks out weaknesses of mental functioning and aims to strengthen them. Even group work in this field cannot hope to cater for the number of people who need it, however, so that many other approaches have been tried. The deployment of Registered Mental Nurses as community counsellors is in principle a sound idea, but their training and experience are often inadequate to deal with people in their homes; they do not seem to realize that interview techniques which may pass muster in psychiatric wards are far too intrusive for use elsewhere. As yet, nothing like enough counsellors have been properly trained for community work to make much impact on the need.

*Hypnotherapy** is attractive as a possible way out of this problem of demand and supply. In skilled hands it provides a short cut to the heart of many problems of mental and emotional function and can quickly restore people to normal. However, only a minority of subjects are susceptible to entering a deep trance, which is far more effective than the deep relaxation that is the best most people achieve. Furthermore, you can never know what a hypnotic trance may let out of the bag, nor whether your therapist will be skilled enough to handle it. Adequate courses of training, which incorporate plenty of tuition and practical experience in clinical psychology, are few and far between.

There are two ways round this. One is to size up a prospective therapist well before you commit yourself to his care. If you rate him at least as mature and experienced in life as you are yourself, you are reasonably safe. The other is to look for a doctor or clinical psychologist who has added hypnotherapy to his skills, on whose basic professional training you can rely. There are not likely to be many near you, but they represent something like a best buy.

*Relaxation** and *Meditation** are safer disciplines, which can be learnt as personal tools for dealing with tension and anxiety. There are many approaches to the latter, some of which derive from Buddhist philosophy. Others, such as *Autogenic Training** and *Biofeedback,** employ 'mono' technology to teach you quickly what would otherwise take years of 'colour' discipline to learn. They are of course more expensive, but more idiomatic for Westerners; you pay your money and you take your choice.

MOVEMENT THERAPIES

Doctors are not accustomed to thinking of movement as therapy, but its value has been incorporated into every culture all over the world for thousands of years. Dancing and singing are not important merely because they are fun; they uplift your spirits by tuning up your 'colour' function generally, and strongly promote your harmony with others. The Sufi dancing and *yoga** traditions of the Indian sub-continent, and T'ai Chi as practised daily for centuries by thousands of Chinese, were consciously developed in those cultures as direct means for maintaining 'colour' health. In Europe the best established comparable tradition is comparatively recent, the special discipline developed by Rudolph Steiner to represent sound in terms of movement, and known as *Eurhythmy.** But singing, speech and drama, ballroom dancing and ballet are all less specific means to the same end.

That covers all the complementary therapies whose principles would be ideologically acceptable to most doctors. The two remaining schools tax most Western minds far beyond their accustomed range, though the first of them is essentially home grown.

HERBS AND HOMOEOPATHY

Doctors dislike herbs for the same reason that they are suspicious of whole foods: they are complex, impure and mysterious. Certainly all natural tissues possess the same 'colour' dimension that whole people do, which introduces properties well beyond the scholarship of chemists. Amongst these are the mechanisms that enable your sensibilities of taste and smell to transcend the crude 'mono' apparatus in your mouth and nose, functioning with a subtlety that baffles physiologists. Just as whole fresh foods kindle these functions which dead and refined foodstuffs fail to arouse, so whole fresh herbs can engage your 'colour' functions in a way refined drugs cannot. When carefully dried for use out of season, they retain the merits of good chemical balance even when most of the 'colour' has gone from them.

Up to a point herbs are entirely plausible for doctors, because many drugs were originally identified in them. *Homoeopathy** is something else again. Yet once you have overcome your incredulity, its principle is very attractive. So are its practitioners, in the main. They listen attentively and at length to your symptoms, because details matter to them. They recognize your individuality, although your nature will still be classified – this time according to remedy, instead of disease. Their reverence for natural order is usually obvious, and corresponds with the respect they show to the remedies at their disposal.

But this cosiness is rather antique, like the tradition from which it comes. It has scarcely changed its image since its foundation 150 years ago, and still relies heavily on the archaic language and ideas of that time. Very few modern practitioners expound it well, although several have introduced new remedies or methods of preparation. But George Vitoukas, a very gifted Greek practitioner and teacher, shows the kind of form required to establish homoeopathy in the bedrock of twenty-first-century medicine.

Many low-potency remedies are available without prescription through chemists and wholefood shops, and you can try them for yourself without risk wherever other good treatment is lacking. But you need to understand the basis of their action and how to use them.

Homoeopaths claim to isolate and intensify the 'colour' of any substance, traditionally by diluting its 'mono' material in a particular way. (Some practitioners now claim to synthesize the 'colour' 'radionically', using electronic apparatus.) Moreover, the result is a 'colour' negative; its properties are exactly the opposite of its 'mono' counterpart. It is just as if the dose-response graph for a drug can be extended backwards through zero into the negative range – something a conventional chemist cannot of course accept.

Since the 'colour' intensity increases as the substance is diluted, potency is expressed this way. When one part of the basic solution in an alcohol-water mixture is diluted in 100 parts of fresh diluent mixture and splashed about a lot, the result (using Roman numerals) has potency C or 1. One part of this, diluted in the same way, takes on potency CC, or 2. Potencies up to 6 are usual; 30 is common, and experienced prescribers may go up in stages to M (1000), CM and MM – potencies which should never be used casually by anyone.

Very low potencies are prepared by diluting one part in 10 – Roman numeral X. Up to 3X these seem to intensify the 'mono' effect of the remedy; higher potencies go into reverse. A practitioner matches your symptoms and general nature with a dictionary of the 'mono' effects of all the substances that have been 'proved' on healthy volunteers, and chooses the substance that matches your nature best. He judges the potency of the remedy according to your case, and may need to adjust the potency or the substance.

The remedy works by adding its 'colour' to yours. If it has been chosen well, it exactly corrects the deficiencies in the 'colour' signature of your disease, restoring the full spectrum. That restores your healthy action-pattern, which sets your disorder to rights over several weeks or months.

Packaging of 'colour' presents an obvious difficulty, and has to be done with great care. It is locked up in tablets, drops or powders of an inert material (often milk sugar), like the genie in Aladdin's lamp. It can be released accidentally by handling or contact with dirt, and is neutralized by food, strong scents and steroid drugs.

You can obtain a simple home guide to common conditions, either from a local stockist or by writing to *Weleda* UK Ltd, who distribute several.

Having selected the low-potency remedy which seems to match you best, take doses separately from food and drink; wait until no trace of their flavour is on your breath. Tip them directly into your mouth without handling; use the lid to toss tablets in. Hold the dose in your mouth to absorb its 'colour' well; after a minute or so you can spit out the blank tablet, or you can eat it.

*Bach Flower Remedies** have a similar principle, but are much simpler to use. They were devised by the English physician Dr Edward Bach as an economical system of treatment that ordinary people could use. Their method of preparation is simple and natural. The best flowers of the kind required are taken in full bloom on the morning of a sunny day, and dissolved all day in the open air and in full sunlight, in a bowl of spring water from a nearby source. The resulting solution is mixed with an equal volume of brandy to preserve it, and stored in glass bottles.

Different personality types are associated with each of the thirty-nine flowers in the Bach repertory; you have simply to select the one most appropriate to your frame of mind. A few drops of the tincture are diluted with spring water and are then ready to be taken with water at regular intervals through the day. They should be savoured carefully by rolling them around your mouth, since their influence enters your 'colour' signature by the same taste route as homoeopathic remedies take. All the advice and supplies you are likely to need are available from the Edward Bach Centre, whose address appears in Part Two.

Anthroposophy* is really a different and more comprehensive system of medicine, based on the philosophy propounded by Rudolph Steiner, one of the great polymaths of the present century. But it embraces homoeopathy and herbs along with minerals and crystals, in an idiom which many modern physicists would be startled to recognize and willing to respect. I have therefore included it here, as the most advanced and sophisticated interpretation of the potentialities of this therapeutic school. It also serves to link it smoothly to the last, which it encompasses just as easily.

Steiner was, like Bircher-Benner, a visionary who was able to sense directly the 'colour' nature of things and their interconnectedness. His contributions to art and sculpture bear witness to this, and eurhythmy was intended to bring out the same sensibilities in others. His lectures on nutrition and medicine translate with difficulty from their original German, and he warned his listeners repeatedly against trying to study his sayings by writing them down. His audiences were spellbound and understood his meaning instinctively; the transcripts are by contrast extremely obscure, even in German.

So his ideas have not yet captured the imagination of English-speaking doctors, as I believe they one day will. Of all the systems of medicine I have so far met, this is the one I most desire to study personally. The first volume of a four-part work, *The Anthroposophical Approach to Medicine*, is now available in English from Rudolph Steiner House, whose address appears in Part Two. I warmly recommend it to professionals of any healing discipline who find themselves perplexed and struggling.

HEALING BY 'COLOUR' ENERGY

Homoeopathy and anthroposophy consciously employ the 'colour' properties of natural materials and movement for healing purposes, but this school uses and manipulates 'colour' without embodiment of any kind.

Acupuncture,* the principal and best known feature of *Traditional Chinese Medicine,** has been baffling Western doctors for some time. They are impressed by its use in anaesthesia and pain relief, but are mistaken in their attempts to relate these observations to the 'mono' mechanisms they are familiar with. Naturally they find Chinese medical philosophy and anatomical charts quaint and unconvincing, and few pursue their curiosity very far.

In fact Chinese doctors work from the most beautifully expressed holistic philosophy I have ever come across – far more accessible than Steiner's. Its practical technique is subtle and highly sophisticated, based on a detailed understanding of human 'colour' physiology. Those quaint charts of acupuncture meridians were never intended to relate to 'mono' anatomy at all, but to its 'colour' counterpart. Consequently it chimes much better with *yogic** philosophy and practice, whose use in healing relies in just the same way on balancing a distorted 'colour' signature.

The most pleasing feature of Traditional Chinese Medicine is its emphasis on the maintenance of health. Once your original problem has been dealt with you are encouraged to return at the turn of each season to be tuned up. The ancient custom was to pay your doctor only for this service, and to expect him to remedy his errors – your illnesses – free of charge! In the West we have a long way to go before we can match a practice already traditional in the Orient for thousands of years. I do not personally aspire to acquiring these skills in their traditional form; but when I need a doctor, it is to the Chinese tradition I always turn first.

Shiatsu is the Japanese equivalent of acupuncture. *Reflexology** is a variant of it which specializes in attending to the rich connections of acupuncture points in your feet.

Finally in this school we come to consider Spiritual Healing, Medical Dowsing, Applied *Kinesiology** (Touch for Health) and Radionics. I have direct experience of all but the last of these, and have no difficulty in appreciating their relationship to 'colour'. What they tell us about the intelligence and power of 'colour' fields is quite startling at first.

The Confederation of Healing Organizations is embarked on a series of studies designed to prove in scientifically acceptable terms the 'mono' efficacy of spiritual healing. Their motives and sincerity are beyond dispute, but I cannot help wondering whether the intelligence behind 'colour' approves of their efforts. If he or she does not, I have no doubt that these well-intentioned experiments will produce a peculiar result, or none at all.

Dowsing, the use of a twig or pendulum to magnify subtle sensations or movements in response to variations in 'colour' fields, is sometimes employed by Water and Electricity Boards when other means of locating their underground pipes have failed. Most people can do it if they try. You may then find you can conduct a conversation with or through your pendulum, provided you only expect simple answers like 'yes' and 'no'. Applied kinesiology is a refinement of dowsing in which the strength or weakness of particular muscle groups reflects the vigour of corresponding bodily functions. The examiner can even use one test muscle like a pendulum, mentally asking questions about the health of that person and getting strong or weak responses from the muscle in reply. This is strong stuff for dentists and doctors to take, yet I have attended enthusiastic seminars of both intent on acquiring this technique to extend their diagnostic ability. Like most skills it improves with practice. And as in all clinical work you have to ask sensible questions in the first place.

Whilst I have no personal experience of radionics, I have several friends who retain a radionic practitioner and are well satisfied. But I was amused and impressed by the tales of a dear old man I used to know, who treated his horses this way. Many of his friends in the racing world had become accustomed over the years to enlisting his aid in treating their charges at a distance, during the journey to the course and immediately before races for which they were entered. However temperamental the animals had been in training, on the day they always functioned at their best, though without transcending their known capabilities. Their trainers and owners – hard-nosed individuals, most of them – were sufficiently impressed to keep my friend sweet with small tokens of esteem, and to return repeatedly for more of the same!

I do not expect anecdotes of this kind to impress the sceptical, and can only encourage you to pursue any curiosity you may have in this area with an open mind. I do not often explicitly recommend any of the methods in this school, but respect them enough to attend a Traditional Chinese doctor myself, and to wish people well consciously whenever I touch them. In that habit I am only cultivating in myself the instinct of every parent who has ever lovingly stroked an ailing child, and every child who has ever comforted a much loved pet – unconsciously, yet somehow knowingly, offering 'colour' energy to heal them.

PART TWO

PART TWO: *Contents*

ACNE, rosacea

Your skin is not just a container but a remarkably sophisticated *organ*** which regulates losses of heat and moisture from your body, can store and excrete surpluses from *metabolism*** and receive sensory impressions. Despite its permeability it is a very effective barrier against *microbes*** and moisture, and can regulate the penetration of sunlight to the tissues inside. It wears tirelessly, and will grow into a form appropriate to the physical work expected of it. Its elasticity enables it to cope with changes over the years in your shape and size.

Hairs are an invariable characteristic of all human skin except the palms of your hands and the soles of your feet. They do not develop to the same extent all over your body: in some places the hairs are scarcely visible, but they are there, rooted deeply at frequent intervals. Only serious and permanent deficiency of your CIRCULATION causes them to disappear.

Hair and skin both require lubrication and sealing against moisture, so each hair root has its own flask-shaped *sebaceous*** gland which trickles out a fatty material it produces, slowly but steadily.

Health provides for the regular flow of nutrients to this gland, and for their manufacture into sebum at just the pace required for its flow to match the rate at which it matures and dries. Sebum is therefore delivered to your skin in prime fresh condition, where its ripening and rancidity are positively beneficial.

This healthy rhythm is easily upset, usually at times of transition in your life. Puberty is the best known, when *steroid*** hormones are actively preparing you for adulthood; but rosacea is the same process at any other time. The '*colour*'* change in both acne and rosacea is evidently most intense around your face, neck and shoulders, for these are the chief parts affected.

A baby may have a similar condition called *roseola*** which affects his whole body but is usually most intense on his face and neck. This happens as his skin adapts its structure to the much drier conditions after birth. Before then he needed lots of sebum to waterproof his skin for life in the womb. Once born he needs far less. The redundancies do not always go smoothly, and acne-like pimples may form. It almost never upsets the child, requires no treatment, and clears without a blemish within a few weeks. Perhaps teenagers who had roseola as babies are more likely to suffer acne too.

These changes all make the flow of sebum more sluggish, so that it can begin to dry and go rancid while still inside your sebaceous glands. These block and swell, forming *blackheads***. The pressure that builds up inside them causes leakage into your surrounding skin, which INFLAMES it. The bacteria which thrive on degenerate sebum are rather aggressive, so that painful BOILS form if they appear and multiply.

Rich fatty food makes matters worse. Your metabolism makes the surplus into extra sebum of second quality, which stagnates into acne very easily.

HELPING YOURSELF

Health Maintenance: Eat the DIET for health. Your skin reflects, stores and excretes excesses in your food and will never heal while they keep coming. Medical assurances that food has no effect on acne are based on very narrow, inadequate research. A clean diet can cure the condition and always improves it.

Brush your skin all over every day with a loofa or grooming brush firm enough to stimulate and clean it without scratching. Then spend about ten minutes with your affected parts naked or very lightly clad, to let your skin breathe.

At another time bathe hot for three minutes, then cold for twenty to thirty seconds; a shower is best for this. You can repeat the cycle several times if you wish, but must end with cold. This opens your skin and relaxes it, then firms and tightens it again. You are not only rinsing it, but wringing it out!

Treatment: Use the cleansing DIET, especially avoiding fatty food – chocolate, chips, crisps, cheese, cream, butter and meat. You will need to persevere with mainly raw vegetables and fruit for at least six weeks, because it takes your skin that long to grow through from its foundations. Rosacea takes even longer than this to improve.

SUPPLEMENTS of Zinc and Vitamins B$_6$ (Pyridoxine) and C are helpful. Take some Brewer's Yeast as well, to balance the Pyridoxine.

Steam your face for twenty minutes daily. Fresh or dried camomile and hay blossom improve the effect; pour the freshly boiling water over a handful of the herbs. Cover your head with a towel and bend close enough to the steam to feel its heat. When time is up, splash or shower your face with cold water and blot it dry.

Avoid using *steroid** creams on the diseased areas, since they contribute to the cause. Salicylic Acid and Sulphur Cream BP is an inexpensive peeling agent you can apply to badly affected areas for an hour or two, then wash off; it opens spots more quickly. No other external applications are worth while in the end; skin must be cleaned and healed from inside.

Tetracyclines are widely used to reduce acne, and work well. But they must be taken continuously and being also ANTIBIOTICS can profoundly alter your colon bacteria and make THRUSH a serious risk; this in turn can make acne worse! Only use tetracyclines if your skin is really bad, and limit yourself to a month; by that time your diet and bathing should prevent further serious recurrence.

Homoeopathic* Sulphur 6 and Carbo veg 6 are often useful in straightforward teenage cases. You can alternate three doses daily of each, continuing for a few days at a time and stopping if you get a satisfactory result. Resume treatment in the same way once the effect of one course has worn off.

ADDRESSES

Al-Anon, 61 Great Dover Street, London SE1 4YF, tel. 01–403 0888

Alcoholics Anonymous, P.O. Box 1, Stonebow House, Stonebow, York YO1 2NJ, tel. 0904 644 026

Bach Flower Remedies Limited, Mount Vernon, Sotwell, Wallingford, Oxon OX10 0TZ, tel. 0491 39489

British Association of **Beauty Therapy and Cosmetology** Ltd, Suite 5, Wolseley House, Oriel Road, Cheltenham, Glos. GL5 1TH, tel. 0242 570284

Beauty Without Cruelty Ltd, 37 Avebury Avenue, Tonbridge, Kent TN9 1TL, tel. 0732 365291

The British **Beekeepers'** Association, National Agricultural Centre, Stoneleigh, Kenilworth, Warwicks, tel. 0203 552404

The West London **Birth Centre**, 33 Colebrooke Avenue, Ealing, London W13 8JZ

Cancer: New Approaches to Cancer, c/o The Seekers Trust, Addington Park, Maidstone, Kent ME19 5BL, tel. 0732 848336

BACUP (The British Association of Cancer United Patients), 121/123 Charterhouse Street, London EC1M 6AA, tel. 01–608 1661

Cancer Help Centre, Grove House, Cornwallis Grove, Clifton, Bristol BS8 4PG, tel. 0272 743216

The British **Chiropractic** Association, 5 First Avenue, Chelmsford, Essex CM1 1RX, tel. 0245 358487

Clinical Theology Association, St Mary's House, Church Westcote, Oxford OX7 6SF, tel. 0993 830209

Counselling: Templegarth Trust, 82 Tinkle Street, Grimoldby, Louth, Lincs LN11 8TF, tel. 0507 82655

Dance: Imperial Society of Teachers of Dancing, Euston Hall, Berkenhead Street, London WC1H 8BE

Dental Kinesiology: Anthony C. Newbury, 72 Harley Street, London W1N 1AE, tel. 01–580 3168

Drama: British Theatre Association, Regent's College, Inner Circle, Regent's Park, London NW1 4NS, tel. 01–935 2571

Environmental Medicine Foundation, 111 Toms Lane, Kings Langley, Herts WD4 8NP, tel. 092 77 65389

The Natural **Family Planning** Centre, Birmingham Maternity Hospital, Queen Elizabeth Medical Centre, Edgbaston, Birmingham B50 2TG, tel. 021–472 1377 ext. 4219

Fileder Systems Ltd, 50 Old Road, Wateringbury, Kent ME18 5PL, tel. 0622 20050

National Anti-**Fluoridation** Campaign, 36 Station Road, Thames Ditton, Surrey KT7 0NS, tel. 01–398 2117

Foresight, The Old Vicarage, Church Lane, Witley, Surrey GU8 5PN, tel. 042879 4500

Gymnastics: British Amateur Gymnastics Association, 2 Buckingham Avenue East, Slough, Berks SL1 3EA, tel. 0753 34383

The Confederation of **Healing** Organizations, 113 Hampstead Way, Hampstead Garden Suburb, London NW11 7JN

The British **Holistic** Medical Association, 179 Gloucester Place, London NW1 6DX, tel. 01–262 5299

The **Homeopathic** Development Foundation, Suite 1, 19A Cavendish Square, London W1M 9AD, tel. 01–629 3205

The **Hyperactive** Children's Support Group 59 Meadowside, Angmering, Littlehampton, Sussex, BN16 4BW, tel. 090 62 70360

The Association for Applied **Hypnosis**, 33 Abbey Park Road, Grimsby, S. Humberside DN32 0HS, tel. 0472 47702

La Leche League of Great Britain, BM 3424, London WC1V 6XX, tel. 01–404 5011 (office hours), 01–242 1278 (any time)

National Institute of **Medical Herbalists,** The General Secretary, 41 Hatherley Road, Winchester, Hants FO22 6RR, tel. 0962 68776

Medion Limited, 4 Beadles Lane, Old Oxted, Surrey RH8 9JJ, tel. 0883 712229

Midirs (Midwives Information and Resource Service), Westminster Hospital, Dean Ryle Street, London SW1P 2AP, tel. 01–834 3240

Arms (Multiple Sclerosis Research) Limited, 71 Grays Inn Road, London WC1X 8TR

The **Multiple Sclerosis** Society, 25 Effie Road, Fulham, London SW6 1EE, tel. 01–736 6267

The **Naomi Bramson** Trust, The Science Park, University of Warwick, Coventry CV4 7EZ, tel. 0203 413671

The **National Childbirth** Trust, 9 Queensborough Terrace, London W2 3TB, tel. 01–221 3833

Nature's Own Ltd, 203–205 West Malvern Road, West Malvern, Worcs WR14 4BB, tel. 0684 892555

United Kingdom Central Council for **Nursing, Midwifery and Health Visiting**, 23 Portland Place, London W1N 3AF, tel. 01–637 7181

Nutrition: The McCarrison Society, 24 Paddington Street, London W1M 4DR, tel. 01–935 3924

ADDRESSES

'Organic' Gardening: The Henry Doubleday Research Association: Ryton Gardens, The National Centre for Organic Gardening, Ryton-on-Dunsmore, Coventry CV8 3LG, tel. 0203 303517

The British Register of Osteopaths, 21 Suffolk Street, London SW1Y 4HG, tel. 01–930 3889

The Pegasus Trust, Runnings Park, Croft Bank, West Malvern, Worcs WR14 4BP

The Organization of Chartered Physiotherapists in Private Practice, 50 Mannering Gardens, Westcliff-on-Sea, Essex SS0 0BQ, tel. 0702 352113

The Podiatry Association, Swaynes Cottage, Fore Street, Weston, Hitchin, Herts SG4 7AS, tel. 046 279 371

The Premenstrual Tension Advisory Service, PO Box 268, Hove, Sussex BN3 1RW, tel. 0273 771366

Psychologists: The British Psychological Society, St Andrew's House, 48 Princess Road East, Leicester LE1 7DR, tel. 0533 549568

The Radionic Association, 16A North Bar, Banbury, Oxon OX16 0TF, tel. 0295 3183

The College of Reflexology, 9 Meads Road, Shenley, Radlett, Herts, tel. 092 76 7192

Relaxation for Living, Dunesk, 29 Burwood Park Road, Walton-on-Thames, Surrey KT12 5LH

Riding: The British Horse Society, British Equestrian Centre, Stoneleigh, Kenilworth, Warwicks CV8 2LR, tel. 0203 52241

Sailing: The Royal Yachting Association, Victoria Way, Woking, Surrey GU21 1EQ, tel. 048–62 5022

The Schizophrenia Association of Great Britain, International Schizophrenia Centre, Bryn Hyfryd, The Crescent, Bangor, Gwynedd LL57 2AG, tel. 0248 354048

Shrubland Hall Health Clinic, Coddenham, Suffolk IP6 9QH, tel. 0473 830404

Rudolf Steiner House, 35 Park Road, London NW1 6XT, tel. 01-723 8219

Templegarth Trust, 82 Tinkle Street, Grimoldby, Louth, Lincs LN11 8TF, tel. 0507 82655

Traditional Chinese Medicine: The Council for Acupuncture, Suite 1, Cavendish Square, London W1M 9AD, tel. 01-409 1440

The Twins and Multiple Births Association, 20 Redcar Close, Lillington, Leamington Spa, Warwicks CV32 7SW, tel. 0926 22688

University of the Third Age, 6 Parkside Gardens, London SW19 5EY

The Open University, Walton Hall, Milton Keynes MK7 6AA, tel. 0908 74066

The Vegetarian Society of the United Kingdom Ltd, Parkdale, Dunham Road, Altrincham, Cheshire WA14 4QG, tel. 061-928 0793

Water Pik, R.C.L. Limited, 42 Earlham Street, Covent Garden, London WC2H 9LJ, tel. 01–240 0385

Weleda (UK) Ltd, Heanor Road, Ilkeston, Derbyshire DE7 8DR, tel. 0602 303151

Westbank Healing & Teaching Centre, Strathmiglo, Fife KY14 7QP, tel. 033–76 233

Wholefood Ltd, & The Wholefood Bookshop: 24 Paddington Street, London W1M 4DR, tel. 01–935 3924

Windsurfing: The Royal Yachting Association, Victoria Way, Woking, Surrey GU21 1EQ, tel. 048–62 5022

Wines: Baker Wines, 74 Tinkle Street, Grimoldby, Louth, Lincs LN11 8TF, tel. 0507 82227
Hinton Wines, Camellia Cottage, Leyswood, Groombridge, Tunbridge Wells, Kent
Clive Edwards, 'Burlton', Shillingstone, Blandford Forum, Dorset DT11 0SP, tel. 0258–860641
Maison Millières, 29 Sydney Street, Brighton, East Sussex BN1 4EP, tel. 0273 676830
Vintage Roots, 88 Radstock Road, Reading, Berks, RG1 3PR, tel. 0734–662569
Eaton Elliot Winebrokers, 15 London Road, Alderley Edge, Cheshire SK9 7JT, tel. 0625–582354
Ilkley Wine Cellars, 52 The Grove, Ilkley, West Yorks LS29 9BN, tel. 0943-607313
Peter Green, 37a/b Warrender Park Road, Edinburgh EH9 1HJ, tel. 031–229 5925
The Lincolnshire Wine Company, Laburnum Cottage, Chapel Lane, Ludborough, Grimsby, S. Humberside DN36 5SJ, tel. 0472 840858

Women's Health Concern, 17 Earls Terrace, London W8 6LP

The Wrekin Trust, Runnings Park, Croft Bank, West Malvern, Worcs WR14 4BP, tel. 06845 60099

The British Wheel of Yoga, 80 Leckhampton Road, Cheltenham, Glos

AIDS, Acquired Immune Deficiency Syndrome

AIDS is the newest epidemic to threaten human beings. It began quietly in Central Africa (especially Zaire and Uganda), where it may have been long established, and was first diagnosed in America and Britain during 1981. Since then it has spread rapidly among the limited group of people who are susceptible, and rather more than half of those affected have since died.

Susceptibility depends on INFECTION with a virus known as HIV, HTLV III, LAV or ARV. It only affects humans, and can only be caught directly into your bloodstream. Once there it arouses an IMMUNE response so that within about three months antibody to HIV can be detected in your blood. If you are healthy you can destroy the virus in this way, before any damage is done.

But this virus is capable of penetrating precisely those blood cells that enable you to make immune responses! If for any reason your immunity is deficient at the time you are infected with the virus, it succeeds in penetrating those white blood cells that are specially programmed by your *primal adaptive system** to recognize threats and start an immune reaction. Once inside these *T-helper lymphocytes** the virus can overprint part of your genes with its own. That blood cell is then enslaved to the virus, no longer responding to your *'colour'** control; it produces thousands of copies of the virus before dying, exhausted. Eventually too few T-helper lymphocytes survive to keep your immune system working. This allows rare CANCERS and infections you can normally prevent to romp freely through your body.

This catastrophic breakdown of your immunity is not inevitable, even if you are infected with HIV. It affects particularly people who may be poorly nourished, have little self-esteem or are poorly regarded by their neighbours and family, or who have little purpose in living. These are the adverse factors common to all the groups in whom the disease has spread fastest, and lacking in the group that has resisted the disease most impressively against great odds – the wives of infected haemophiliacs. Statistics bear this out in their bald and colourless fashion. Two years after exposure sufficient to cause an antibody response, three out of four people remain quite healthy; they have destroyed the virus, prevented it from penetrating their blood cells or resisted its effects once inside those cells. The immunity of three fifths of the others (15% overall) has come under strain. The remaining two fifths (10% overall) have full-blown AIDS and about half of these have died from its effects. Individual experience varies widely; some victims quickly contract AIDS and die, whereas others stay healthy or survive much longer than these averages forecast – because their immunity stands up to the virus.

Exposure to HIV seems set to spread rapidly through homosexual and bisexual men, then through their female partners to their children. It has already reached more than half the haemophiliacs in Britain, through the regular blood transfusions they need; that exposure has now ceased, but its legacy remains. Drug abusers who inject are rapidly sharing the infection; up to one-third now have antibodies. It will eventually reach a sizeable minority outside the present high-risk groups, despite every sexual precaution.

HELPING YOURSELF

The only positive protection against AIDS is to maintain your general IMMUNE function at a very high level. If your general health is good this means maintaining the DIET for health, SUPPLEMENTED with Honey Cider Vinegar or the Egg Nog RECIPE for minerals, and Vitamin C.

If your general condition is poor or you are in one of the risk categories listed below, supplement the diet more intensively as for immunity.

The only sexual partnerships that are absolutely safe have been exclusively monogamous since 1980 or before. Heterosexual intercourse is not safer than homosexual intercourse. Regular correct use of sheaths offers some protection.

Ordinary social contact with an HIV or AIDS victim is quite safe, but you should not share toothbrushes or razors. Wash their used crockery in detergent water hot enough to require rubber gloves, which will kill any virus there may be. Launder their clothes and bed-linen with an ordinary hot-wash cycle; it is quite safe to use a public launderette.

Spillages of blood, vomit, faeces or urine from a victim should be cleaned up carefully, by its owner if he is fit enough. Dampen the cloth you use with a strong chlorine disinfectant diluted one part in ten with water; wear rubber gloves yourself. The virus is very easily killed by disinfectant or heat and cannot survive outside the victim's body.

Further guidance is available if you call or send sae to:

Terrence Higgins Trust, BM AIDS, London WC1N 3XX. Telephone 01–833 2971
Welsh AIDS Campaign 0222–464121
Scottish AIDS Monitor 031–558 1167
Haemophilia Society, PO Box 9, 16 Trinity Street, London SE1 1DE for 'Advice on
    Safer Sex'
Healthline, 0345 581151
Royal College of Nursing (UK), Publications Department, 20 Cavendish Square,
    London W1M 0AB, for 'AIDS guidelines for health professionals'
London Lesbian and Gay Switchboard 01–837 7324
Standing Conference on Drug Abuse 01–430 2341
Any Special Treatment or Venereal (Sexually Transmitted) Disease Clinic
Department A, PO Box 100, Milton Keynes, MK1 1TX – for a copy of the booklet
    'AIDS: What Everybody Needs to Know'

Supportive COUNSELLING, meditation, relaxation or visualization can greatly boost your self-esteem and purposiveness if you already have AIDS, or are antibody positive. The St James Centre for Health and Healing, Piccadilly, London, offers an experienced holistic team approach to this which has helped many a great deal.

ALCOHOL

Fermentation to wine has for thousands of years been the only available means of preserving the nutritional value of the plentiful fruit harvest in hot climates, and incidentally of providing a WATER supply safe to drink; but it has always had its drawbacks. Alcohol is a *metabolic** poison, attacking your liver and kidneys as well as making exceptional demands of them. When fortified and purified by distillation it is separated from the vitamins and minerals in the original fruit or grain which you need to metabolize the alcohol as fuel; you steal these from other food sources to alleviate the STRESS as quickly as possible. Spirits and chemically refined beers and wines are therefore a drain on your nutrition. This is why sherry and cocktails are such effective aperitifs – they steal trace nutrients and lower your blood sugar, making you hungry. In excess, of course, the alcohol itself and this HYPOGLY-CAEMIC effect combine to stupefy your palate and general sensibility, thoroughly spoiling your meal.

Dr Carl Pfeiffer of the Brain Bio Centre (ADDRESS) has contributed much to our biochemical knowledge of alcoholism; several of his BOOKS are in print. He recognizes four types of alcoholic. First there is the chronic DEPRESSIVE, overstimulated with the brain sedative *histamine,** who slowly drinks himself to death because of his depression. In direct contrast stands the overstimulated individual who has too little brain histamine to relax and breaks his periods of TENSION by alcoholic binges at weekends. Then there is the cerebral ALLERGIC, who becomes dependent on alcohol and over-indulges but is embarrassingly hypersensitive to intoxication. Finally, there are probably a few pre-diabetics with HYPOGLYCAEMIA who use alcohol as a handy means to satisfy their frequent carbohydrate cravings.

Once dependence on alcohol is established, for any of these reasons, it enters the adaptation phase of stress disease for anything up to several years. Provided you can get alcohol regularly it cheers you up, keeps you functioning and makes you quite confident you can give it up whenever you want. But if you cannot get it you become irritable and nervous, gloomy and unable to concentrate or function well. Eventually the periods of good cheer shorten, and you need to drink earlier in the day and more heavily to keep going.

By this time your mineral and vitamin nutrition are gradually deteriorating with secondary effects on your APPETITE and metabolic organs. Your liver in particular is poisoned by every drinking bout. *Cirrhosis** is the fibrous INFLAMMATORY healing process that patches up wounds in your degenerate liver. At first it may swell as a result, but eventually the fibrous tissue shrinks and strangles its CIRCULATION and *bile** passages.

Total exhaustion of your response to alcoholic stimulation heralds the end stage of your illness, in which structural disorders of your liver and kidneys predominate. Even at this stage, however, a lot can be reclaimed if you decide to try and take appropriate corrective action.

HELPING YOURSELF

If you wish to enjoy alcohol safely, choose 'real ale' and wines made by traditional chemical-free methods, preferably from 'Organic' fruit or grains – those grown on naturally composted soils without chemical pesticides. Hinton Wines (South East) and Baker Wines (Midlands) import an excellent exclusive range of traditional wines from France; Wholefood (London) and the Lincolnshire Wine Company purvey fine 'organic' wines, some of which are suitable for DIABETICS.

Spirits are more dangerous, especially to young people; consume them rarely. Avoid establishing any daily drinking habit, and avoid getting drunk.

If you intend to drive within a few hours, do not drink at all.

If you abuse alcohol, you must accept and realize this before you can even begin to get better. So long as you think you are in control and could give it up any time, nothing can help you. When the truth dawns, join Alcoholics Anonymous (ADDRESS).

If you are close to an alcoholic who will not admit it, join AL-ANON (ADDRESS).

The alcoholic who can still function normally needs urgent help with a healthy DIET emphasising whole protein foods a little – fish, milk or yoghurt, peas and beans. To combat HYPOGLYCAEMIA he should avoid refined starchy snacks and sugar of all kinds.

The sick alcoholic, who probably has significant liver degeneration already, needs instead a low protein diet for health so as not to overload his weakened capacity for protein metabolism.

SUPPLEMENTS should include a Strong Vitamin B Complex (eg Nature's Own Ltd), which incorporates Vitamins B_3 (Niacin) and B_6 (Pyridoxine) in high dosage – 150–300mg of each. Vitamin C (500mg) and Vitamin E (100–200IU) three times daily consolidate this. Zinc 15mg, Dolomite 2500mg and Chromium 3mg are important minerals to supplement: these and Vitamin C together will correct the excessive Copper and deficient Magnesium levels found in many alcoholics.

In skilled hands, *Traditional Chinese Medicine** (Acupuncture) can help very much to reduce alcohol dependence. *Hypnotherapy** makes similar claims, but should only be put in the hands of a therapist mature enough to cope with the complex and deep-seated psychological problems hypnosis may reveal. A *Psychiatrist** or *Clinical Psychologist** should ideally be involved in the process (ADDRESSES).

ALLERGY, hypersensitivity, intolerance

If your IMMUNE system is perfectly balanced, it is also elegant and economical. You recognize each threat accurately and with complete confidence, and defend yourself just vigorously enough to neutralize it. There is the same poise and grace about this as you expect in the POSTURE of a dancer or the hands of a musician.

Though there are diseases like AIDS in which the immune response is insufficient, they are hard to survive because they so drastically undermine self-maintenance; your body is taken over by other organisms or CANCER. In the survivable nuisances and diseases that can arise in your immune system errors show up as clumsiness or exaggeration of the effort put into overcoming a challenge, simply because the system is having to work too hard. Consequently the commonest symptoms are exaggerations too, caricatures of the normal defensive reactions at your body's key entry points – *rhinitis** and ASTHMA, VOMITING, DIARRHOEA, COLITIS and ECZEMA. Once the challenge gets into your blood, new possibilities arise – RHEUMATIC pains, MIGRAINE or HEADACHES and HYPERACTIVITY or other disturbances of mood and behaviour. And the struggle to get it out of you again may challenge your liver and kidneys and reactivate the original disturbances in your lungs, nose and skin – they are equally vulnerable from inside and out.

You may have inherited this problem but *atopic** people, who seem to possess a bodily defect which makes them unable to cope with a few perfectly natural *allergens*,* are uncommon. Nor does atopy account well for a new wave of sensitivity problems that were first recognized in the middle of this century. At first these appeared to be allergies in the traditional sense. However challenge tests gave variable results that were hard to reproduce and seldom corroborated by positive skin or blood tests. The lists of substances reacted to were so long and unreliable that doctors incredulously rejected the whole phenomenon.

Its explanation is simple. Your immune system is not defective as in true allergy but simply overwhelmed by STRESS. There are thousands more unnatural and irritant chemicals in our environment than there used to be before industrialization, with current additions running at around ten every week. These heap increasing challenges on your immune system, so that it fails generally as your health declines. The problem in this case is not in you but your surroundings.

Intolerance of this kind is now forcing itself increasingly on doctors' attention because it is rapidly becoming very common in all developed countries. Government medical advisers still hugely underestimate it because they rely on a science that cannot cope with '*colour*'* phenomena. Perhaps they also dread the implications of admitting its validity. Your experience is all you need to convince yourself, however. And you do not have to put up with it.

HELPING YOURSELF

Commence the special DIET for cleansing, SUPPLEMENTED for your immune system. If your symptoms are not severe, the diet for health may be sufficient on its own.

If after three weeks you are no better for this, try to identify what sort of things are still upsetting you. These could include foods still included in your diet or chemicals with which they have been grown or treated. Details of how to find out are given in Mansfield's BOOK *Chemical Children*, which you may need to consult; the special DIET for allergy gives basic directions. You will need to classify your foods into similar families and strictly exclude one whole family from Monday to Friday afternoon of one week. Re-introduce it at teatime on Friday, and watch for any effect. Worsening of symptoms during the weekend will suggest you are intolerant of that food family at present. Remember to check your drinking WATER, cosmetics and household chemicals – including medicines, where possible.

If you draw a blank on food families, alter the basis of your approach and try a salicylate-free special DIET for six weeks.

Avoid in any case things you do not need which may be irritant – artificial food colourings and preservatives, sugar, refined flour and tobacco. See Lawrence's BOOK for further guidance on food chemicals.

Try a week without coffee, Indian or Sri Lankan tea, cocoa, chocolate, cola or tobacco to check whether the xanthines they contain aggravate your problems. If they do you may feel dreadful during that week and better on Saturday after resuming them. If so you need a cleansing DIET for three weeks and will need to avoid consuming them regularly ever again.

Your doctor will be able to arrange skin tests for allergy to things you cannot easily exclude yourself – house dust, dogs and cats, moulds and spores. Take hairs from your own pets for him to test you with – they vary as much as people do. Preventative medication may be available to suppress over-reaction to any of these you cannot totally avoid.

THRUSH infestation can play havoc with your immune system, giving symptoms which fail on some of these tests. Consult that topic for advice.

A beard or moustache greatly increases your exposure to dust, smoke and fumes. Shave them off if you are desperate enough. It solved my problem.

ANGINA

Wherever arteries are heavily stressed they age faster, because ARTERIOSCLER-OSIS proceeds more rapidly. This gradually narrows them, slowly strangling the blood supply beyond.

The arteries of your heart are particularly susceptible to this kind of degeneration because they bear the brunt of its pulsations. The maximum power your heart is capable of depends ultimately on the blood supply it receives, and dwindles gradually over the years as the blood vessels become narrower. In developed countries people rarely exert themselves fully, so the limitation is very advanced before you begin to notice it. Then you feel a tight gripping pain in the centre of your chest, or down the inside of your arms or in your jaw, whenever you exert yourself beyond a certain limit. It quickly eases when you rest and is predictable so that you learn to recognize the limit of what you can do. This lessens after meals, in cold weather and when you are angry or under pressure. You can do more in warm weather, with nothing to digest. Provided you keep within the pace dictated by the pain, you can get on with your life normally. The condition can remain very stable over decades but your STRESS tolerance is permanently hindered.

Other disorders commonly coexist with this, such as DIABETES and high BLOOD PRESSURE, because they also make your arteries age faster. Shortage of red blood cells (anaemia*) makes matters worse, and can cause angina while your arteries are still quite healthy if the shortage is severe enough.

Arteries elsewhere can be similarly involved, most commonly in your leg. Pain then arises in your calf after brisk walking. It is identical with angina in origin but was named intermittent claudication* after Claudius, the limping emperor of ancient Rome.

Angina makes it more likely that you will have a CORONARY at some time, because narrowing of your coronary arteries is the usual background for this. Nevertheless, many people with angina who settle to a comfortable and measured pace of life defy this risk, because their disease teaches them to manage stress and to keep within their capabilities.

When all this has been said, remember too that your body constantly seeks to conform to your 'colour'* pattern, and that your arteries slowly grow and change their shape even when they are diseased. People sometimes manage to reverse the progress or effects of their disease, if they are determined about it and persevere doggedly enough. They are in effect intensifying their 'colour' blueprint and encouraging their arteries to rally to it after a period of disarray.

The same intensity of living can prevent your decline in the first place, and remains available to you at any stage in the disease. You can choose to relax into decline, so making it inevitable. Or you may find the enthusiasm to gracefully defy decline and come alive instead. Angina is a symptom that gives you the time to go through all this, and monitors your progress.

HELPING YOURSELF

Relief of angina attacks can be accelerated by holding your breath and sucking hard for a count of five. Then BREATHE with your abdomen, slowly and deeply, for a few minutes more. This draws down your *diaphragm*,* which elongates your heart and lungs and expands your coronary vessels slightly, massaging and drawing blood into them. It complements rest and reduces your need for medication. Abdominal breathing for a few minutes each day has a cumulative effect which will extend your exercise limit.

More cumulative relief results from the regular habit of bathing your forearms, first in hot water for three minutes and then under the cold tap for thirty seconds. This cycle can be repeated three times, finishing with cold. It eases the tone of the nerves to your heart, making you less susceptible to TENSION and STRESS. Ten minutes of this twice daily is well spent.

You should be able to stem or reverse the progress of your condition by adopting the cleansing DIET and SUPPLEMENTING it as for *arterial disease*.* After a few weeks' perseverence you can afford to relax on to the diet for health, but maintain the supplements. If you are OVERWEIGHT take steps to reduce, slowly but surely. If you SMOKE, make it an urgent priority to stop.

If you are a naturally COLD person, consider the advice on that topic.

With all these measures in hand, you can afford to exercise well up to your limit. Walk for half an hour, clothed lightly but warmly, on a disciplined daily basis. This intensifies the 'colour' pattern of your defective part, challenging its blood vessels to expand along all available routes which by-pass the blockage. In this way tiny arterioles gradually enlarge in a permanent structural fashion and your exercise tolerance expands – sometimes even to the point where your angina completely disappears. This will take courage, and perseverence for at least a year. Then maintain the habit, to celebrate and sustain your condition.

Keep a bright outlook on life, take a keen interest in everything around you and pursue consistent purposes of your own. This intensifies your 'colour' pattern, and keeps your IMMUNE system busy living up to it.

However silly you may feel, spend a few minutes each day relaxing and imagining what it is like inside your damaged arteries. Then visualize fish, or soldiers, or blood cells, cleaning out the rubbish and healing the damage. The image does not matter – great things can be done with imaginary flue-brushes. Repeat this interlude every day, each time seeing the results accumulate. You are exercising the power your mind was always supposed to have over the *'mono'** substance of your body. With constant practice, you can regain that power. Your disease will give you all the time you need.

ANTIBIOTICS

Antibiotics are chemical substances which kill *bacteria** or stop them multiplying. Many of them are made by other kinds of *microbes** such as fungi as part of their IMMUNE mechanism. Chemists have extracted these, altered some, and manufactured them for medical use. Others have been invented that do not occur naturally.

Their discovery nearly fifty years ago revolutionized the treatment of bacterial INFECTIONS and greatly enhanced the standing of medicine in Western society. But it involved removing a natural mechanism from its proper context and increasing enormously the scale of its use. This called for a high degree of responsibility and discretion, which has unfortunately not been exercised. Consequently antibiotics are used far too often, mostly when bacteria are not even involved in the disease being treated.

Particularly unfortunate is their routine use in low doses to promote the growth of animals for food. You consume these antibiotics with their meat, but in doses too low to eradicate the bacteria in your *colon** or on your skin. Instead, with a generation time measured in minutes rather than years, bacteria adapt much faster than animals and people. As a result many are now resistant to destruction by the simplest and safest antibiotics. Resistant varieties thrive at the expense of the non-resistant, altering the kinds of bacteria that live alongside you and contributing to COLITIS. *Gastro-enteritis** resistant to any form of antibiotic treatment arises in the same way and has caused some lethal epidemics in residential institutions.

Meanwhile habitual assistance from antibiotics is making us lazy. We give ordinary hygienic precautions too little attention, instead expecting anti-biotic treatment as soon as we ail. Our defences are therefore challenged insufficiently to establish adequate immunity to those bacteria we do encounter, so that next time we meet them we are still vulnerable. What is more, every course of antibiotics encourages the growth of fungi like THRUSH, which are not affected by antibiotics and multiply unopposed during anti-biotic treatment. Their ability to transform into a *mycelium** is particularly worrying, as this makes FUNGAL INFECTIONS much more troublesome and difficult to get rid of in their turn.

The long-term result of continuing like this exactly resembles personal *habituation** to any other drug. If you take SLEEPING medicine very occasion-ally, the benefit is reliable and the side-effects few. But habitual consumption enables your body to decode the medicine and neutralize its effects. Conse-quently you need more and more to achieve the same benefit and suffer increasingly from the side-effects of higher dosage. Eventually you find yourself dependent on a regular high dose to achieve sleep no better than before you started medication – all you get are its complications!

With antibiotics we are seeing an historical version of the same thing. Habituation has now taken place; a generation has grown up accustomed to depending on them. By next century we shall have rendered antibiotics useless unless we stop using them casually now. Doctors should give a much stronger lead, but everyone must learn for themselves to rely on simpler defences.

HELPING YOURSELF

Look on antibiotics as a precious capital reserve, to be drawn on a few times only in your life, if at all. Do not assume they will always remain as readily available as they are now.

When a SORE THROAT is accompanied by a runny or congested nose, the cause is probably a VIRUS. Use antiseptic lozenges or gargles for at least three days before seeking more drastic treatment. Red sage leaves make a very useful gargle or drink. Use one teaspoon of dried leaf per breakfast cup, brewed in freshly boiled water for three minutes. Alternatively the garlic lozenge RECIPE is a powerful natural antiseptic, and Vitamin C in large doses (1000mg hourly to begin with) helps to reduce the upset of the condition; it will sometimes stop it in its tracks.

Most EARACHE is caused by pressure from trapped CATARRH, not INFECTION at all. If you consult the doctor for it, make clear that you understand this and would prefer to avoid an antibiotic until treatment for the catarrhal blockage has been tried.

Hold out even against *bacterial** infections for three days if you can. That ensures that your defences are properly alerted, so that adequate *antibody** protection is built up for the future; you will then not need any treatment next time you encounter this particular germ. During this time you will find that garlic and Vitamin C are powerful aids to your general defences; both are antiseptic to most microbes including bacteria. Local treatment with antiseptics such as Hydrogen Peroxide, dilute Potassium Chlorate or Permanganate solution or 1% Gentian Violet (Crystal Violet) in water is very effective – Gentian Violet keeps the best but is rather colourful! After three days only change to antibiotic treatment if that is still necessary to shorten the incapacitation or illness.

Delay is only unwise for seriously ill children or anyone with severe HEADACHE or stiff neck. Even then you can put the matter in your doctor's hands, waiting for results of the proper tests before pressing for treatment. You will rarely need to do this; doctors usually exercise much better judgement when pressure is withheld.

If you accept an antibiotic course, take it meticulously as instructed. Vitamin B_5 (Pantothenic Acid 50mg twice daily) helps to prevent side-effects.

If side-effects occur, consult your doctor before stopping the course of antibiotic treatment. You may need to follow it with another kind without a break.

Follow the antibiotic course immediately with live yoghurt RECIPE at each of three meals daily, on its own or with cereals or fruit. This reintroduces *Lactobacillus aerogenes* into your intestine, to restore digestion and discourage fungi such as thrush. The *Lactobacillus* culture will usually over whelm this, but prolonged treatment or several different antibiotics in close succession make this less likely; look up THRUSH for further advice.

APPETITE

Millions of years of simultaneous natural evolution of human beings and their food supply have enabled you to sense the value of your food by its 'colour'.* Your 'mono'* senses of taste and smell are crude by comparison, capable of a very limited range of sensations; yet up to now, our scientific knowledge of appetite is based entirely on these. We have never before been able to understand how a year-old baby can select just what he needs from a range of whole fresh foods without any nutritional knowledge. He simply hungers for the 'colours' lacking in his own signature and craves foods offering these 'colours'.

That experiment does not work with modern refined, processed and preserved foods because they no longer have a 'colour' signature. The child is forced to depend on his 'mono' senses, craving for the sweetness, saltiness, acidity or bitterness which is all they can tell him. These isolated 'mono' tastes only switch off when he is thoroughly glutted, sick of the food bearing them; by then he has had far too much. Anything less obviously tasty is dull by comparison; he will not show any inclination to eat it, however nourishing it may be. The result resembles an addiction; unbalanced nutrition makes the child crave for chemicalized food in huge quantities – his taste buds are briefly gratified but his hunger never is. Nutritional balance is lost, along with physical and mental health. If this includes CATARRH or Zinc deficiency his sense of taste is further impaired, which makes matters worse.

Food manufacturers have taken full advantage of all this. Never in the forefront of fundamental nutritional research, their chief concern is with microbial* safety, cosmetics, simplicity of manufacture and taste. They vie with one another to synthesize ever more tantalizing flavours. Sugar, salt, acids and bitters are heavily used as primary flavours and to enhance what little characteristic taste the food has left. Newer flavour enhancers have since been added to this battery, and a long list of secret flavourings is treasured by each chef to give his product that extra edge. Sales now depend so much on 'mono' taste, colour, texture and marketing that nutritive value had become a very poor second – until people began to notice what was going on.

We now know that HYPERACTIVITY, ALLERGY, OVERWEIGHT and anorexia nervosa* can sometimes be traced either directly to chemical food additives, or to the faulty nutrition that results from dependence on the counterfeit refined foods created around them. Widespread public awareness of chemical additives has made their absence from a manufactured food product a strong selling point.

'Organic'* agricultural methods are our next target, to replace the 'mono' chemicals in fresh foods with real 'colour' substance to which our finer faculties can learn to respond. But it takes a long time to regain the use of senses long neglected. Meanwhile we must continue to fly out of the chemical murk relying chiefly on our 'mono' instruments, but encouraged by gradually lengthening glimpses of the 'colour' sky.

HELPING YOURSELF

Go through your larder and take stock of the food you buy. Note how much of it is really fresh and alive until you eat it, and how much is dead and preserved unnaturally; how much is still whole in its natural form and how much refined and chemically processed. Decide not to buy a few of the most refined and chemicalized dead items next time.

Do not simply leave these out but substitute something tasty and better. Replace sweets with nuts and fruit, sugary cereals with porridge or whole wheat, white sugar with black molasses or malt. They cost more, so buy and use less of them; they are much more nourishing and tasty, weight for weight.

Keep up the pressure once you have started, replacing each week a few of the worst remaining items. Learn as you go along how to serve them to best advantage. You are gradually changing over to the DIET for health.

Do not make an issue of the changes with your husband; let him have some old favourites but gradually meet new options.

Be much firmer with your children, and make the change quickly. The secret is to let them get really hungry, if necessary. Tell them what you are doing, and go right ahead. Serve three fresh wholesome meals a day, withholding all sugar and salt to start with. Replace squashes and cordials with diluted juices and sweets with fruit. Show no concern at what they leave on their plates but refuse any snacks between meals. Within a very few days they will be properly hungry and begin to notice the subtle satisfaction proper food offers.

If they do not, they may need mineral or vitamin SUPPLEMENTS; deficiencies can disturb their taste sensibility. Zinc (15mg daily), Brewer's Yeast (3–6 tablets daily) and Vitamin B_6 (Pyridoxine, 50mg daily) are the most useful to start with; but they may eventually need more, under guidance from a *Naturopath,* *Nutritionist* or Dietitian.

Do not then expect them to empty every plate. Respect their appetites for good quality food, they will not need so much of it.

Ban chemical food treats at home; they will get quite enough at other children's parties, and you may be surprised at the disturbing effect they then have on them. If they feel bloated or ill, or are actually sick, it is worthwhile sympathetically pointing out the connection with the counterfeit food they are usually spared. Other children are adapted to this STRESS because they are regularly exposed to it. Better fed children resist the stress properly because they meet it seldom and recognize its threat to their IMMUNITY.

ARTERIOSCLEROSIS, atheroma, hardening of the arteries

Your heart is a very remarkable organ. It beats 100,000 times daily throughout your life, expanding and contracting through a considerable range of size with each beat. This is punishing enough for the muscle of your heart, but consider the amazing resilience of the thin glistening skin which lines its chambers and the walls of all your arteries in one seamless streamlined sheet. This too is being stretched and crumpled 100,000 times every day – treatment no plastic or leather would stand up to for seven days, never mind seventy years!

Your heart lining has the advantage of being alive and able to sustain itself. Its blood supply is exceptionally rich, coming not only from the small blood vessels that feed the wall of the artery but from the blood flowing past it as well. Provided this contains what the skin cells require they can maintain a perfectly smooth elastic surface of supple cells firmly cemented together at their edges, new cells forming to replace each exhausted veteran as it harmlessly disintegrates.

Any imperfections in this supply system quickly make the skin cells and their cement more fragile so that they tear more often. This mostly happens near your heart, where the stresses with each heart-beat are much greater. The same imperfections make healing prolonged and difficult, during which time the tiny open wound is readily soiled with any surpluses your blood is burdened with. Many of these dissolve back into your blood when it is cleaner, but this continual silting process distorts the 'colour' form the skin is trying to resume, leaving a grotesquely deformed and thickened scar in place of the inconspicuous seam your nature intended. Worst of all, the turbulent blood flow around these scars makes fresh tears more likely, which add to the deformity and narrow the calibre of the artery.

This is the nature of arteriosclerosis, which in developed countries affects almost every child from birth and gradually accumulates throughout life. It affects the tiny arteries in the muscle of your blood vessels too, so that they degenerate into rigid pipes that can no longer elastically absorb the energy of your pulse-beat; high BLOOD PRESSURE may show this, or unfolding of the crook of your *aorta** (visible on your chest X-ray). The COLDNESS of thyroid insufficiency greatly accelerates it. SMOKING magnifies its effects. It is the basic weakness in ANGINA, CORONARIES, STROKES and many other CIRCULATION problems.

It is not inevitable, being virtually absent in less developed peoples who have held to their traditional ways. Even in quite advanced cases it can be stopped, and perhaps reversed. That doctors neglect these possibilities, steering all our medical resources into the SURGICAL treatment of its effects instead, is obviously foolish and wasteful. It remains for you to help yourself, and impress your doctor into paying some attention to your methods.

HELPING YOURSELF

Stick to the DIET for health, which cannot unleash huge surges of sugar or fat into your bloodstream to stress the nourishment of the skin surrounding it or interfere with any wounds in the skin's surface.

SUPPLEMENT the diet with Vitamin C (Ascorbic Acid 1000mg 3 times daily), Vitamins B_5 (Pantothenic Acid 50mg daily) and B_6 (Pyridoxine 50mg twice daily), Zinc (15mg daily), and Dolomite (500mg three times daily) if you know you have heart disease or aortic unfolding already. Balance up your total Vitamin B intake with 3–6 additional tablets of Brewer's Yeast daily.

Vitamin E (200–400IU twice daily) and Selenium (200 microgm twice daily) are more expensive, but well worth while if you wish to stem the tide of further degeneration.

If the level of fats in your blood is too high Lecithin (1000mg 3 times daily) can reduce this and may be capable of emulsifying fatty deposits for proper disposal.

Give up SMOKING, or at least cut it down drastically.

EXERCISE regularly for at least ten minutes each day, energetically enough to make you mildly breathless throughout that period. Extend this to thirty minutes at least three times weekly if you are also OVERWEIGHT.

BREATHE deeply with your diaphragm five to ten times, at least once or twice daily. This massages your heart and great blood vessels, keeping them supple and giving your nutritional measures more of a chance to work.

If you are COLDER than you feel you should be follow the guidance given on that topic, which is especially important for younger people.

If you get ANGINA, try the additional measures discussed under that heading.

Whether or not these steps are supervised by your doctor, seek his guidance and blessing in undertaking them, and keep him informed of your progress. Some of the tests he can make may show changes that impress him, and he may offer the programme to other patients. He is often now able to recognize people whose risk for heart disease is high but cannot offer them much positive help. Your willingness to take the initiative makes it much easier for him to explore the possibilities. That is how progress is made.

ARTHRITIS

Your JOINTS are specialized for hard mechanical work. An ordinary circulation would be torn or crushed whenever you moved, so each joint is bathed in a fluid that oozes out of blood vessels in its capsule and is massaged back and forth as it moves. This is much slower than the arrangement elsewhere in your body and cannot cope with rapid metabolism or healing. But it refreshes and nourishes the joint surfaces quite fast enough to cope with the modest demands of healthy *cartilage** that is not being abused.

Any habitual derangement of your POSTURE or movement throws extra strain on the joints involved, which may call for healing nourishment beyond their means. Many people with flat FEET walk badly enough to strain their ankles, *knees,** *hips** and BACKS excessively over many years. Why as many as one in ten seem to have this problem from birth is still a mystery to me. Nevertheless most osteo-arthritis, or joint wear and tear, probably arises from it.

COLDNESS affects joints more drastically than any other part because it makes the fluid in them flow more slowly. Since it also diminishes the pain which might otherwise warn you of abuse, you are doubly vulnerable to wear and tear until it is corrected.

*Rheumatoid arthritis** stems from the same weakness. Your joints are a metabolic backwater, and whenever you are congested with waste acids they tend to be dumped there; severe THRUSH sometimes contributes to this. At first these deposits are only semi-solid, easily taken up into solution whenever opportunity arises, as in MIGRAINE. But if the deposit becomes permanent it hardens into crystalline incrustations which are much denser and less bulky. At first they are insignificant, and you tolerate them. But after years of accumulation they begin to irritate – they are poisons, after all. Your joints inflame against them, perhaps quite acutely; conventional medical treatment may suppress that INFLAMMATION but cannot remove its cause. So you are liable to relapses whenever your tolerance breaks down.

Meanwhile the accumulating deposits, and your frustrated inflammatory energy, chronically disrupt the joint's *'colour'** so that it cannot maintain its proper form. Grotesque deformities are the most striking and visible *'mono'** consequence of the disease. PAIN, weakness and handicap are more likely to preoccupy its victims.

Few people die of arthritis, though some are killed by BLEEDING caused by their treatment. Instead they linger on, dogged increasingly by pain and handicap, more and more dependent on others. Medical researchers pretend to seek a cure but refuse to look in the only profitable direction. Evidently it is too cheap and easy, or not clever enough to appeal to them. They avoid it by choice, not ignorance. Bircher-Benner's methods were tried successfully on twelve 'incurable' arthritics at the Royal Free Hospital in 1937 (see p. 40), but nothing more was heard of it. Doctors carry a heavy responsibility for consistently ignoring the obvious, at their patients' expense.

Take seriously repeated or chronic pains in your joints, especially if they also swell and stiffen. Plan a special DIET for long-term cleansing to reverse the basic process. Tell your doctor you are doing it, and seek his cooperation in avoiding pain-killing medicines that will spoil its effect.

SUPPLEMENT this with Zinc (15mg daily), Vitamin C (Ascorbic Acid 1000mg three times daily), and Vitamins B_5 (Pantothenic Acid 100mg twice daily) and B_6 (Pyridoxine 50mg twice daily) supported with 6 tablets daily of Brewer's Yeast.

If you feel unnaturally cold or your normal temperature is low follow the advice given on COLDNESS.

Use heat to increase the traffic of healing in your joints. Ideally soak them in hot water for three minutes, then tone them up with cold water for half a minute; repeat this cycle up to three times on each occasion. This gives relief lasting up to a few hours and can be repeated whenever you wish.

For some joints an infra-red lamp is a more convenient source of heat, which can be applied for five to ten minutes at a time. Shorter times are better, alternated with cold water or ice packs as above.

Low Melting Point Wax BP gives a comfortable heat for your hands. Melt it in an old pan and let it cool until the surface skins over. Dip your hands in it, peel off the solid wax, and repeat. Finish after 5–10 minutes with a fifteen-second rinse under the cold tap.

Comfrey helps joints heal faster and is safe provided you keep the joint moving. Do not take tablets of comfrey root all the time; plant a few in your garden and use their leaves and stems in season as salad or tea. They also make excellent poultices, macerated and bound onto a painful knee or elbow with a cold damp cloth, then bandaged. This can be kept in place for an hour or two.

Green Lipped Mussel Extract has produced remarkable benefits for some arthritic people. Take it exactly as directed for a full six months. If you are elderly or severely affected, persevere for longer.

Gentle *yoga** exercises help to remobilize stiff joints after the worst inflammation has settled. Contact an experienced teacher for help with major joints, but treat fingers and toes yourself. Work each joint through its full range of movement with your other hand, leaving all the muscles around that joint relaxed. Give ten minutes to this daily and your dexterity will rapidly improve.

An *Osteopath** can very much extend the range of treatment possibilities open to you. Consult one to discuss what he can offer and what you should expect. If there is none locally, look for a *Chartered Physiotherapist** with post-graduate experience in manipulative treatments. If his reputation is not clear on this point, ask the therapist directly.

ASTHMA

The millions of tiny bubbles at the business end of your lungs are amongst the most specialized *tissues** in your body. In order to permit fast exchange of gases between your blood and your breath these bubbles consist of only two skins, each no more than a single cell thick. This makes them extremely delicate and vulnerable, but so absolute is their dedication to their one function that they can do nothing else, least of all defend themselves. The merest whiff of solvent, acid, detergent or smoke can destroy them totally.

So they are carefully guarded by a series of defences stationed at intervals along your airways. Your nose not only conditions air to your lungs' liking, but is your most discriminating sentinel. Smells alert you to many airborne threats and may trigger extra *'mono'** defences – secretions, sneezing and nasal congestion indistinguishable from a COLD – as well as *'colour'** offence that makes you want fresh air. These defences are perfect for peaceable times, a screen through which essential traffic passes without impediment. They are overwhelmed by sustained challenges, and by-passed altogether by newly-invented chemicals whose 'colour' we have not yet learnt.

Your wind-pipe and its rigid branches then do their best with rather ineffectual COUGHING and INFLAMMATION. Your smaller airways, muscular and capable of shrinking their calibre almost to nothing, add this last desperate ploy to the defence of your vital gas-exchange skin. Except in very brief encounters this is futile, but their purpose is clear.

This is the basic process of asthma, which is mobilized in anyone by a challenge strong enough. *Atopic** people are peculiarly sensitive to a limited range of particular *allergens** as personal idiosyncracies, but all of us react in some way to obviously irritant or poisonous fumes, even in very small amounts. Thousands of chemical irritants are already widely prevalent, and ten new ones are being introduced each week. Some of them, like the organochlorine insecticides, accumulate in your body fat and reduce your IMMUNE resistance to everything else.

If you are well defended your nose bears the brunt, as *rhinitis** or *sinusitis.** Stubborn COUGHING means challenges have penetrated as far as your voice-box and wind-pipe. Asthma implies the deepest encroachment, all the way down to your smallest bronchial tubes. Any of these symptons can also be provoked from within. Your bronchial muscle and nasal skin react in their characteristic fashion to any kind of challenge. They do not appear to discriminate between airborne allergens and irritants and those that CIRCU-LATE in your blood stream.

Medical treatment to suppress asthma is quite effective, so that few wonder what causes the condition in the first place. Doctors are ready to admit that many more people suffer from asthma than used to be the case. But they are not as concerned as they should be to find out why or to take a definite stand on the environmental issues the answers provoke.

HELPING YOURSELF

Make sure that all gas and paraffin heaters and cookers burn efficiently and are properly ventilated to the outside. Draw fresh air from the least polluted windows of your home. Avoid using pressurized aerosol spray-cans – even most medicines come in alternative forms. Get SMOKERS to use a room separated from the rest of your house by a ventilated lobby. These precautions minimize your exposure to irritant gases.

An *ionizer** will efficiently clean and recharge the electrical quality of the air in your bedroom, car or living room. It would be hard pressed to cope with a kitchen or mains electronic appliances. Larger units are available to install in workplaces.

Learn to BREATHE efficiently, and always through your nose. During attacks inhale quickly and exhale very slowly; forcing your breath out only tightens your tubes more.

Most attacks can be relieved by a hot pack treatment you can give an asthmatic without any expert knowledge; but attend carefully to the details. You will need two good dry towels, and three good face-cloths in a basin of very hot water. Strip the victim to the waist and sit him facing away from you. Rub a little cold-pressed vegetable oil up and down either side of his spine. Wring out one of the face-cloths quickly and spread it over his back, covering it immediately with several thicknesses of towel to keep in the heat. Replace it with a fresh hot face-cloth every half minute, for 15 applications in all. The sixteenth should be cold; drench the cloth under the tap, not in the basin. Wash off the oil with soap and water, dry, and rest the victim for half an hour. You can repeat this if required, obtaining up to 50% relief each time.

Check yourself for ALLERGIES to foods and chemical additives, using the special DIET for allergy.

Keep to a diet for health, avoiding any food family you react badly to and falling back on the special diet for cleansing if you have a bad spell.

SUPPLEMENT this for IMMUNITY if the results are disappointing.

Conventional medicines for asthma suppress symptoms very well but do nothing to remove their cause or build your resistance. An *Osteopath,** *Homeopath** or *Traditional Chinese Medicine** practitioner may be able to cast fresh light on any riddles you and your doctor cannot solve (ADDRESSES).

WHAT HAPPENS

The twenty-seven bones that make up your spine get far too much attention because they show on X-rays and can be preserved hygienically enough to display as a hinged skeleton for study and display purposes. But this skeleton has very little stability on its own, sacrificed in favour of the suppleness and flexibility provided by the JOINTS, cartilages, ligaments, muscles and tendons attached to them. These are the really important parts, for which the bones are just a hard core. Doctors misunderstand this, which is why they deal with backache unimaginatively.

Your spine is therefore only the axis, anchorage and load-bearing part of your back. Its various other components weave together so harmoniously that you cannot dissect out their separate functions; they work as a whole. Your limbs, ribs and skull are not separate either; their muscles and ligaments interweave with their counterparts along your back, gracefully extending your form and faculties in smooth continuity.

'Mono'* physiology is a very inadequate way to understand a form like this, which has to flow as a whole in response to rhythmic changes in your 'colour'* signature. Brain, NERVE and muscle can execute your movements, but your 'colour' function creates and directs them – just as elaborate 'mono' processes digest your food under the direction of APPETITE.

So when your back aches, changes will not usually show on X-rays, and structures are seldom seriously disturbed. The pain signifies strain in the structures most abused by your unbalanced action-pattern. They may not even be INFLAMED, but congested with a backlog of metabolic waste your circulation cannot reach – your muscles are contracted so much of the time that blood is almost permanently squeezed out of them. Often the contraction in turn protects an over-stressed joint or ligament by gripping it firmly like a living splint; the pain of the part is small by comparison with the spasm of the much bulkier muscles protecting it.

Another kind of problem arises more suddenly and hurts more sharply, when one of the small joints at the side of your spine is dislocated. You can often feel it happen during some awkward movement. The dislocation is far too slight to show on X-ray, and your doctor is likely to recommend anti-inflammatory drugs. The joint really needs manipulating back into place, the sooner the better. Happily, some doctors are now taking an interest in manipulative treatments and a few are learning these skills for themselves.

A slipped disc* is quite another feeling, like a sharp stab which may shoot down your leg. It can happen in your neck too, giving HEADACHE or PAIN down your arm. In either case INJURY has torn the cushion joint between two spinal bones, letting some of the stuffing pout against a nerve. This is the condition conventional doctors understand best, though they have been slow to realize the potential of osteopathy and manipulative physiotherapy to accelerate healing of the injury.

HELPING YOURSELF

If you may have slipped a disc, consult your doctor. He will suggest rest in bed. Ask him to cooperate with an osteopath or chiropractor if you have one; he may even recommend one. Gentle manipulation by an expert can very much improve your healing.

Otherwise accept your doctor's assurances that you have no structural damage in your back and seek your remedy elsewhere. If you accept pain-killing or anti-inflammatory drugs, use them briefly and sparingly.

Heat always relaxes muscles by establishing a digestive mood and encouraging your CIRCULATION. Soak in a hot bath for ten minutes in a comfortable position; lavender oil helps the relaxing effect.

If massage finds muscles that are tender and tense, get your masseur to knead them for ten minutes with his fingertips. Any caring relative can feel instinctively what he should do, and is rewarded as the muscles soften and your discomfort is eased.

Arnica ointment can be applied after the massage or bath, to reinforce their effect and soothe any bruising which may partly account for the spasm.

Magnetic foil strips have been devised by various manufacturers to exploit the undoubted healing properties of magnetic fields. But you need enough information to apply the correct polarity to your skin – north, or south. If you have repeated problems of the same kind, it may be worth your while to invest in a piece of foil and experiment with it according to the instructions. Some are delighted, others disappointed with their results.

An *Osteopath,* * *Chiropractor* * or *Chartered Physiotherapist* * should be at home with chronic or recurrent backache and treat its structural aspects particularly well. *Alexander Technique* * is better for re-learning your posture, preventing recurrence in the first place, but you may discover lots more about yourself in the process. *Traditional Chinese Medicine* * can correct the 'colour' impulses which underlie your postural problems but may not remedy structural disturbances. A *Podiatrist* * can tell you if your walking is at fault, and by correcting it will remove a cause which stubbornly recurs otherwise (ADDRESSES). If you use a 'bonesetter', choose carefully by reputation.

A simple back strengthening exercise is worth repeating night and morning. Lying on your face in bed, lift your chin and your knees off the mattress simultaneously for a count of ten; then relax for ten. Repeat this a few times at first but increase the number as your back muscles get stronger.

Learn to make all your powerful movements at your ankles, knees, hips and arm joints with your spine rigid and straight. Never lift with your spine bent or use movement in your spinal joints to do the work.

Yoga, * dance and eurhythmy (Steiner) develop graceful movement well, which protects your back; look for local instructors through ADDRESSES.

Swimming, cycling and walking give safe EXERCISE.

BED-WETTING, enuresis

You are born already able to save up your urine for hours at a time, gradually filling your bladder. An automatic reflex is tripped when it gets to a certain size and your bladder empties itself completely. As a baby you do not control this, and may not even notice; but your emptying reflex can be trained to respond to promptings other than size from quite an early age. However, during your third year of life you make the NERVOUS connections which enable you to over-ride the reflex by a conscious effort. By stages you become aware that you are wet, then that you are wetting, and finally that you want to go. By that stage you are ready to control your voiding when you are awake; dryness at night follows a little later, usually with only a little encouragement and no special training.

Any structural defect of your bladder can interfere with this, especially if it makes you more susceptible to INFECTIONS of your urine. But difficulties of that kind are unusual; your doctor will check you for infection from time to time, but even that is unlikely if your urine does not smell strongly. If you have ever had a single dry night or reasonable daytime control, and your urine is not infected, then your apparatus is basically sound.

So the problem lies at some stage in learning to control it. This is often more difficult for a child who has at a younger age been conditioned to wee to order. He often appears to relapse into wetting for a few weeks or months while he gets his conscious control mechanism together. It can take a lot of patience to wait for the function to return. Otherwise, a serious upset of any kind during that crucial third year may be enough to distract you and spoil your progress. Admission to hospital, separation from mother while a new baby is born or moving your home to a strange part of the country are typical circumstances.

Generally poor health that persists for months at a time should be avoidable, but may continue undermining your alertness until a fundamental cause is corrected. ALLERGY is a common example. DEPRESSION is probably a more common cause of bed-wetting than we realize, because the most usual medication for bed-wetting happens to be effective against depression as well.

You may lapse back into wetting or never really learn. Either way, gaining control is harder once that third birthday is long past. By then you are choosing other things to learn, and always succeeding. Bed-wetting is probably your only failure and it nags at your pride. You become ashamed of yourself, feel hopeless and begin to evade the issue. That only confirms the problem, since by now you need to concentrate your effort to overcome it.

For very small children, a parent's obvious displeasure at their failure to wee in the pot is extraordinarily impressive. It gives them a great sense of power, and they may deliberately exploit it. Shrewd parents can usually spot this and make a point of losing interest in failure. To show positive pleasure at your child's success is often the only change required.

HELPING YOURSELF

You should not be rewarded for dry nights, nor punished or threatened for wetting your bed; but it should be a perfect nuisance to you. You must get up, bathe, change your pyjamas and your bed and get back in it, with the least possible help from your parents. You should help do the washing you cause. All this inconvenience will concentrate your mind on improvement without making you anxious.

Drink lots on the mornings when you are at home; when your bladder fills, practise holding on for as long as you can. Then drink nothing flavoured after lunchtime. If you are thirsty, drink WATER – preferably bottled or filtered. That gives your body a chance to get rid of its waste long before evening, by which time your urine will be less. To make sure, get a grown-up to take you to the toilet when they go to bed; this need not even wake you up.

Draw up yourself a calendar for each month, with five columns of seven rows each; make each box big enough for you to draw a face inside it. Each morning draw one for last night, smiling in red if your bed was dry, and sad in yellow if not. Add up the smiling faces in each weekly column, then for the whole month, and watch your progress. Do you seem to wet on the same nights each week? If so, why do you think that is? Arrange with your doctor or health visitor to show them your progress calendars every month.

Get checked out for ALLERGY. Avoid colourings in sweets, squashes, tinned peas and fish fingers anyway; perfectly good brands are available without these unnecessary irritants. Stop using fluoridated toothpaste to clean your TEETH; you probably swallow it. Improve your DIET, with help for your APPETITE if necessary.

If your success does not quickly make you keen and hopeful, take *Dr Bach's** Gorse *Flower Remedy*.* Clematis suits dreamy uninterested people, Wild Rose helps if you have just given up the effort to improve. Chestnut Bud deals best with slow learners. Someone locally may prescribe them, or you can write direct to the ADDRESS.

If none of this helps and you sleep very heavily, take your calendar cards back to your doctor and ask for medicinal help for a few months; but keep everything else going too!

Several *Homoeopathic* remedies may help you. Belladonna 3, taken 4-hourly, is appropriate if you sleep heavily. Sepia 6 8-hourly fits better if you are wet early in the night. If these do not work there are many other possibilities; consult a reputable practitioner for further help (ADDRESS).

Persevere. Late learning takes six months at least before you are reasonably safe; you may still have accidents on holiday or under stress for many months longer. Everybody manages eventually.

BITES, stings

The insects that pester you in summer do not bite, but probe you with a specialized hypodermic mouthpiece to feed from your blood. This is not designed to irritate you, which would be very self-destructive on the insect's part. Unfortunately for the insect, it must inject a trace of saliva to prevent your blood from clotting before it can be drawn. Eventually you react to this saliva with an ITCHY red INFLAMMATORY swelling which makes you aware of your passenger, whom you then set about deterring. Some enviable people are naturally repellant to insects. Some others who appear to be may simply tolerate their bites, which is not quite so desirable.

Wasps, honey-bees, hornets and ants are rather different. They have no interest in feeding off you and only sting in self-defence. That is unusual unless you unwisely try to swat one on your skin, tread or sit on one or bite it on your apple. Bees flying about their business will not normally worry you provided they do not get tangled in your hair or clothing. But some hives are particularly aggressive and may attack you if they scent or sense your fear.

The bee is not well adapted for hard-skinned opponents and often cannot withdraw its sting; you may therefore see the insect trying to unscrew itself. The usual outcome is that the sting is left behind, complete with its venom-sac still pumping; the insect escapes, fatally wounded. Wasps do not have this problem, but are easily distinguished in any case by their larger size and brightly striped yellow bodies.

Dogs, cats and rodents are capable of inflicting quite serious INJURY, and may INFECT you through their toothmarks and scratches. Rabies is so far an exceedingly remote risk in Britain but should be thought of if the animal is particularly aggressive or salivating heavily. If you are bitten abroad by an animal that may be infected protection is urgent; consult a doctor or hospital immediately. Tetanus is only an appreciable risk if the wound is dirty, deep and bleeds little, but a bite may serve to remind you to renew your IMMUNIZATION.

Jelly-fish and other sea creatures produce powerful venom which can hurt exceedingly. When large areas of skin are poisoned simultaneously the dose is large, and the accompanying *shock** may be severe.

Nettle-rash is very irritant, but only dangerous if it is very extensive.

The Giant Hog-weed produces an alarming reaction in some people. You will know if this affects you and that you should seek prompt medical attention whenever you are exposed to it. On many others it produces a rather irritant rash which responds to the same treatment as nettle-rash.

HELPING YOURSELF

Do *not* use insect repellents impregnated with chemical insecticides. These accumulate in your body fat and can have serious long-term effects. Derris, pyrethrum, tobacco powder or crumpled cigarette ends make the basis of much safer alternatives for your garden, described in detail in L. D. Hills' and Juliette de Baïracli Levi's BOOKS. Sticky fly-papers are usually safe but read their small print carefully.

Rosemary, rue, sage and summer savory are all very effective *insect repellents.* * Use them in *pots pourris* or infused as a body lotion. Prepare for an outdoor event on a still summer evening by burning any of these herbs in a metal dust-bin, with paper and a little paraffin.

Make a strong lotion of fresh elderflowers in spring and preserve it by mixing with an equal quantity of surgical spirit. Label it carefully 'for external application only' and keep it well away from children. This lotion is an excellent first aid for all insect bites and stings.

Treat *animal* * bites as INJURIES.

Cover *ant* * bites immediately with a crushed garlic clove or sliced onion.

If a *bee* * stings you, first give it a chance to remove its barb. If it fails, scrape the barb out yourself with the edge of a knife. Do *not* attempt to grasp it with tweezers or fingers; this usually squeezes the remaining venom out of the sac and into you. Suck out what you can, then dab the wound with whitewash (slaked lime), moistened wood ash, domestic ammonia or (failing all else) saliva. Take one tablet of *homoeopathic* * Apis mel 30 every few minutes if you are in severe pain or shocked, especially if stung in your mouth. After an hour wash the alkali off your skin and dress it if necessary with a piece of bruised dock leaf or a sprig of parsley.

As soon as possible after a *wasp* * sting suck as much venom out of the wound as you can and dab it with vinegar. Take *homoeopathic* * Arnica 6 or 30, repeating this every 15–30 minutes if the pain or shock is severe.

Give a *jelly-fish* * victim *homoeopathic* * Arnica or *Bach Rescue Remedy* * immediately, then apply oil of wormwood, rue or rosemary, or a pulp of crushed sage or rue leaves in hot water. Otherwise bathe the rash with vinegar diluted with an equal amount of hot water.

For nettle stings take homoeopathic Urtica urens 3x every 2–4 hours and rub the area with a dock leaf. *Hog-weed* * may need medical attention.

ITCHY bites respond to antihistamine medicines, but take time to do so if treatment has been delayed. If none of the above remedies is practical or satisfactory, keep some antihistamine tablets by you and use them as soon as you are bitten. They may make you drowsy or increase the effect of ALCOHOL.

If a sting becomes red and starts to throb after a few days, it is probably INFECTED. Try cold bathing, antiseptics and a firm bandage first, but seek ANTIBIOTIC treatment if it worsens or you become FEVERISH.

BLEEDING: eye, nose, womb, wounds

WHAT HAPPENS

When you tear an artery or vein its muscular wall immediately contracts, narrowing the breach and slowing the leak of blood. The damage attracts millions of *platelets* * – tiny cells circulating in the blood – which stick to the wound in clumps, helping to plug it. Meanwhile the spilt blood, prompted by contact with your damaged flesh, clots with dense insoluble fibres which begin to darn the tear within about ten minutes. That is usually well before the muscles relax, by which time the leak is blocked but vulnerable. The darning fibres eventually shrink, wringing fluid out of the clot to make it hard and strong. In a day or two repair work is well under way, soundly knitting the tear and dismantling the clot within about a week.

Only if you have one of the uncommon major defects of this complex array of defences are you in much danger of bleeding to death, except from very large blood vessels. These are mostly deep inside your body, vulnerable only to disease or serious INJURY. If you neglect severe or protracted INDIGESTION a *peptic ulcer* * may eventually puncture a stomach blood vessel; by the time you vomit blood (altered to a black curdled mess by your stomach acid) you are in serious trouble. *Steroid* * medication or the CONTRACEPTIVE pill make you more liable to this; take coincidental stomach pain seriously.

A woman bleeds most often from her womb. Menstruation occurs every time PREGNANCY fails, which is about five hundred times in your life. You may control your ovaries better than that, releasing eggs almost to order or not at all and menstruating seldom. This seems very sensible but worries a lot of the women it happens to. Even if you want to conceive, think very carefully before asking a doctor to unlock this perfectly natural economy mechanism. Not only is bleeding tedious, wasteful and hazardous; medicinal hormone adjustment and CONTRACEPTIVE pills can unbalance you in ways that do not reverse easily and may make future PREGNANCY more difficult.

There are many other places where small blood vessels are easily wounded. Bleeding from exposed blood vessels on the eye looks alarming but is harmless. Nose-bleeds can be heavy but are usually easy to control. Blood in your urine is a nasty shock but may only indicate CYSTITIS; a urine test can confirm this, and other tests are available if the problem recurs. If you have recently eaten beetroot you are probably seeing the purple pigment, which some people excrete unchanged; you can test this by eating some more. There are also some medicines, vitamins and food colourings that stain urine, and you should mention what you are taking if you seek advice.

A slight trickle of fresh blood from your bowel when you empty it usually indicates PILES or a *fissure*; * but if the blood is dark in colour, mixed with your faeces or accompanied by mucus, COLITIS is more probable and should be taken up with your doctor.

Frequent occurrence of any or several of these may be your only hint of raised BLOOD PRESSURE, which your doctor will be glad to check if you ask him. If everything is normal your blood-vessels may be uncommonly fragile.

As soon as possible press firmly on any surface wound with a compress, either very cold or as hot as you can bear. Ten minutes will stop the bleeding and minimize bruising. Then dress with Arnica Ointment unless your skin is broken, when Calendula Ointment is better. Antiseptic is less useful.

For surface bleeding of the *eye,** spray cold water on your eyelids for ten minutes, then leave them alone.

If your *nose** bleeds blow it to expel clot, then pinch it firmly between finger and thumb for at least ten minutes. A cold compress may be helpful on the back of your neck or across your brow and the bridge of your nose. If the bleeding is drastic, sprinkle cold water from a can or shower over the head and back of the victim, then put him to rest.

If your PERIOD floods, go to bed firmly padded with a towel, and with a small ice-pack (crushed ice in a face-cloth, inside a polythene bag) in the cleavage of your buttocks. If this does not quickly control it, call the doctor. If you succeed, work on measures to reduce your tendency to heavy PERIODS over the next few months.

Stop bleeding from your bowel by sitting with an ice cube against your anus or spraying it with cold water from a bidet, for a few minutes in either case. Pat yourself dry and massage Calendula or Hamamelis (Witch Hazel) Ointment well into your anal passage. Your doctor can supply Bismuth Subgallate Suppositories, which are harmlessly effective; it is better to avoid anything containing steroids.

Bleeding into your urine can sometimes be stopped by cold compresses or deep massage over your spine just below your shoulder-blades; or by contrast bathing between your legs just in front of your anus and behind your scrotum. Sponge with hot water for one minute, cold for a half, two or three times, finishing with cold. Follow the next advice as well.

Fragile blood vessels benefit from Vitamin C (500mg) and Rutin (50mg) three times daily after meals. Persevere with dosage for at least a month, as it takes time to heal and reconstruct even the tiny vessels usually involved.

A rash of striking red spots suddenly appearing all over the body, often of a young person, is usually caused by a toxic or allergic reaction and often coincides with drastic but temporary reduction in the blood platelets. Doctors seldom find a specific cause for this, though it sometimes seems to occur in small outbreaks within a locality. INFECTION can sometimes be blamed but not always. It is possible some of these outbreaks result from chemical pollution incidents or pesticide spraying operations, neither of which is at present monitored sufficiently closely to rule out. Full recovery is the rule but medical supervision is essential.

BLOOD PRESSURE, hypertension

WHAT HAPPENS

Your blood pressure is the nearest thing you have to a barometer. It varies according to the resistance of your CIRCULATION to the blood flowing through it and is the net result of many contrasting influences.

The simplest is the thickness of your blood itself. Watery blood flows freely whereas blood congested with animal fat, sugar or waste acids creeps round reluctantly.

Common salt goes further. By interfering throughout your life with part of the chemical machinery that regulates your blood pressure, it raises this gradually. Only in countries where salt is scarce do most elderly people still enjoy naturally youthful blood pressures.

The varying demands of physical, mental and digestive effort determine the rise and fall of your blood pressure with activity throughout the day. These show off the mechanism at its healthiest, serving most directly the purpose for which it evolved. You can often maintain the balance of your circulation, and your sanity, by letting off steam through effort contrasting with the cause of your exasperations. Motorists would vent their frustrations more safely if they could tear about on bikes sometimes.

Anxieties and passions that are not relieved in this way accumulate to affect your nervous TENSION, which is reflected in the tension of muscles that control the size of small arteries everywhere in your body. When these tighten their resistance rises disproportionately, pushing blood pressure up. This may be temporary and relatively harmless, or more permanent if tension begins to bias the climate of your life.

None of this would matter if your heart and arteries did not wear faster under higher pressure. Their efforts to compensate for this only make matters worse. Extra pressure makes the muscles of your small arteries thicken, which increases their resistance further. They stretch under constant press-ure into tortuous curves which have the same effect. Premature ageing eventually stiffens them, so that they can no longer absorb the shock of your heart's violent pulsations but receive their full force. Tears develop in their lining skin which heal imperfectly as ARTERIOSCLEROSIS. Worse still, small arteries may crack right through, so that you bleed under high pressure into the nearby tissues. *Subarachnoid haemorrhage** and *strokes** arise in this way from arteries near to or within your brain. One of your eyes may be blinded suddenly in a similar fashion by rupture under pressure of a brittle blood vessel inside it.

Moderately raised blood pressure does not cause such catastrophic changes quickly, which gives you plenty of time to reverse it and prevent them. But very high pressure in a young person is a serious matter which can do damage in only a few years, rising all the time. Get yourself medically investigated and under adequate control before exploring more fundamental cures. You may have a small benign tumour that SURGERY can cure. Conventional diagnosis and treatment give you valuable time to explore causes at your ease.

Use your raised blood pressure to monitor how you deal with its causes. Medical treatment may postpone complications but only tinkers with the meter readings and may cause side-effects. Regard it as a temporary tactic and aim to undermine your need for it eventually.

Adopt for three weeks the special DIET for cleansing, avoiding meticulously all meat, fish, dairy produce and stimulants – especially coffee and SMOKING. Garlic powder or a potassium chloride condiment (eg Ruthmol) replaces salt. Thereafter follow the DIET for health, still avoiding animal fat except a little butter and soft cheese, one or two eggs a week and a little fresh fish if you want them. Keep off salt and all kinds of sugar faithfully. The more sugar you eat, the more salt you retain, and the higher your blood pressure will be.

This diet deals coincidentally with OVERWEIGHT. Loss of excess weight lowers your blood pressure usefully on its own, regardless of any other benefits.

Rue tea is a therapeutic and non-stimulating drink. Mistletoe (four berries twice daily on an empty stomach) soothes an overdriven heart and the underlying tensions. Garlic reduces blood pressure directly. Ginseng eases the causes of hypertension and increases generally your tolerance of STRESS.

Use good BREATHING, *recreation** and EXERCISE to counterbalance your other exertions. If *relaxation* is difficult practise it with a relaxation, *meditation** or *yoga** teacher (ADDRESS) if necessary.

Correct the quality of your SLEEP.

If these simple measures do not complete the job within six months, SUPPLEMENT your diet for three months with Blackcurrant Seed Oil (500mg twice daily half an hour before food) plus Vitamin C (1000mg on each occasion) and Rutin (an extract of rue, 50mg twice daily). Vitamins B_3 (Niacin, 50–100mg twice daily) and B_6 (Pyridoxine, 50mg twice daily) and Inositol (300mg twice daily) all have useful effects on raised blood pressure, but you should balance them with six tablets daily of Brewer's Yeast.

Garlic Oil may work when whole garlic fails, but take a good multimineral supplement with it to offset accidental losses of nutrient minerals.

Consultation with a *Homoeopath** or practitioner of *Traditional Chinese Medicine** may prove worthwhile at this stage.

Give yourself time regularly to reflect how your life is going. Are your objectives realistic and are they fully satisfying your needs? Are you too attached to distant goals and enjoying too little the process of getting there? Honest answers to questions like these will uncover the fundamental causes of unease you cannot get rid of, which is keeping your blood pressure up. Action bold enough to correct what you discover may require courage, but is within your scope and worthwhile or else the pressure would not be there.

BODY ODOUR, bad breath

Chronic infection in nose or throat, rotten TEETH or *bronchiectasis** used to be thought the chief cause of malodorous breath; doctors do not seem to regard offensive sweating as a medical condition at all. Both impressions were probably misguided, even when chronic infection was much more common than it is now. Centuries ago, naturally vegetarian natives of the new European colonies were able to scent a meat-eating white man a hundred yards away and track him in the dark. Newly-converted non-SMOKERS are often horrified to rediscover the rank odour of stale tobacco on another's breath, an offence of which they were oblivious when still themselves addicted. Most doctors eat handsomely, and few are vegetarians; only those who rid themselves of dietary odour can begin to be aware of it in their patients.

The root cause of persistent body odour is the burden of offensive chemicals your body is forced to carry, and tries to get rid of very hard. Some of these arise from environmental pollution, some from medication, others from metabolism of meat products eaten to excess. A few, such as *trimethylamine,** build up because you cannot break them down for disposal.

These make their way out of your body as best they can. Any that will vapourize, like ammonia and solvents, pass out through your lungs; this probably accounts for the greater part of what you successfully excrete. Rather little dissolves in your sweat, since most that could go that way is dealt with by your kidneys.

Nearly all organic chemicals such as pesticides dissolve readily in fatty material, which is why they mount up in your body fat and cannot easily escape through your kidneys. These fat stores are laid down deep inside you, and there the pollutants tend to stay; but a small amount spills over from these deep stores into the *sebaceous** material produced to lubricate your skin and hair. This may cause ACNE or may simply be secreted with the sebum and dry onto your skin. It does not easily rinse off without soap, which you cannot use often without destroying your skin's protective sebaceous film. Even when you do get rid of it, there is plenty more stored up inside to take its place. So if stored pollutants are your problem a persistent chemical odour is practically inevitable, worst in the hairy parts of your body, especially your armpits.

Sometimes the problem is entirely external and easily solved. A BED-WETTING child who does not wash properly before he gets dressed or carries on wearing underwear stained with urine is bound to smell at school. Sometimes a whole family smells of stale tobacco because one of them SMOKES heavily. Embarrassment deters their friends from telling them; the 'friends' are therefore few.

Offensive VAGINAL DISCHARGE may result from INFECTION, particularly with *anaerobic** germs that thrive best in the absence of air. This smell is very conspicuous and you really do need a friend to tell you about it because you cannot detect it for yourself.

If your best friend summons up the courage to say that you have BO, don't be offended or incredulous; be grateful.

If you have CATARRH, work on getting rid of that.

If you SMOKE, give up. Nicotine chewing gum will solve your immediate odour problem but nor your addiction.

If your TEETH are in poor shape, get them attended to.

If you regularly cough up phlegm you have chronic BRONCHITIS; see under that topic how to deal with this.

Adopt the special cleansing DIET for several weeks, then relax onto the diet for health; but beware of eating much meat or dairy produce.

Some unfortunate individuals possess a strikingly offensive smell whatever they do. Try avoiding foods rich in choline, which is metabolized to trimethylamine – a strong-smelling substance you may not be able to break down further. These include especially fish, eggs, liver and legumes (pea and bean family). Your body odour will vanish within a week if trimethylamine accumulation is your problem.

SUPPLEMENT your diet for cleansing. Zinc, Magnesium, Para-aminobenzoic acid, and Vitamin B_6 (Pyridoxine) are sometimes dramatically effective at relieving odour, either alone or in combination.

Do not use antiperspirant cosmetics, which merely frustrate your body's legitimate business.

If you are treating ACNE with a cream or lotion containing Benzoyl Peroxide, this may be the cause of your odour. In this case your odour will vanish very quickly when you stop using it.

Shower frequently, first hot to encourage perspiration and then cold to close your skin pores. Use soap very seldom, substituting a little cold cream if necessary. Try to air your body naked for ten minutes each day, invigorating your skin beforehand with a shower or a brisk rub with a dry towel or loofa. If you begin to shiver, shower again or dress quickly.

Roll-on deodorants can be irritant; dab your armpits instead with a cotton wool ball dampened with cider vinegar or sodium bicarbonate (baking soda). Scent your fresh underwear in advance by keeping sachets of pleasant herbs amongst them in the drawer.

Get candid progress reports from that best friend, but you'll know you're there when you can easily detect odour from other people. Your experience may give you a turn as a tactful 'best friend' to one or two of them!

BOILS, carbuncles, septic spots

Your skin is not just a container but a remarkably sophisticated organ which regulates losses of heat and moisture from your body, can store and excrete surpluses from metabolism and receives sensory impressions. Despite its permeability it is a very effective barrier against microbes and moisture, and can regulate the penetration of sunlight to the tissues inside. It wears tirelessly and will grow into a form appropriate to the physical work expected of it. Its elasticity enables it to cope with changes over the years in your shape and size.

Your skin can appear healthy when you are not. Its attention is directed outwards, and it is up to six weeks out of touch with events inside you because of the time its surface layer takes to grow. This remoteness makes it particularly easy for *microbes** to take up unopposed residence in your skin whenever your IMMUNE system weakens its vigilance against encroachment.

Boils occur when your health is rallying again, as a means of banishing pus-forming *bacteria** which have taken these liberties during low periods of your life – COLDS and other STRESSES such as menstrual PERIODS often let them in. They may arise anywhere, but most commonly appear around your face, neck and shoulders or on your bottom and thighs. The most familiar condition is an almost continuous rash of numerous tiny dull red pimples which rarely point and yield very little pus if they are squeezed. They are unsightly but give little trouble.

Small boils like these that start in your skin commonly originate in *Staphylococcus** colonies lodged in your nostrils and ears and *Coliform** bacteria from your bowel. They are always ready to take advantage of these conditions, which are very much to their liking. FUNGUS INFECTIONS, especially *Candida,** may co-exist with these or occur separately. Anyone with chronically unhealthy skin, ACNE, ECZEMA or impaired IMMUNITY is likely to pick up one of these microbes eventually and carry them somewhere on their body for months or years at a time.

Larger boils are less common but tend to occur in crops over a period of months. They may not originate in your skin at all but deep inside, from your body's efforts to wall off and get rid of INFLAMMATORY or INFECTED material. These *abscesses** can migrate under 'colour' guidance and surface under your skin. They may appear to be forming there, and doubtless some do. In either case your skin inflames and breaks open to let the abscess burst. A healthy body will sometimes in this way shed fragments of stitching and debris for several years after an operation or penetrating wound.

Crops of boils may begin during a cleansing DIET or period of improving health and be quite troublesome for months; they stop when no longer required. Rather than be dismayed by their appearance, take encouragement from them. When they pass, you will be vividly aware of the great improvement in your health they have helped to engineer.

Encourage a boil to burst and resolve by poulticing it twice daily with cotton wool or gauze soaked in hot water or Calendula lotion. Handle it with dry gauze or in the bowl of a wooden spoon if the boil is on your face. Refresh the poultice frequently in the hot water for up to five minutes. Rinse briefly with cold water, then dress the boil with gauze and Magnesium Sulphate Paste, which dessicates the skin and 'draws' the boil more quickly. It runs easily at body temperature, so take precautions against leakage.

Start a cleansing DIET or persevere with the one that caused the boils.

A Vitamin C SUPPLEMENT and Comfrey tea or tablets (two with each meal) speed up your healing and may enable you to absorb inflammatory material rather than form abscesses. Sometimes Zinc deficiency underlies a tendency to boils; try taking 15mg daily for a few months. Extend this to the full SUPPLEMENTS for IMMUNITY if you suspect that your health is generally run down.

*Homoeopathic** Belladonna 12 helps early abscesses before they swell if given frequently; Apis mel 3x is better for swelling. Merc sol 6 or Silica 6 are worth trying in more advanced cases.

If you have repeated crops of small boils or pimples on your face, try massaging a little antiseptic cream (eg Naseptin) up each nostril three times daily. This will weaken and eventually wipe out any colonies of Staphylo-cocci that you are carrying, and the boils will stop.

ANTIBIOTIC treatment is unwise and usually ineffective; your doctor is only likely to give it under pressure from you. He may however by taking swabs be able to identify reservoirs of Staphylococci which can be reduced with suitable antiseptics; this is safer and altogether more useful.

BOOKS

Airola, Paavo: *Stop Hair Loss*. Health Plus (Arizona) 1965

Barnes, Belinda and Irene Colquhoun: *The Hyperactive Child*. Thorsons 1984

Barnes, Broda: *Solved: The Riddle of Heart Attacks*. Cancer Control Society 1985

Bentov, Itzhak: *Stalking the Wild Pendulum*. Wildwood House 1978

Bircher-Benner, M.: *The Prevention of Incurable Disease*. James Clarke & Co. 1959

Bircher, Ralph (ed.): *Bircher-Benner Nutrition Plan*
- *For Headache & Migraine*. Nash 1972
- *For Skin Problems*. Nash 1973; Pyramid 1977

BMA: *The Medical Effects of Nuclear War*. Wiley 1983

BMA: *The Long-Term Environmental and Medical Effects of Nuclear War*. BMA 1986

Bohm, David: *Wholeness and the Implicate Order*. Routledge & Kegan Paul 1981

Bryce-Smith, Derek *et al*: *The Zinc Solution*. Century Arrow 1986

Cannon, Geoffrey: *Fat to Fit*. Pan 1986

Cannon, Geoffrey and Hetty Einzig: *Dieting Makes You Fat*. Century 1983

Capra, Fritjof: *The Tao of Physics*. Wildwood House 1975

Capra, Fritjof: *The Turning Point*. Wildwood House 1982

Clarke, Jane: *Multiple Sclerosis*. New Age Science Press 1983

Cleave, T. L.: *The Saccharine Disease*. Wright (Bristol) 1974

Conservation Society: *Lead or Health*. 1980

Diamond, John: *Your Body Doesn't Lie*. Warner Books 1980

Dowding, Hugh: *Many Mansions*. Rider 1944

Dowding, Hugh: *Lychgate*. Rider 1945

Ehret, Arnold: *The Mucusless Diet Healing System*. Ehret Literature Publishing Co. 1983

Forbes, Dr Alec: *The Bristol Diet*. Century 1984

Fredericks, Carlton *et al*: *Low Blood Sugar and You*. Ace 1979

Grant, Doris and Jean Joice: *Food Combining for Health*. Thorsons 1984

Hills, Lawrence D.: *Organic Gardening Month by Month*. Thorsons 1983

Hoffer, A. and H. Osmond: *How to Live with Schizophrenia*. See Schizophrenia ADDRESS

Homoeopathic Development Foundation: *Homoeopathy for the Family*. See ADDRESS

Howard, Sir Albert: *Farming & Gardening for Health or Disease*. Faber & Faber 1945

Hume, E. Douglas: *Béchamp or Pasteur?* C. W. Daniel & Co. 1963

Husemann, Friedrich and Otto Wolff: *The Anthroposophical Approach to Medicine*. Anthroposophical Press 1982

Lawrence, F. (ed.): *Additives: Your Complete Survival Guide*. Century 1986

Levy, Juliette de Baïracli: *The Illustrated Herbal Handbook*. Faber & Faber 1982

Lindlahr, Henry: *Natural Therapeutics* (3 vols). C. W. Daniel & Co. 1983

Lovelock, J. E.: *Gaia: A New Look at Life on Earth*. Oxford University Press 1979

Kenton, L. & S.: *Raw Energy*. Century 1984

Kidman, Brenda: *A Gentle Way With Cancer*. Century 1983

Kübler-Ross, E.: *On Death and Dying*. Tavistock 1970

Kunz-Bircher, Ruth: *The Bircher-Benner Health Guide*. Woodbridge Press 1980

McCarrison, Robert: *Nutrition and Health*. McCarrison Society 1982

MacManaway, Bruce and Johanna Turcan: *Healing*. Thorsons 1983

Madders, Jane: *Stress and Relaxation*. Martin Dunitz 3rd edn 1981

Mansfield, Peter: *Common Sense about Health*. Templegarth Trust 1982

Mansfield, Peter and Jean Monro: *Chemical Children*. Century 1987

Mellor, Constance: *Natural Remedies for Common Ailments*. Granada 1975

Melville, Arabella and Colin Johnson: *Persistent Fat and How to Lose It*. Century 1986.

National Radiological Protection Board: *Living with Radiation*. HMSO 3rd edn 1986

Nilsson, Lennart *et al*: *A Child is Born*. Faber & Faber 1977

Oakley, Ann *et al*: *Miscarriage*. Fontana 1984

Odent, Michel: *Primal Health*. Century 1986

Pearce, Innes and Lucy Crocker: *The Peckham Experiment*. Scottish Academic Press 1985

Pfeiffer, Carl: *Zinc and Other Micro-Nutrients.* Pivot Original 1978

Pfeiffer, Carl and Jane Banks: *Total Nutrition.* Granada 1983

Pickard, Barbara: *Eating Well for a Healthy Pregnancy.* Sheldon Press 1984

Picton, L. J.: *Thoughts on Feeding.* Faber & Faber 1946

Rowe, Dorothy: *Depression: The Way Out of Your Prison.* Routledge & Kegan Paul 1983

Sheldrake, Rupert: *A New Science of Life.* Granada 1983

Templegarth Trust: *What is Health?.* See ADDRESS

Templegarth Trust: *Starting Life Well.* See ADDRESS

Volin, Michael: *Challenging the Years.* Harper & Row 1979

Waerland, Are: *The Cauldron of Disease.* David Nutt 1934

Waldbott, Dr George *et al: Fluoridation: The Great Dilemma.* Colorado Press 1978

WHAT HAPPENS

Birth entails novelties of every kind, far wider ranging than you will ever face again. Within a few seconds your first breath introduces you to air, and to other forms of life which challenge your personal IMMUNITY. All your senses are bombarded simultaneously with new impressions, and your skin is confronted with the phenomenon of temperature. Your CIRCULATION is radically revised, and you are suddenly aware of the weight of your limbs.

Sorting this out takes your whole infancy, and centres on rediscovering your mother from the outside. You have to piece her familiar heart-beat, warmth and altered voice together with novelties – her touch and appearance, taste and smell. To begin with you have no 'mono'* means for connecting all these; you cannot comprehend that these separate impressions arise in one being. But you still sense the same loving 'colour'* climate that has pervaded your life from its conception and are profoundly reassured. This frees you to explore the novelties with serene curiosity, while your body settles into the new terms of its existence.

Your feeding at mother's breast is the epicentre of all this. It conveys ideal food of precisely the character you are familiar with, and commissions your digestive functions gradually, without fuss. It directly protects you against INFECTIONS from mother's past and helps you to cope with present challenges new to you both. It automatically caters for your increasing appetite and changing needs, coping even with your extra thirst on hot days.

Its subtlest function is to simplify your task in dealing with the alien creatures that jostle you for space to live their lives, some of whom are ready to colonize you if you let them. It is easy for you to distinguish these from your food, because mother's milk retains characteristics familiar to you since before you were born. So you confidently reject anything you do not recognize, without compromising your nourishment. Only later, when you have learnt the rudiments of how to maintain your IMMUNITY, do you choose to explore those other creatures as possible foods themselves. This much more subtle judgement – do I kill it or can I digest it? – is not enforced before you are ready. Consequently you far more seldom make mistakes during WEANING that could result in ALLERGY, COT DEATH or susceptibility to INFECTION.

Besides all of these advantages bestowed by feeding exclusively on breast-milk, mother's love surges and flows with it, effortlessly and directly. The satisfaction she derives from being suckled passes directly back to you. It sparkles in the eyes you gaze into, tones the endearments that fall on your ears and motivates her hands and body as they caress and warm your skin. Even the scent of her armpit, unlovely to her, is wonderful to you.

All these delights powerfully reinforce your personal wholeness and profoundly motivate and gratify hers. They kindle your appetite for living and refresh your mother's, whatever disappointments her past may have held. This is your access to the purposiveness and confidence that enable you to live without fear, whatever odds you may be challenged to overcome.

HELPING YOURSELVES AS PARENTS

Get your new baby home from hospital as soon as you can. Unfamiliar surroundings and routine are very unsettling and undermine your confidence in coping. Simple things that come easily at home are difficult elsewhere.

Suckle your baby early and often. His instinctive desire to explore your breast is strongest from about twenty minutes after his birth and certainly within the first hour of his life, when his suckling can help to deliver your afterbirth and stop your womb BLEEDING. Thereafter impose no timetable or deadlines; simply relax into exploring each other.

Avoid using scented soap or deodorant, at least above your waist.

Get your suckling technique right, from the beginning. He can move his head to and fro if you support its weight, so balance it on your forearm. Poise your breast so as to point your nipple prominently. As you cradle him in towards it, aim his nose at your nipple; this prompts him to lift his mouth towards it, arching his neck slightly and freeing his nose to breathe. Then press his chest close to yours and keep his head poised on your forearm while he chooses for himself the most comfortable angle at which to settle.

Do not let anyone give him anything else. Your milk flow takes two days to begin and will correspond in quantity to how hard and how often your baby sucks your nipples meanwhile. If any part of his appetite is satisfied otherwise, your milk supply will fall that far short of his needs.

If he is nervous or fretful handle him more, not less. Have him in bed with you, skin to skin. Massage him and speak soothingly, the way you would like for yourself. Intimacy with you reassures him as nothing else can, and reaffirms your self-confidence. You cannot spoil an infant, and can easily train him to SLEEP alone when that time comes.

After a few weeks, feeding settles into a confident routine. You may seem to be short of milk occasionally if his appetite suddenly increases; two days' unruffled perseverence sets that right. Then just keep going until he starts to wean himself, around six months. Don't be put off by prejudices, even professional ones: most ailments do not call for early WEANING.

La Leche League and National Childbirth Trust are the best ADDRESSES for experienced self-help, though many health visitors and midwives are excellent too.

Twins and super-twins do *not* rule out breast feeding automatically. It is much more convenient, since you can feed two at a time. You are perfectly well equipped to succeed, and can eat lots more yet still lose weight!

Premature, feeble and underweight babies need your milk more, not less – by cup and spoon or tube at first, if need be. Jaundice is seldom a reason to stop either. The kind that is caused by breast feeding is quite harmless.

Adoption and artificial feeding do not make second-class families! Every other means remains open, to cultivate your loving intimacy to perfection.

BREAST PROBLEMS

WHAT HAPPENS

There is very little behind the nipples of either boys or girls, and nothing to distinguish them until *pubescence*,* when breast tissue develops in both sexes. This may not happen on both sides at once and can be very tender and lumpy for a few months, resembling an *abscess** or tumour. It is a great relief to realize the truth, even though the tenderness may make contact sports and even heavy clothing very uncomfortable for several months.

Most of a young woman's breast is fat, formed around rudimentary glandular tissue. That is in principle a series of tubular passages arranged round your nipple like the spokes of a wheel. Each tube is highly tortuous and ranges through a segment of your breast like a slice of cake, centring on your nipple. The segments under your armpit extend up into it, so that your breast is comma-shaped, not circular.

Every time you *ovulate* your body begins to prepare for a PREGNANCY that seldom comes. In your breast, the CIRCULATION to each tubular segment gets richer, and the tube dilates and twists in an even more elaborate fashion. Yet within two weeks you are dismantling these preparations. This wasteful monthly cycle of activation and deactivation may be repeated five hundred times in your life and gives plenty of scope for *ageing** and mistakes. Cysts form easily, in small *culs de sac* of glandular tubing whose necks shut off although their secretory *cells** have not shut down. Secretions then accumulate in the second half of each monthly cycle and cannot get away. In general, women with fuller breast development are more liable to the repeated heavy engorgement that strains your elastic *ligaments*,* eventually making them slacker and more pendulous.

PREGNANCY changes your breasts most radically of all. The glandular segments expand enormously, and the fat recedes to make space for its tightly packed convolutions. Nevertheless the gland increases considerably in size, and so do its blood vessels.

When *lactation** begins a few days after your baby is born, your breasts at last come into their own. For the next year or so the glandular tissue will turn over huge quantities of nutrient fluid, each cell engorging between feeds and emptying promptly in response to suckling. It is correspondingly vulnerable to excesses of food and *waste acids** in your blood, which easily stagnate in bloated vessels. This unbalances milk production and flow through the cells and tubes of your breast, which become congested and liable to obstructive kinks. The consequent back-pressure and engorgement can disorganize whole segments of your breast with cystic swellings you can feel for the rest of your life.

When this hectic activity subsides the fat does not return for some years, leaving your breasts flatter and more nodular than before. But several healthy and prolonged lactations leave them less liable to CANCER, whereas suppressed lactations and oral CONTRACEPTION frustrate their purpose and make mischief considerably more likely.

94

If your food is faulty, your breasts suffer for it monthly when you are not pregnant, and daily when you are. For a breast problem of any kind go straight on the DIET for health; if it is bad enough, use the more drastic special DIET for cleansing throughout at least one periodic cycle. Avoid especially coffee, strong tea, SMOKING or nicotine chewing gum, and lots of cola or chocolate.

Modest SUPPLEMENTS of Vitamin E (200IU twice daily) are helpful for simple cysts in your breasts, but only use it once your doctor has ruled out CANCER.

Never leave a hot bath without splashing your breasts thoroughly with cold water. This tightens their blood vessels and tubular glands, making congestion and obstructive kinking much less likely. This habit protects you powerfully against *premenstrual tenderness** each month, and slows down or even stops the gradual accumulation of breast *lumps** throughout your fertile life.

Leave your breasts unclothed for five minutes daily. Wash them with tepid water or brush them lightly but briskly with a dry towel or soft brush. Stroke from the periphery towards the nipple.

Let no debris accumulate in crevices of your nipples, and massage them lightly to keep them supple. If they erect inwards, reverse this sometimes with gentle peripheral pressure.

After each period, when ordinary lumps are least conspicuous, watch in a mirror how your naked breasts lift as you raise your arms above your head. Show any puckering, distortion or new assymmetry to your doctor.

*Engorgement** is best attended to by contrast bathing in your bath or shower. Sprinkle or immerse the breast in hot water for three minutes, then apply a very cold pack for half a minute. This can be a cloth wrung out under the cold tap or even a few ice cubes wrapped in a cold damp cloth. This cycle can be repeated several times, always ending with cold. Before reapplying heat, stroke the engorged segment gently several times, from its periphery towards the nipple. Wipe off surplus water with your fingers and allow the breast to dry by evaporation while you dress the rest of you. Support it with an ample and well-braced bra. If your problem is acute you can usefully repeat this every two hours.

If you are *lactating** and become engorged, contrast bathe before each feed. Finish the bath with a long ice pack to numb the anticipated pain. At all costs keep on feeding your baby – things only get worse if you stop.

Prevent him chewing your nipple by filling his mouth with it; little or no dark skin should show. Treat any nipple sores or cracks with Calendula or Witch Hazel (Hamamelis) Ointment; avoid antiseptics unless they actually get INFECTED.

BREATHING

You can survive weeks without food, and days without water; but you can last only minutes without air. Breathing is your most immediate vital function. Its efficiency determines how fast you can refresh your body with oxygen and clear away exhaust gases, so it directly determines the maximum power available to you for any kind of living. Yet you can control how you do it, which provides you with a great opportunity to improve your health directly.

Although you have the option to use your mouth when breathing hard, your nose is obviously intended to moisten, clean and warm the air you breathe in and to sense its quality. Your outer defences against airborne poisons, *microbes** or dust include CATARRH or a COLD, sneezing, an overwhelming urge to get fresher air and COUGHING if your vocal cords are challenged.

Beyond the passages resemble a hollow tree suspended upside down from your vocal cords. The trunk divides into two, a main branch for each lung, where each forks repeatedly into smaller and smaller twigs, each bearing a multitude of tiny bubbles instead of leaves. These bubbles are the business end, packing ninety square metres of gas exchange skin into about five litres of lung.

That leaves no space for defences, which are all higher up. The branches are braced open with rings of cartilage, but their skin makes a film of mucus and possesses thousands of tiny feet which sweep this mucus up-hill out of the twigs. The smaller twigs are not braced open but soft and muscular, able to shut themselves almost completely in emergency. These are your inner and ultimate defences against corrosion of the delicate skin in the bubbles.

Air is sucked in or blown out of your lungs by a bellows action of your ribs and *diaphragm,** a sheet of muscle stretched across the rim of your bell-shaped rib-cage; your wind-pipe enters where the handle of the bell would be. Your lungs try to empty like a balloon, but only succeed in sucking your diaphragm up into your chest like a dome; then the elastic pull of your ribs and diaphragm just balances the pull of your lungs, still one-third inflated. However inflation is not perfectly even; some bubbles are collapsed at this resting volume. Only with your lungs fully inflated is every bubble full.

You can breathe in with your ribs, with your diaphragm, or both. Tight corsetry or waistbands cut out diaphragmatic breathing, but Westerners mostly use their ribs anyway because they prefer a trim-waisted image.

Speech and singing set up vibrations in different parts of your body according to the kind of sound you make. Good voice production maximizes these vibrations and harmonizes them, which not only economizes on effort but helps everything about you to cohere as a whole, from your *primal adaptive system** down. Chanting, poetry recitation and singing have been used to promote health in this way since time immemorial.

HELPING YOURSELF

Breathe in always through your nose, however you exhale. Persevere during a COLD or a spell of CATARRH, whenever congestion permits. Before you exercise hard and need to by-pass your nose, give your passages time to acclimatize to the conditions they will have to cope with.

Wear loose and elastic clothing around your waist, so that you can push out your belly when you want to and explore the shapes you can be. This simple gesture liberates you quite remarkably.

Learn to breathe exclusively with your diaphragm, lower or upper rib-cage at will. Each one exercises a different part of your bellows mechanism and inflates your lungs into various shapes; learning them greatly increases your awareness of yourself. A few breaths daily by each mechanism sweep air through every corner of your lungs, keeping each bubble in prime condition however little EXERCISE you take.

Practise slow deep diaphragmatic breathing in particular. Hold your breath in for as long as you comfortably can – usually five to ten seconds. Ten of these breaths twice daily, or whenever you panic or feel tense, can have a powerfully calming and clarifying effect on your whole outlook. They balance your 'colour'* energy evenly above and below your solar plexus,* a nerve centre near your spine just under your diaphragm. Moreover the piston movement of your diaphragm massages the soft organs in your chest and abdomen, toning up their functions in particular and your CIRCULATION in general.

Sing without restraint whenever you can – it almost redeems the exasperations of travelling by car. Discover where different vowel sounds resonate and try different postures of your tongue and throat. This will always refresh you, brighten your mood and raise your spirits. You are exercising the extraordinary power of sound vibration – fundamental to harmony of every kind, including yours.

If you find these manoeuvres difficult on your own, you probably have a problem of TENSION around your throat or chest which may in turn stem from NERVOUSNESS or STRESS disease. It would be worth while getting help from a speech therapist,* singing* or yoga* teacher. Check the ADDRESSES to discover which is available in your area.

The quality of the air you breathe is very much improved by running an ionizer* in rooms you occupy for long periods, such as your bedroom.

BREATHING: THREE WAYS

Thoracic or rib breathing (middle level)

Lungs

Rib cage

Sternum, on front of chest

Diaphragm

Sternal breathing – raising sternum (top level)

Spine

Lung

Abdomen

Diaphragmatic or abdominal breathing (lower level)

BRONCHITIS, chest infection

If COUGHING and your other defences against VIRUS INFECTION break down, a COLD may spread to involve your lung passages in some degree. Involvement of your wind-pipe and its mains branches is quite common, especially if you SMOKE.

The skin of these tubes INFLAMES just like your nose – with congestion, irritability and mucus production. These restrict the airspace in them, making you feel tight and BREATHE noisily. You may feel sore behind your breast-bone and cough uselessly at the least provocation. But mucus needs to be expelled sometimes, especially after accumulation overnight, when coughing is more productive and satisfactory. Expectorant linctuses trade on this by giving you something to cough up; you feel as if you are getting somewhere whether you are or not.

*Acute bronchitis** of this kind does not make you feel ill in yourself, unless the virus then spreads further as in 'FLU. But after several days you may begin to feel you are deteriorating for another reason. Although you can only have one VIRUS INFECTION at a time, any number of *bacteria** can take advantage of your disarray and colonize the skin already INFECTED. Pus then becomes more copious and you may be FEVERISH for the first time.

Pneumonia is then more likely, involving the smaller tubes and bubbles of tissue at the business end of your lungs. But with some bacteria and viruses this can happen from the start. You cannot survive pneumonia affecting the whole of your lungs, because then you could not breathe; but scattered patches (*broncho-pneumonia**) or solid infection of a whole branch or lobe of your lung (*lobar pneumonia**) can still be a serious illness. In either type, *double pneumonia** means that parts of both your lungs are involved; this does not necessarily mean that your condition is more serious. Doctors do not use this term as much now as they used.

*Chronic bronchitis** is much commoner now, provoked especially by SMOKING and air pollution if your DIET does not adequately repair the damage done. The skin of your bronchial tubes thickens permanently and its escalator mechanism (the feet that sweep mucus uphill) is damaged or paralysed by tobacco smoke. Consequently pus accumulates in the defenceless bubbles. If the walls between them break down, the bubbles get bigger but gas exchange skin is permanently lost overall; that is what *emphysema** means. Drastically reduced gas exchange makes you breathless and blue, and tightness or wheezing makes hard work of getting your breath back. Some badly affected people lose weight on the effort it costs them simply to breathe.

For this condition you will be offered various forms of medication, perhaps including continuous ANTIBIOTIC treatment to prevent or reduce INFECTION. This raises the possibility that THRUSH will take over where bacteria leave off; FUNGUS INFECTION of your lungs is insidious and can be just as destructive as anything bacteria can do.

HELPING YOURSELF

Build up your IMMUNITY to VIRUS INFECTIONS generally, to keep them local if they must occur at all.

Eat raw live vegetables daily, especially in winter, for their 'colour'* protection. Avoid mucus-forming and rich foods like meat, cheese, sugar and confectionery. The fewer difficulties you make for yourself with your food, the better you can heal your lungs.

The garlic lozenge RECIPE is very helpful, used for two hours daily at a socially convenient time. You can take tablets of Comfrey Root 400mg two three times a day for a few months during the winter; but use tea or eat the fresh herb for most of the year. No harmful effects in people have ever been demonstrated but any risk is in any case confined to the root and its products.

Practise BREATHING to keep your lungs fully efficient. Get rid of pus regularly by tilting yourself head down so that trapped mucus can drain out, encouraged by deep regular breathing. Get someone to drum lightly on the uphill part of your chest and move every few minutes to give every part a chance. Productive coughing confirms your success.

Avoid tobacco SMOKE, your own and other people's, so that your escalator mechanism can start working again. Filter the air in polluted living- or bedrooms, preferably with an *ionizer** or an air filter incorporating one.

If you are disappointed by the results of all this effort, take SUPPLEMENTS of Vitamins C (1000mg three times daily) and E (200IU twice daily), Essential Fatty Acids and Trace Minerals including Selenium and Zinc. Persevere for three months at a time, especially in anticipation of winter.

*Homoeopathic** Bryonia 6 is worth trying, but may not fit your condition exactly. If not, take advice from a homoeopathic practitioner about other possibilities.

Despite all this, if your condition is far advanced you may still require occasional help with an antibiotic course. Credit yourself with an advance of any kind – getting off long-term treatment or reducing the frequency of bad attacks. Make your aspirations clear to your doctor and he will be encouraged to share them with you.

If repeated antibiotics seem to lose their power or you become unaccountably sore and breathless during a continuous preventative course, consult your doctor. Infection with THRUSH or other fungi may be hard to prove and needs to be thought of and deliberately looked for. This is worthwhile as treatment is available.

BURNS, scalds

Your skin is quite distinct from the body it clothes, except for a few anchorage points where blood vessels and nerves can also reach it. In health you can pick up large folds of skin over most parts of your body and stretch them about quite elastically like the pelt of a cat or dog.

Its distinctive outer proofing layer is thin and vulnerable to ECZEMA and INJURY, but heals in a few days so long as enough healthy remnants of its foundations survive. Those which form your sweat glands and HAIR roots usually do, since they shelter deep within the main layer of your skin. This is the tough fibrous and elastic foundation of its strength and flexibility, and contains all its vital blood vessels, LYMPH passages and NERVES. These mount a second line of defence against INFECTION and further injury while the proofing layer heals.

Extremes of heat and cold are the most searching forms of INJURY, and destroy everything exposed to them. If heat penetrates vertically through the depth of your skin it leaves nothing viable over the entire area exposed; even the elastic fails, and the wound *ulcerates** – gapes like the hole in a damaged nylon stocking. This is disastrous; you have no defences there until the hole heals inwards from its edges, which may take months.

Consequently your skin has evolved to prevent this. Whenever it is heated severely it tries to dissipate the heat sideways, sharing a cooler temperature over a wider area of skin. Its arteries work like hydrants to achieve this, coming straight up from within and scattering branches out sideways. Blisters can quickly form in the surface layer of your skin as fluid barricades, diverting heat sideways before it can penetrate to that layer's foundation; damage there amounts to full-thickness destruction. Seared nerves make you withdraw automatically, ending the threat from a hot or frosted surface in a split second. A freezing wind, steam or a naked flame may be more dangerous since they spread over a wider skin area and reach out further from their source, which makes them harder to dissipate or escape.

Only ELECTRICITY defies these defences totally. The high resistance of your skin to an electric current makes it flow all the hotter, and forces it to choose the shortest route across its thickness to *tissues** like muscle that conduct electricity more easily. In consequence electrical burns, however small, invariably punch holes right through your skin.

ALCOHOL, fatigue and neurological disease such as MULTIPLE SCLEROSIS slow your reactions, and may prolong disastrously your exposure to thermal injury. This is particularly dangerous because you are unlikely to realize at first how seriously you are injured. For up to an hour your skin may look fairly normal, though discoloured and blistered. Then it begins to shrink and disintegrate, leaving a massive ulcer through which you lose a great deal of fluid and let in every available *microbe.** It is vital that you, or someone, realizes this possibility if the circumstances warrant it, and gets you urgent medical attention.

100

Take all the obvious and well-publicized precautions – fire-guards, fences around cooker hobs, pan handles turned out of the way. Avoid standing radiant electric heaters anywhere but in a guarded grate, even if no children are around.

Treat a burn or scald as soon as possible with cold water, sprinkled from a watering-can or shower nozzle if possible. Hold it under the cold tap while these are organized. Immerse your whole body, fully clothed, if necessary. *Twenty minutes under a cold spray immediately after the burn or scald will usually prevent injury altogether.* Your skin can cope with intense heating if it is not prolonged; urgent cooling makes all the difference.

If you keep *homoeopathic** Arnica 6 or 30 in the house, take a tablet onto your tongue as soon as cooling is begun, and every fifteen minutes until your composure returns. *Bach Rescue Remedy** is equally suitable; take two or three drops neat, then sip frequently at half a glass of water containing three drops more.

Meanwhile weigh up the risks. A light touch on a hot surface is much less dangerous than a blast of flame or steam, contact with burning clothes or treading on an ember. Numb, tired, drugged or drunken limbs burn worse than alert ones. Burnt skin that can still sense a heat or cold contrast, or a pin prick, has its nerves intact – its deeper layers have survived.

If the burn is electrical, or took you at one of these great disadvantages, assume that it will damage the whole thickness of your skin. Its appearance in the first hour is not reliable; if it cannot detect the prick of a sterilized pin, cover it with a dry clean dressing or fresh handkerchief and consult a doctor *urgently.* Do not attempt to remove burnt clothing.

Otherwise apply a non-stick dressing, with Ointment of Comfrey, Witch Hazel (Hamamelis) or Calendula if you have it. The insides of banana skins, or thin slices of fresh raw potato, are very satisfactory alternatives. Keep blisters intact as long as you can.

Use as little adhesive tape as possible, to leave access to the air. Do not bandage over the dressing. Raise the affected part above the level of your heart and rest it, continuing to keep it cool. Persevere with doses of Arnica or Rescue Remedy, lengthening the intervals gradually.

Renew the dressing daily, disturbing the skin as little as possible. Show any ugly or foul-smelling patches to your doctor. Otherwise use Calendula or Comfrey until it is soundly healed.

SUPPLEMENTS of Vitamins B_5 (Pantothenic Acid), C and E all help to consolidate your recovery and reduce complications.

CANCER, growth, malignancy, tumour

WHAT HAPPENS

Your personal integrity is maintained by the constant wilful effort of your *primal adaptive system,** which generates your IMMUNITY. This unifies the separate efforts of all the cells in your own body, and establishes relationships of high mutual regard with all other organisms in your vicinity. When you eat any of them as food, your IMMUNE system is responsible for the *'colour'** change which dismantles their own integrity and establishes their allegiance to yours.

This is a highly dynamic function, like a juggler keeping all his clubs in the air at once. It can be upset by anything that distracts your attention, dashes your hopes, injures your primal adaptive organs, undermines their motivation or starves their lines of supply. Your self-maintenance then breaks down in some degree; you stand up to STRESS less well, *microbes** INFECT you more easily, and your authority over everything in your body is weakened.

Accidents of cell division conspire with chemical pollution and RADIATION damage to produce a small proportion of new repair cells that are deformed, or else lack self-discipline. Normally your immune system destroys every one of these immediately, but a few may pass unnoticed when your system is upset. The unruly cells then get a chance to multiply into an outlaw *tissue** that grows more or less aggressively according to its type.

This cancerous growth will continue to prosper so long as its causes are unrelieved. These causes may operate at any level of your being:–

Body: *'mono'** pollution, INJURY, nutritional imbalance that deprives your immune system of essential resources;
Emotions: unrequited yearnings, unexpressed passions, unresolved anger, shock or grief;
Self-esteem: failure to love yourself *as well* as you love others, or to claim sufficient space and time in which to live your own particular life;
Life purpose: having no purpose large or inspiring enough to animate the whole of your life.

Doctors generally behave as if the causes of cancer were not known, and spend their whole effort on refining and administering treatment to destroy the growth. They are trying to establish cures parallel to the great success of antibiotics in dealing with infections. Sometimes they succeed, at least for a time; often you can make use of what they have to offer, along with other things. But this approach fails to deal effectively with your natural question – how can I stop it coming back?

The answer is to correct its cause, which frees you to re-establish order. This will be hard work, in 'colour' healing as well as INFLAMMATORY 'mono' curing. You are never beyond healing, so long as you are still alive; but your cancer may by then have weakened you too far to be capable of cure by the means available to you. That brings you face to face with the positive process of DYING with dignity, your WELLBEING intact to the end.

HELPING YOURSELF

Cancer is above all a disease to prevent. Once a growth is big enough to diagnose, it is already months or years old; by then it has already begun to undermine the reserves you need to draw on to get well.

Therefore make it a practice consciously to review each level of your being from time to time, in a periodic overhaul of your life process. This habit can make New Year resolutions worthwhile and meaningful. Do it together, within your marriage or circle of confidants; it goes more easily as a co-counselling session. Templegarth Trust (ADDRESS) has been developing Stress Analysis and Health Overhaul for uses of this sort.

Restore your body with a healthy DIET including fresh live food daily, and SUPPLEMENTED with Vitamin C at least. If your resistance to other diseases calls your IMMUNITY in question, SUPPLEMENT this energetically.

If your feelings are regularly at odds with your reason, find ways to act on or express them adequately – you cannot afford to put up with NERVOUSNESS or STRESS disease. You may need help of the clinical psychologist based at your local hospital, otherwise a voluntary or private counsellor, a teacher of relaxation or yoga; but a sensible and confidential friend or relative may be all the help you need.

Make sure that you esteem yourself highly enough to receive a fair share of love, time and attention. You can be too unselfish. If you are constantly deferring to the needs and demands of others, have some changes made.

Think about the meaning and purpose of life. Too few people do, or else suppose glibly that it has none. Whether or not you wish to recognize a supreme life principle in nature, you absolutely require a purpose of your own. Ambition is dangerously fickle and temporary: set up a comprehensive and fundamental personal moral code by which to decide your ambitions, and review your code regularly as further experience of life deepens your insight.

For cancer go on a SUPPLEMENTED cleansing DIET, whatever else appeals to you. Conventional treatment seeks only to destroy the 'mono' growth. SURGERY and radiotherapy can be skilfully focused and certainly have their place, saving you many months of hard healing work which you may be too ill to manage for yourself. But immunotherapy, or cytotoxic drugs, usually damage your IMMUNE system along with your tumour. Their use is one of the few points of direct conflict between conventional and new approaches to cancer treatment; in all other respects they are genuinely complementary.

Doctors are uneasy with cancer, and may be evasive in answering your questions. BACUP will help you to work with the established medical system; New Approaches to Cancer can put you in touch with additional 'colour' options, including doctors who can advise you personally taking both approaches into account. Contact both ADDRESSES, and make your choice.

CATARACT, lens opacity

The lens in each of your eyes lie immediately behind its pupil, the dark circle of variable size in the middle of the iris, which is a colourful shutter of muscle. If it is transparent, as it should be, your pupil will appear pink in a flash photograph with you looking at the camera. Cataract, which is frosting over of your lens, diminishes this pinkness and eventually changes it to a dense white.

The function of your eyes makes contradictory structural demands that would baffle the cleverest engineer. They require precise construction, with perfectly transparent and elastic corneal skin and lenses that must be able to bounce back to exactly the same shape without permanent harm after considerable and repeated deformation, over many years. The transparent parts must resist degeneration by ultra-violet sunlight, but manage without the brisk CIRCULATION otherwise desirable for this purpose – blood vessels would spoil their transparency.

So your lenses, like your JOINTS, put up with indirect nourishment and drainage, conveyed with the watery fluid that circulates through the front part of your eye, between small arteries on the front of your iris (the coloured part of your eye) and veins arranged all round the lens, amongst the muscles that hold it in place. This watery fluid flows slowly around your iris through your pupil (the dark hole in its centre), and only comes into contact with the front surface of your lens. But changes of its shape (to enable you to focus near or far) help to wring spent fluid out of it and let fresh air and nourishment in. Nevertheless its metabolism is restricted to a low level, and it is very susceptible to the same *colloidal** and crystalline deposits of waste acids that cause RHEUMATISM and ARTHRITIS.

Your lenses are therefore liable to degenerate in response to the same dietary factors which set off this crystallization in other parts of your body – heavy meat consumption in particular. But their exposure to sunlight makes them particularly liable to *free radical** damage, which not only stiffens their substance directly but promotes crystallization of any dissolved materials concentrated there – waste acids in particular. This only increases the degenerative tendency which shows as stiffening, irregularity of lens surfaces and loss of transparency.

All this was known by natural healers a century ago, but has been utterly rejected in favour of the exclusive use of SURGERY to remove the lens, once it is past repair. Degeneration to that point is regarded as inevitable once it has started – so much so that cataract was recently chosen as a fair test of the effectiveness of spiritual healing.

Eye surgery is a brilliant success, but expensive and imperfect. It is as foolhardy to discard simple eye hygiene in its favour as to stop washing cars just because neglected bolt-on bodywork can so easily be replaced!

HELPING YOURSELF

If the optician or your doctor notices that you have cataract or confirms your own suspicions, take remedial steps forthwith – even though the changes do not yet seriously affect your vision. You should be able to stop further deterioration, and may actually heal the damage you have already. Your main aims are to improve nutrition and cleansing, to stimulate your eye circulation, and to prevent further damage by ultra-violet exposure.

Start with a cleansing DIET to reduce drastically your protein and fat intake. After the first month you can temper this to the DIET for health.

SUPPLEMENT this with free radical scavengers – Vitamin C 500mg, Selenium 100microgm and Vitamin E 200IU, three times daily – to protect your eyes from ultra-violet damage. Additional Zinc 15mg (150mg of Zinc Orotate) and Manganese 20mg (150mg of Manganese Orotate), with one Strong Vitamin B Complex daily, make good the deficiencies common in cataract that can prevent recovery.

Bathe your eyes frequently and thoroughly in cool or tepid water containing a little sea salt, or use a tea made of Aloe Vera or Rue. You need to open your eyes under the water and roll them through all directions of gaze, to expose every part. Repeat this four to six times daily for a minute or two.

To encourage the circulation of fluid in the front of your eye, follow this bath twice daily with a strong shower jet of cold water directly at the closed lids of each eye in turn, until your eyeball begins to ache with the cold. Then massage it firmly for one minute through your closed eyelids with the tips of two fingers, making a brisk vibratory or trembling movement. Finish with a few firm rubbing strokes across the eye from the inside corner, then in the opposite direction, moving your upper lid under the stroking finger. Repeat the entire sequence on the other eye. Do not be afraid of damaging them – eyes are a lot tougher than most people think.

If you wear sunglasses, make sure that they cut out ultra-violet light. Otherwise they widen your pupils to admit even more ultra-violet than usual, doing more harm than good. If they tint everything on the brown side, they are probably satisfactory. You may need to consult the salesman or an optician if they are blue or black. If you are unsure of your present glasses, use an opaque eye-shade or broad brimmed shady hat as well or instead.

Never use a sun-bed or ultra-violet lamp without full eye protection.

CATARRH

Catarrh is a discharge of the skin of your digestive and breathing passages, and is very little understood for something so common. It results from INFLAMMATION or arousal of the skin, which responds to lubricate and protect itself; COLDS are a common example. But it can go on happening long after obvious irritation has ceased; then subtler principles apply.

In the first place, catarrh may be used by your body to excrete something you cannot otherwise cope with. It may be excess protein, as Arnold Ehret claims in his BOOK; his special cleansing DIET, freely adapted, works very well.

Secondly, all the catarrhal skins have deep kinship and sympathy with each other, dating back to their origin from the same source in your embryonic development. This kinship expresses itself largely through a fine mesh of nervous connections built into the skins' foundations. If one part of this network is irritated, the ripples spread to all the others. So your nose may get congested when your bowel is loaded and needs emptying; your faeces irritate the skin they touch and your nose picks up the influence. As your bowel empties itself naturally you feel a wave of ease pass through your whole body, reaching your nose within seconds. In CONSTIPATION this emptying never occurs properly, so your nose is never relieved; you seem to have HAY FEVER, but all the year round. Irritation from pollens or pollutants may aggravate the condition without being its fundamental cause.

The usual seat of catarrh is however not your bowel but your stomach. This is commonly drawn in the shape of a kidney bean, as it appears in dissection and at operations. In life it adopts quite another form, clearly visible on X-rays, and handles different foods very selectively. Its top half takes on the form and function of a hopper, holding your swallowed mouthfuls in layers exactly as they arrive. So your first mouthful forms the outer skin of an onion-like mass, to which each fresh arrival adds a new heart.

This gives your saliva a chance to break open starch grains in your food and start digesting them. Once a meal passes down into the acid bath in your lower stomach, all that is stopped. Any grains left intact cannot be digested there, but serve as grit to irritate the lining of your stomach as it churns. At first it responds with more acid, but this turns to mucus as reserves are exhausted; a chronic catarrhal condition is the result.

The chief cause of all this is white bread, cake, buns and biscuits. This consists of a protein sponge with starch grains embedded in it. It scarcely needs chewing, so gets very little salivary treatment. Many of the starch grains therefore survive to irritate your stomach, whose chronically catarrhal state ripples through the rest of you. Catarrhal bowels are also prone to THRUSH and CONSTIPATION, which only reinforce the whole tendency.

Sinusitis* and EARACHE are particularly troublesome results. In these catarrh formed in caves in your skull gets trapped and builds up a terrific pressure.

HELPING YOURSELF

Stop eating baked floury food of any kind. The special DIET for cleansing is ideal. Dry toasted wholemeal is permitted because starch grains are burst and chemically altered by toasting; its dry bulk forces you to chew it well. Add a SUPPLEMENT of Vitamin C, 1000mg three times daily.

Stop using catarrh medicines. They have only a temporary effect and are habit-forming; confine them to any attacks of sinusitis and EARACHE you may suffer before the catarrh stops. Even then, use them only on three days in any week. You can use one of the remedies listed below on the other days.

Garlic is remarkably helpful in acute bouts of catarrh, so long as you can cope with the BODY ODOUR it causes. Minimize this by using the Garlic Lozenge RECIPE at socially acceptable times of day.

*Homoeopathic** Merc. Sol., Aconite, or Nat. Mur. may be beneficial, and are safe substitutes for other medicines.

Check yourself for ALLERGY. Food from the cow and wheat commonly provoke catarrh in susceptible people. Avoid them if they affect you, at least until the catarrh is thoroughly cured. You may then be able to tolerate occasional portions without trouble.

Contrasting views of stomach function

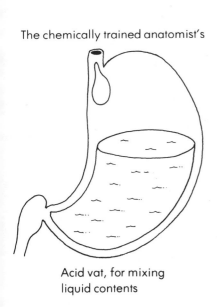

The chemically trained anatomist's

Acid vat, for mixing liquid contents

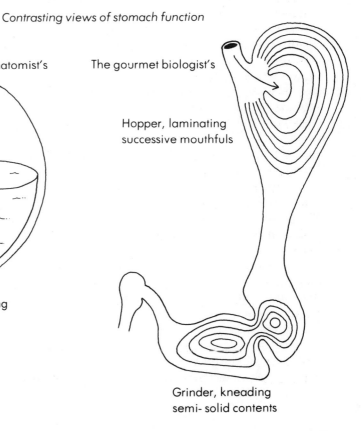

The gourmet biologist's

Hopper, laminating successive mouthfuls

Grinder, kneading semi-solid contents

CHICKENPOX, varicella, herpes

WHAT HAPPENS

Pox viruses are related to the herpes family, all of whom have a particular liking for your skin. But unlike *genital herpes** and *cold sores** poxes cannot get there direct; they must pass the defences of your nose and throat and reach your skin through your bloodstream. Viruses as aggressive as that can theoretically be very dangerous to life. Smallpox was, and killed a high proportion of its victims until it was eradicated in 1980. Happily it is not now so vital to distinguish chickenpox and smallpox from each other.

You become infected by inhaling or swallowing droplets of saliva, blister fluid or scabs from an infected person. You will not notice this, but may be a little off colour while the virus is multiplying inside your *cells.** After two or three weeks' *incubation** these cells burst releasing millions of virus particles, and the disease breaks out in earnest – sometimes with FEVER and a mild illness. Your saliva and breath are INFECTIOUS at this stage, and remain so for a week.

Simultaneously or next day a crop of small blisters appears, each one in the centre of a small red patch of skin. New crops appear successively for several days, concentrated mostly on your body and head. The extent of the rash is very variable, and seems to be determined by your general IMMUNITY before-hand; some individuals can prove very hard to infect at all, even by nursing other members of their family who get it badly.

If chickenpox catches you at a bad time, you may get blisters in your mouth and throat as well. This is very uncomfortable and interferes with swallow-ing, which gets most victims down badly. Or very occasionally the virus may get in your brain, making you ill and irritable with a terrible HEADACHE, very intolerant of light in your room; this is *encephalitis.**

Each blister eventually bursts releasing very infectious fluid, and a mildly infectious scab forms on its base. The blisters are within the thickness of your skin, which only has to close over to heal them without any scarring. The chief hazard arises from ITCHING of the scabs as they heal, which may tempt you to scratch unconsciously during your sleep. Scratching may pierce your skin right through, forcing it to heal more laboriously and form a scar, just as after a full-thickness BURN of your skin.

Chickenpox recurs sometimes, or can remain dormant for many years to be rekindled as SHINGLES when you are re-exposed; how this is supposed to happen stretches conventional theories of INFECTION well beyond their normal limits. The virus evidently survives in several of the NERVE junction-boxes alongside your spinal cord, to rekindle during a fresh outbreak of chickenpox later in life. Whatever the correct explanation may be, it is likely that your IMMUNITY was below par when you were originally infected, so that you never completely healed. Careful convalescence from chickenpox there-fore seems well worthwhile.

*Cold sores** (a different virus) survive between bouts in just the same way. They too can break out afresh whenever another illness weakens you.

Foster the IMMUNITY of everyone in the house when chickenpox is about. Large SUPPLEMENTS of Vitamin C (1000mg three times daily) are well worthwhile.

Once a member of your family has chickenpox, give him his own towel and face-cloth of a different colour and get him to keep it in a separate place. Change his bed carefully, to avoid dust billowing off it around your house; keep all his laundry in a sealed plastic bin-liner until it can be washed hot.

Precautions like these are mainly to protect adults and debilitated children; let young healthy children mingle with victims to acquire natural IMMUNITY. If they are really well you may have quite a job infecting them.

*Homoeopathic** Aconite 3 is helpful during fever at the onset; Antimony tartrate 6 is more use once the blisters have begun. Both can be given every two hours. Merc. sol 6 may be useful four hourly once the fever is over.

For the ITCHING, dab on neat Cider Vinegar, or Calamine Lotion BP containing 1% Liquefied Phenol BP. The latter is mildly corrosive, so avoid getting it on eyes, lips or genital skin.

At night give a full dose of an antihistamine medicine such as Phenergan or Piriton rather than risk unconscious scratching.

If severe irritability, *delirium** or HEADACHE accompany chickenpox, consult your doctor urgently. Even if its course is straightforward notify him for record purposes that you have the disease. Consult him in any case if you suspect SHINGLES.

*Cold sore** virus needs air as it settles into hybernation between attacks. If you seal each sore meticulously with vaseline for a month after each outbreak, you will successively weaken them until they are finally eradicated.

Your doctor can provide you with a paint which, applied from the very first sign of a *cold sore** outbreak, may succeed in aborting it altogether.

*Genital herpes** requires the attention of your doctor. Consult him if you have reason to suspect it.

CIRCULATION poor; anaemia; cramp; chilblains

WHAT HAPPENS

Your main blood vessels, conspicuous though they are on anatomical charts, are only the means for refreshing your blood and getting it back as quickly as possible to the business end of your circulation. That is the massive network of microscopically fine capillaries, many of them only just big enough to admit a blood cell, distributed inconspicuously through every *tissue** you possess. They are not permanent but grow and expire with the tissue. Some are renewed every few weeks, most within months; in two years none will remain of those you have now.

This means that the layout, size and nervous regulation mechanism of your blood capillaries are determined in part by the physical conditions in your body at the time they are growing. If your body is clean and well supplied you recreate perfectly the *'colour'** pattern of every part, though the exact *'mono'** layout varies at random – just like the twigs and branches of a tree, which manage even so to perpetuate its characteristic form overall. You can even adapt constructively to your circumstances, such as prolonged periods in the open air. But when you are out of order you cannot manage any of this perfectly, and lay down a generation of inadequate capillaries which function unreliably.

This is how your complexion can so faithfully reflect your general health and customary circumstances. But the way your circulation works has other implications too. Muscles congested chronically with waste acids are served sluggishly with blood, and much more prone to RHEUMATISM in consequence. *Cramp** is caused by temporary failure of your muscle release mechanism under STRESS. This arises in a sluggish circulation which may also be insufficiently supplied with the minerals that enable your muscles to work properly.

*Chilblains** are a more prolonged and complicated local disturbance of your whole skin, not just of the blood vessels there. Its reaction to cold includes inappropriate release of *histamine,** and weakly resembles ALLERGY. *Cold urticaria** is a more violent and widespread version of the same thing which is much less common.

*Anaemia** is a different kind of problem, in which the *oxygen**-bearing red blood *cells** are either too scarce or contain too little *haemoglobin,** the red iron-containing protein which stores oxygen in them. This condition is well understood generally by doctors, and a medical success. But emphasis on iron supplements is illogical. Most anaemic people already consume enough iron but fail to absorb a large enough proportion of it. Organic acids such as Vitamin C increase that proportion if eaten along with meals containing iron, treating your problem much better than excessive doses of iron. Moreover the problem is sometimes not iron deficiency at all, but lack of other trace minerals such as zinc and molybdenum, and occasionally of vitamins. Broadening the scope of anaemic treatment in this way deals with it much more adequately.

To check that your circulation is healthy, press the tip of your big toe firmly for a few seconds and watch how long it takes to flush pink again after you let go. Anything over two seconds suggests deficiency.

Maintain the DIET for health, to give your blood vessels a chance to correct themselves.

Make full use of them regularly in sustained physical EXERCISE.

SMOKING narrows your blood vessels chronically. If your legs are getting cold and painful, stop it urgently.

COLDNESS can cause poor circulation, or result from it. Follow the advice given on that topic.

Intermittent circulation problems respond to *contrast bathing.** Immerse your whole body (or the affected part) in hot water for three minutes, then in cool or cold for thirty seconds; repeat this for up to three cycles, finishing with cold. You will glow and feel larger than life for a couple of hours afterwards, and easily get warm in bed.

A tendency to *cramp** usually responds to daily mineral SUPPLEMENTS. Kelp is cheap, but if two tablets a day for a month at a time are ineffective try a more carefully formulated preparation such as Nature's Own Multimineral (see ADDRESS), which can be taken indefinitely. Brewer's Yeast may also be worthwhile; if so, the effect is quickly obvious.

Chilblains* often improve dramatically with Tamus Ointment, or *homoeopathic** Tamus Communis 6. Nicotinamide SUPPLEMENTS (50mg once or twice daily) may be helpful, and will not make you blush in the way Nicotinic Acid does. Add Vitamin E (200IU twice daily) if you do not seem to benefit from the less expensive items alone. After the chilblains have gone tone up the affected limb with contrast baths, but make the cold phase only tepid to start with. Correct your DIET, and EXERCISE regularly if you don't already.

Most chronically *anaemic** people consume plenty of iron, unless you are on an unbalanced vegan diet. What you need is ample Vitamin C, to let in more of the iron you eat already. Other minerals are involved as well, zinc being foremost among them. If you are not getting anywhere with your present treatment and do not seem to be BLEEDING chronically from anywhere, revise your DIET and SUPPLEMENTS. Zinc (15mg daily) or a good multimineral, together with at least 500mg Vitamin C with every mineral dose and meal, will usually solve a stubborn anaemia problem.

Consult a practitioner of *Traditional Chinese Medicine** if after all this you are still in trouble and your doctor can find nothing wrong that he can help you with.

COLDNESS

Your body works best in a narrow band of temperatures centred on 37°C, to which all your chemical apparatus is tuned for optimum performance. Your skin thrives best a little cooler, and the temperature of your limbs is usually rather less. Occasionally you employ FEVER to out-run illness. Otherwise, despite all but the most extreme weather, your body keeps close to this ideal so long as sufficient food is available and you can burn it fast enough. Only a misguided starvation DIET to reduce OVERWEIGHT, some medicines, over-exposure to cold weather and thyroid insufficiency are likely to prevent you.

Medical knowledge of thyroid function began to suffer in the middle of this century, when chemistry gained supremacy over biology as a tool for investigation; doctors have never since then been able to stand back and see *metabolism** as a whole. Medicine consequently makes two false assumptions. Firstly, it associates thyroid function too closely with the levels in your blood of the chemical hormones supposed to control it. This is rather like using a fuel gauge and the manufacturer's performance figures to decide how far your car can go without refuelling. It ignores all circumstantial factors and takes no account of idiosyncracies in your particular car. There is no substitute for a trial run. In your case that means some measure of the actual rate at which your metabolism proceeds. That used to be determined by monitoring the rate at which you released heat or use up *oxygen;** but both of these measures were slow, expensive and unreliable. It turns out however that the humblest measurement of all works well in most circumstances – your body temperature when at rest. This indicates the tick-over rate of your metabolism, which is largely determined by your thyroid function.

Secondly, one purified hormone (thyroxine) is now supposed to represent the output of your whole thyroid gland, as if its three other hormonally active products only get into your blood by accident. At least one of them is actually more potent than thyroxine, though it is normally present in smaller quantities. It is more logical to replace inadequate thyroid function with whole thyroid glandular tissue, which is cheaper than the refined hormone. This fell from favour because it deteriorates in storage and is therefore of unreliable potency. But its pharmaceutical properties are different, and much longer lasting. In particular it can permanently lower blood *cholesterol** to normal, whereas thyroxine only does this for the first three months of treatment. This has eclipsed the relationship between ARTERIOSCLEROSIS and thyroid insufficiency, correction of which was in the 1940s shown to convey a ten-fold protection from premature CORONARIES and STROKES. The modern purified hormone probably lacks this property, though nobody is trying to find out.

If you feel cold in conditions which would toast most people, your doctor can quickly rule out all medically respectable causes. Even if he accepts what I have said, desiccated whole thyroid (Thyroid BP) is no longer routinely available to him because the licence to manufacture it has been withdrawn. Science has in this instance thrown out the baby with the bath-water, and misinformed a whole generation of physicians.

If you are unaccountably affected by cold conditions, or close relatives have had *tuberculosis*,* STROKES or CORONARIES quite young, check your *basal temperature** – that is, your body temperature at tick-over. This is best measured first thing in the morning after a restful night's sleep, twelve hours or so after your last meal. Have the thermometer ready by your bed to minimise your effort in using it, and keep it under your armpit for a full ten minutes before stirring from your bedding. Repeat for three consecutive mornings, discounting any following a restless night. The result should be consistently above 36.6°C (97.8°F), except for women around *ovulation** time. You may record around half a degree less before ovulating than after and plummet even lower on ovulation day. You should however be able to keep your basal temperature higher than this minimum throughout your monthly cycle.

Consult your doctor if this basal temperature is low, and refer to this account if you wish. I will gladly send him a summary of selected scientific references if he sends me a stamped addressed envelope. Broda Barnes' BOOK is available through libraries and gives full details. Even if he feels unable to cooperate, it is important to keep him informed.

Check the other members of your family. This will convince you that the thermometer is working, and may discover others with low temperatures – the tendency runs in families.

To correct your temperature try first the effect of one or two Kelp tablets daily, or a generous daily portion of fresh water cress, to provide plenty of the iodine your thyroid requires. Sometimes this harmless measure is sufficient to set your thyroid function right. Children in particular may improve dramatically on it, with correct temperatures within a few days. If improvement is not obvious re-check your temperature after a month and reduce your dose to one tablet daily.

If it is still sub-normal and you are taking no other regular medication, obtain from Lamberts mail order ADDRESS some tablets of Thyroid Glandular Concentrate 150mg. Take *a quarter of one tablet* after breakfast daily for two months, and check your temperature again before doubling this. You may increase your dose by a quarter of a tablet every two months until your temperature reaches normal or your dose reaches one whole tablet. *On no account proceed further or faster without medical supervision*, and stop in any case if you experience *any new symptoms at all*.

Whole thyroid is still the basis of homoeopathic treatment for thyroid insufficiency, so a *Homoeopathic practitioner** may help you if your doctor cannot. *Traditional Chinese Medicine** may reveal a treatable hindrance to your thyroid, and a *Yoga** teacher can help you promote its energy.

COLDS

Virus particles capable of INFECTING you are constantly present in the air you breathe; hundreds enter every time you inhale. It is not so remarkable how many VIRUS INFECTIONS you get, but that you get so few. To achieve this you have maintained a defensive policing operation ever since your very first breath, focused in the first place on your nose.

This is your air monitor and conditioner. Through it you can appreciate the 'colour'* scent of your immediate atmosphere and can detect and react to tiny traces of poisonous fumes mixed with it. Air which is cold or dry is moistened and warmed to a condition your lungs can cope with; their specialized function makes them very vulnerable to BRONCHITIS otherwise. SMOKE and dust is filtered out by a dense web of hairs, then washed off and made harmless with antiseptic mucus loaded with white blood *cells** – your body's cleaners and police all in one. They move in according to a regular shut-down schedule, one nostril at a time. Normally you are not even aware of the contra-flow arrangements; business carries on as usual in the other nostril.

To cope with the tremendous turnover of work required of it your nose needs a lot of maintenance, which you automatically provide. A rich CIRCULATION nourishes it lavishly so long as you eat food of good enough quality in the first place. You can then meet every new challenge with a flawless skin, well lubricated with potently protective mucus.

Anything which interferes with this – exhaustion, prolonged COLDNESS, heavy smoke pollution, inadequate food – can let a virus breech your defences and colonize you. Once established in skin cells anywhere in your nose it is free to take its course there but you can still limit its further spread. Local INFLAMMATION generates a brisk mucus response loaded with protective white blood cells. The normal shut-down procedure is intensified, and becomes apparent as congestion or blockage if the schedules for each nostril overlap.

If in this first few hours you rally resources quickly, you can contain the problem and stay well. Otherwise the virus breaks through to your lymph GLANDS and takes on your general IMMUNE mechanisms. Your inflammatory discomfort by now involves your neck, and you may begin to feel FEVERISH and ill.

In this case you are committed to a period of disease lasting at least a few days while your body creates immune *antibodies** against the virus. This preoccupies your effort, and leaves you little energy for everyday living unless you deliberately fortify yourself with the extra resources called for in these circumstances.

Medical claims that Vitamin C SUPPLEMENTS do not prevent colds arise from a misunderstanding of what to expect, and from looking for 'mono'* effects where 'colour' change is what matters.

HELPING YOURSELF

As soon as you detect the least soreness in your nose, start taking Vitamin C SUPPLEMENTS, 1gm hourly for several hours. Pure crystals are the most economical.

Keep a clove of fresh raw garlic, in all its coverings, in your cheek as a lozenge. Its 'colour' energy and gentle reek are powerfully antiseptic and dramatically reduce CATARRH.

An alternative to garlic is *homoeopathic** Aconite 6 or 30, taken frequently from the very first cold feeling at times other than the Vitamin C doses. This is particularly appropriate for the kind of cold that starts with frequent sneezing.

Infludo (Weleda UK Ltd) is an *anthroposophic** remedy formulated for colds and influenza taken as drops every two hours. It is available on an NHS prescription. Use it in combination with rest, in bed if necessary.

The vapour from a dish of very hot water containing a teaspoonful of Menthol and Eucalyptus Inhalation BPC is very soothing to an irritable throat; inhaling it for five minutes is the best first aid for COUGHING. If you go out, carry in a warm pocket a second clean handkerchief impregnated with a few drops of neat Inhalation and breathe deeply from this whenever you feel the need.

Eat light meals only, avoiding rich meat dishes. Fresh fruit and raw salads are ideal, with baked potatoes or wholemeal bread.

Gentle deep BREATHING through your nostrils, whenever they are open, will help reduce congestion. Really fill your lungs three or four times, taking 15–20 seconds over each breath. Pause with your lungs full before exhaling slowly. On the other hand, begin your next breath as soon as your lungs are empty.

Hum and sing the sounds 'mmm' and 'nn' to vibrate your sinuses, which helps to keep them clear – and raise your spirits!

For preventive measures see VIRUS INFECTIONS.

For Cold Sores see CHICKENPOX.

COLITIS, irritable bowel

Your large bowel acts as a sewer for your whole body, voiding not only the unwanted remains of what you eat but whatever your liver and intestines have excreted in *bile** and CATARRH. But if you can once clean your body enough to make little sewage in the first place, your bowel then contributes positively to your health in quite a different way.

In health, no *bacteria** of any kind survive your stomach to occur in your small intestines, where most of your food is absorbed. But residues discharged from there into your large bowel abruptly meet the bacteria that thrive there on its cellulose fibre content. Two of these, Bifidus and Acidophilus, never produce disease. The third type, known as Coliforms, only do so if they are forced to survive on meat residues instead of cellulose.

The first part of your large bowel is shaped like a cauldron, with your *appendix** dangling from its lowest part. Here the bacteria ferment fibrous residues into acids, running their metabolism on the proceeds. This releases minerals from the fibres which failed to soften in your stomach. The bacteria eventually die releasing valuable minerals, vitamins and other nutrients in just the right organ to absorb it. This mechanism saved millions from starvation in post-war Europe, and enables modern life-long vegans to make up their dietary needs. New vegetarians acquire these bacteria gradually.

The acid residues from cellulose fermentation are not absorbed but make your faeces very inhospitable to disease-forming bacteria and THRUSH. Enough fibre remains to cocoon the sewage and keep your faeces plastic and bulky so that they are voided promptly – two or three times daily, after most meals. Your whole colon (except its cauldron) remains empty, clean and supple throughout your life.

Things go badly wrong if you eat too much meat and too little fibrous vegetables, cereals and fruit. Meat is more chemically polluted than most food, which may cause damage to your intestines and intoxicate your blood. Damaged intestines discriminate less well, absorbing toxins they would otherwise reject. More of these arise from inefficient digestion in a sloppy liquid, lacking its stabilizing gel of swollen fibres. That gel would have scoured your stomach and prevented polluted digestive effluent from irritating your large bowel. Instead, coliforms and THRUSH overgrow there and Acidophilus and Bifidus die off. Meat residues fester into poisonous alkaline nitrogenous products including gases like ammonia. Much of this toxic material is reabsorbed to interfere everywhere through your blood and paralyse your bowel muscle. Putrid faeces can hang around for days between bouts of *diarrhoea* – bloating your colon, congesting your veins, bladder and womb and straining its own ligaments. Your whole colonic apparatus stiffens gradually over the years, with fibrous repairs from repeated strains and tears.

Colitis is your bowel trying to work against these odds, inflamed by its poisonous contents. Help it succeed, or worse will eventually follow: diverticular disease probably, CANCER perhaps.

HELPING YOURSELF

Use the special DIET for cleansing, but without the preliminary fast. Avoid all meat, fish, hard cheese, tinned produce, eggs and dairy products for the first three weeks. Eat only vegetables and fruit until your tongue is clean and pink; then never again use refined flour or cereals routinely. Only use bran as in the brose RECIPE.

Replace coffee and Indian tea with camomile, elderflower or lime-blossom (linden) teas, cider vinegar and honey and home-made barley water RECIPES, with watered fruit juice by turns. Drink plenty, half a pint before each meal.

Chew your food long and thoroughly. Never eat in haste or under pressure.

EXERCISE well in fresh air, BREATHING deeply. Bathe afterwards while still perspiring; finish with generous splashes of cold water or wrap your belly tightly with a cold damp cloth and go to bed.

*Homoeopathic** treatment frequently helps. Try Chamomilla and Arsen. alb. for yourself, then seek expert help. Alternatively consult a practitioner of *Traditional Chinese Medicine** for a completely different approach.

CONCUSSION, head INJURY

Of all tissues, your brain and spinal cord are the best defended against INJURY. Their structure is so completely committed to their highly specialized functions that they are slow to repair themselves and rely on being cushioned from harmful vibration and jolts by their shock-absorbing suspension. This is provided by the bath of *cerebro-spinal fluid** in which they float, loosely anchored by a web of undergrowth to the tough waterproof lining of your skull and spinal bones, which form a hard flexible casing. This protects you better than several pairs of woollen socks inside an over-sized reinforced Wellington boot, an arrangement which makes it hard to damage your feet.

But your brain is much more vulnerable, and needs all the protection it can get. Its complex pulsatile ELECTRONIC activity is easily unsettled by blows far too light to tear, bruise or INFLAME its flesh. This happens any time you bang your head or fall on your spine heavily enough to be dazed or see 'stars'. It can make you more irritable, disoriented, forgetful and easily fatigued for several hours without producing any structural damage your doctor can demonstrate. And there is one kind of subtle damage doctors do not yet recognize, which can cause serious POSTURAL problems and stubborn HEAD-ACHES for decades afterwards if it is not adequately treated.

Your head bones are not rigidly locked together but hinged like a piano lid, so that they can move very slightly on each other. The movement of each joint disturbs all the others, so that your skull bones do not move independently but as a whole. The result is that your skull can either elongate from front to back and get narrower, or shorten and get wider. This enables your skull shape to pulsate very slightly, from one extreme to the other and back, six times each minute. From their origin in your skull, these pulsations ripple gently down your spine and through your limbs. You can see this for yourself in someone else who is lying relaxed on his back on a flat surface. His feet will pivot very slightly on his heels as his legs roll to and fro, even if he holds his breath.

These movements hinge internally on a stout fold in the tough lining of your skull, which hangs across it from side to side like a tight curtain. But it is strong enough to behave more like a girder, bracing the fixed axis around which these changes of shape occur – rather like the pivot of a see-saw.

How these pulsatile movements originate is unknown. I suspect that they arise ultimately from your *primal adaptive system** as a medium by which you can influence the whole of your body at once. If so, they probably act like the carrier wave used in radio, which you can modulate to broadcast through-out your body *'colour'** coordination of your POSTURE and movement.

Injuries too slight to fracture bones or bruise your brain can jam these movements and frustrate their function. If my speculations are correct, this can have much more profound long-term effects on health than grosser physical damage. Since concussion is the general disruption to brain function that accompanies such structural injuries, it should now be extended to include these more common, subtle and debilitating functional effects.

HELPING YOURSELF

Relax your routine after a heavy blow to your head or spine to give yourself latitude for restful RECOVERY. You may not need it, but will prolong your debility if you leave yourself no room for the rest you require. It will vary from a few hours to a few days, depending on the weight of the blow.

Homoeopathic Arnica 30 can be taken every half hour at first, then less frequently. *Bach Rescue Remedy** is an alternative, two drops in half a glass of water sipped and savoured every few minutes. Either will help you overcome the initial shock.

A cold damp cloth pressed firmly over any tender lump for twenty minutes will limit the swelling; refresh the cloth every minute or so. Then apply Arnica Ointment 10% if your skin is unbroken, otherwise neat Witch Hazel (Hamamelis) extract.

After a hot bath wrap a cold damp cloth tightly around your body from your ribs to your pelvis, pinning it at short intervals to make it fit closely. Wear a woollen sweater over it. This will alter the balance of your CIRCULATION, effectively diverting blood from your head to your abdomen and relieving congestive HEADACHE or irritability. Wear it for two hours, or go to bed in it. Elderflower or lime blossom (linden) tea reinforces the effect.

The weariness and lack of concentration that lasts for days deserves a special DIET for cleansing, SUPPLEMENTED generously with Brewer's Yeast, Vitamin C and home-made lemon barley water RECIPE. The RECIPES for egg nog and Honey Cider Vinegar are occasional alternatives to make up as a hot beverage.

The remedies for STRESS apply, notably SUPPLEMENTS of Ginseng and Vitamin B_{15}.

For any stubborn pain or disorientation which seems to stem from a past INJURY to skull or spine – including difficult forceps or breech delivery or extreme skull moulding at birth – it is worth seeing a *Cranial Osteopath** (ADDRESS). He will have a basic osteopathic qualification with additional postgraduate training in his speciality. His examination and treatment are very gentle, and aim to identify strain or limitation of your cranial pulsations, and to manipulate them back to normal. Go with a companion who can drive you home in case you are temporarily disoriented and confused by sudden correction of faulty movements you were accustomed to. Several treatments may be required.

CONJUNCTIVITIS, pink eye

See also VIRUS INFECTIONS, COLDS

WHAT HAPPENS

Your eye is covered with a special kind of skin called conjunctiva, which is very thin, smooth, sensitive and transparent, revealing the white fibrous eyeball and providing a good optical surface to the cornea. It starts at the margins of your eyelids and drapes in one continuous and closely fitting vacuum-moulding across their insides and the front half of your eyeball, with deep folds into the farthest recesses of the space between them.

This elaborately moulded conjunctiva is flexible and its outside surfaces are very slippery, lubricated by a continuous thin film coating of tears, and nourished from inside by a tracery of fine blood vessels all over the eye and both eyelids. The arrangement seals your eye from the outside yet enables it to move freely inside your eyelids, whether open or closed, by sliding two conjunctival surfaces over each other.

But there are snags. The outside surface of the conjunctiva is like the inside of an irregularly shaped bag, with its neck open to the air outside your eyelids. This bag is empty but for the lubricating film of tears, and is kept at body temperature. This makes it a very comfortable incubator for the airborne microbes* that find haven there. So the tears also have an antiseptic function and, with the assistance of IMMUNE factors available from your CIRCULATION, patrol the bag continuously to prevent microbial growth.

During any prolonged period of eye closure debris from this patrolling function accumulates as a harmless sticky pus-like blob that you can rub from the inside of your eye. There tends to be more of it when you are unwell, because the patrolling is clumsier and less efficient; more effort is required to achieve the same result. Occasionally even in health you need to make a greater effort than usual, to subdue a correspondingly larger or more aggressive colony of bacteria.*

In this way you may often have more than usual of the familiar debris, but runnier and less sticky for having less time to dry out. So long as your conjunctiva is still white and comfortable, you should regard this as a healthy variation of the normal pattern, not as a disease.

If a microbe becomes established in your eye, plentiful watery tears will run from an irritable conjunctiva, reddened by INFLAMMATORY swelling of the blood vessels underlying it. If the microbe is a virus, as is more usual, your nose will soon become involved if it is not already: otherwise, suspect that a bacterium is responsible. The tears are teeming with microbes in either case, and highly INFECTIOUS. They may settle down to the more purulent character reminiscent of health, but the eye will still be pink and feel gritty.

Chemical irritation, smoke or a speck of dirt in the eye will produce a very similar response, but the cause is then more obvious. Continual exposure to tobacco SMOKE can make your eyes chronically irritable and dry. Chronic INFECTION is rather different, and affects your eyelid margins rather than your conjunctivae. They become thickened, encrusted with fine scales, dusky pink and irritable. Your eyes feel TIRED and water easily.

Never use hot water or soap on your face unless it really is dirty. The skin of your eyelids is particularly sensitive to these, which can make them chronically irritable.

Cold water is a powerful tonic if sprayed on your closed eyelids until they just begin to ache. Then massage the eyeballs by rolling them under firm finger pressure through closed eyelids. This procedure is helpful in any chronic eye complaint.

Rue tea makes an excellent eye-wash for general purposes: fresh flowers are the most potent.

A fresh milk eye-wash is easy to organize quickly if chemical gets in your eye. It blots up most of them and relieves chemical irritation safely and well. See a doctor within a few hours if it fails.

Pain from a welding accident or after any fragment has hit your eye at high speed may mean that debris is embedded in your cornea or under your conjunctiva. You will need to see a specialist eye doctor. Bandage a patch over your eye to protect it, and attend a hospital Accident and Emergency Department in the first place.

If your eye remains white but becomes pusy, simple bathing with tepid salty water (a teaspoon in a cupful) is safe while you await developments, and is usually enough to get it better. If it becomes red and runny during a COLD, in the first place treat the cold.

For any other pain or redness or a chronic pusy discharge, see your doctor.

CONSTIPATION and diverticular disease

If *diarrhoea** or COLITIS fails to rid you of the sluggish alkaline products of your faulty DIET, its consequences continue to accrue. Rather than fluctuate between violent expulsive pangs and periods of congestion and stoppage, your bowel fatigues into a more permanently constipated pattern. This is much less trying and is regarded as normal by millions of people in the developed world. Your bowel acts only once a day or less, to pass a few firm faeces each composed of separate nuggets compacted together. Pushing them out is slow unless you urge or strain a bit, and can still take time; reading in the toilet is a modern institution!

*Colic** is the rhythmic pang you get in your lower abdomen when your bowel is trying to move hard faeces along. Children may have it regularly, often together with CATARRH and sometimes seepage or soiling of their underwear. Their appendix is constantly under threat of obstruction; grumbling *appendix** is the occasional painful crisis that supersedes colic when that threat materializes, subsiding after a supreme healing effort or a dose of opening medicine.

But by now unhealthy bacteria are well established generally in your bowel and are probably encroaching into the lower part of your small intestine. If during a grumble one of these bacteria gets a hold, a less easily reversible acute *appendicitis** follows. If your appendix bursts the infection spreads all over your abdomen; that is *peritonitis.**

Whether or not you lose your appendix in this way, the underlying problem progresses. The congestive effects on your circulation produce PILES or VARICOSE VEINS; straining out a hard motion can tear your anus, producing a *fissure.** Reabsorbed toxins poison your metabolism, fouling your BODY ODOUR and causing HEADACHE.

Chronic severe pangs strain your bowel, weakest where blood vessels pass through the muscle layers; the unsupported skin there can pout back during a pressure wave, like a bicycle wheel inner tube through a hole in the tyre. Once a bubble of skin has been forced through a hole like this it gets bigger with every pang. These bubbles are diverticula, which can get as big as Brussels sprouts after a lifetime of constipation. Faeces get in and cannot easily get out. Sometimes they putrefy and discharge painfully into your bowel, giving slimy diarrhoea; this is *diverticulitis;** occasionally an infected diverticulum bursts the other way, giving you another chance of peritonitis.

Without constipation and excessive meat eating, bowel CANCER would probably not occur at all. Thirty years of active resistance to irritation provides many opportunities for the skin of your colon to make mistakes. The usual places are exactly where faecal toxins persist the longest – the cauldron at its very beginning, where your appendix is attached and your faeces are formed; and in the last quarter leading to your anus, where constipated faeces linger before you get rid of them. If you are to prevent this from happening, you must start many years before.

HELPING YOURSELF

You may need an enema to get your bowel moving in the first place. Your doctor can arrange this through your district nurse, if your problem is severe enough.

Otherwise, stop using stimulant medicines to make your bowel act. Half a cup daily of crushed or puréed linseed, or two dessertspoonsful of linseed oil on an empty stomach can be substituted for a time, and is safer in pregnancy.

Brew herbs like camomile and mint instead of coffee and Indian tea.

Start a cleansing DIET, emphasizing fresh and soaked dried fruit and raw green vegetables. Use wheat sprouts and brose made according to the RECIPES.

Drink one pint of water before breakfast, or as much of it as you can manage.

Never take bran dry or on its own. If you use it at all, mix it thoroughly with more than its own volume of whole-grain cereal. Otherwise it may swell into sticky lumps, like badly made porridge, and clog you up worse than you are already.

Vigorous daily EXERCISE is important, followed by a shower while still perspiring. Finish with cold water all over your abdomen and massage it firmly in clockwise circles. Massage a child's stomach in this way during every bath before you dry him.

Four weeks' perseverence should cure you, but refined floury foods and white rice may start a relapse if you slide back into eating them. It should be obvious what is at stake; always keep your diet well within safe bounds.

If your problem persists stubbornly and you are abnormally susceptible to COLDNESS, look up that topic. If you are not, try taking a teaspoon of cider vinegar with or after meals. If this does not make you uncomfortable, increase the dose. Settle eventually on the amount which just avoids discomfort; it will vary according to the meal. This may improve your digestion, reduce GAS and ease your bowel action at last.

To improve your bowel emptying technique, follow the advice for PILES.

CONTRACEPTION, the Pill

In your loins at the embryo stage of your development were two loaf-shaped pieces of tissue with special survival functions. The adrenal and sex glands which derive from them make for you a series of *steroid hormones** whose chemistry shares the same basic structural pattern. Production of these is controlled by another range of hormones from the pituitary gland, a key junction box in your *primal adaptive system** suspended between your nose and your brain.

This control system works on a negative feedback principle. Too much steroid hormone reduces your pituitary output of control hormone, which dampens the steroid gland's over-production.

All varieties of the oral contraceptive pill take advantage of this negative feedback mechanism. The usual form contains a pregnancy-hormone (progestogen) combined with a woman-hormone (oestrogen), to trick your brain into believing that more than enough sex hormone is circulating already. So the pituitary stops producing the control hormones, and your ovaries cease working. That is why it is such an effective contraceptive.

In effect, the pill puts you back to the stage before you started menstruating. The loss you see each month is not a period but a withdrawal bleed, deliberately contrived by the pill-free week. In market research surveys before the pill was launched, many women expressed misgivings about having their PERIODS abolished altogether, despite their inconvenience. Imitating a menstrual loss overcame this market resistance and appeases you for loss of a normal function. It is in any case safer not to continue medication relentlessly, which further justifies the pill-free week.

That alone does not make the pill safe. Despite decades of use, that remains controversial. There is a good deal of commercial interest riding on the issue, so that scientific considerations get blurred and confused. Animal research cannot be trusted for such a widely used long-term medication, and few human studies have met all the criteria of good science; researchers cannot treat masses of people as experimental animals.

But any continuous mass-medication that profoundly alters a basic function must introduce risks. The pill alters BLEEDING, over-distends veins which can cause MIGRAINE, chronic leg discomfort and VARICOSE VEINS, and can alter IMMUNE function enough to precipitate ALLERGY. By disturbing mineral balance, reducing zinc and raising copper levels in particular, it can predispose you to SCHIZOPHRENIA. It makes THRUSH more likely. It may increase a young woman's risk of CANCER in the neck of the womb (cervix) or breast when she is older, though this is hotly disputed.

The *progestogen-only** pill takes advantage of the feedback mechanism that prevents you from conceiving again when you are already PREGNANT, by making your secretions and womb lining hostile to sperms and fertile eggs. The side effects are fewer and your ovaries still function, but more erratically.

HELPING YOURSELF

Contraception cannot abolish risk, but exchanges one kind of risk for another. As methods go, the pill minimizes your risk of pregnancy, but converts it into exceptional risk of unwanted effects. Be sure you need its guarantee, or choose something less risky.

Ovaries whose function is already precarious may give up altogether after pill use. Avoid it if your cycle is long or irregular, especially if you may later want a child.

The long-term risks are greatest if you start very young.

The continuous pill (progestogen only) is both less effective and less risky because it does not stop your ovaries working; but it sometimes upsets menstrual rhythm and causes erratic bleeding.

Take SUPPLEMENTS of Zinc (15mg daily) and Vitamins B (Brewer's Yeast 6–9 tablets daily) and C (500mg twice daily) to cater for increased needs and losses while on the pill, and add Vitamin E (200IU twice daily) when you come off it.

The intra-uterine contraceptive device (IUCD,* Coil) is a piece of plastic inserted into your womb cavity which makes it much more hostile to pregnancy. Insertion and removal can scratch your womb lining, which may spoil a later pregnancy; sometimes people conceive with a coil in place. Go for the all-plastic type that does not have to be changed at intervals. You may get many trouble-free years from one, but do not depend on conceiving again after long use – low-grade INFECTION or INFLAMMATION may by then have made this impossible.

The cap* and spermicidal cream can be very effective and user-friendly, if used every time. It does not prevent sperm getting to your womb but makes their journey much longer and more hazardous. Have it fitted properly, and check the fitting after each PREGNANCY and if your weight changes in either direction. Wear the cap all the time, except briefly every evening to clean and cream it, and of course during your period. Do not take it out within eight hours of making love. Check it for pin-holes and tears every day, and get a new one every six months.

The sheath serves many couples faithfully for years, but should be backed up with spermicidal pessaries since tears are rather common. Most couples prefer something safer and less intrusive.

The least artificial contraceptives are high dosage Vitamin C SUPPLEMENT (1000mg or more three times daily) taken continuously, which enhances the effectiveness of any other method; and fresh yeast taken with Pennyroyal tea at period time, which stimulates womb activity and makes menstruation more certain. They are not fail-safe, even when combined. Take barrier precautions during your fertile phase, which you should learn to recognize from a competent instructor. Full advice is available at your Family Planning Clinic, or from the Natural Family Planning Association (ADDRESS).

CORONARY, heart attack

Most people in economically developed countries have ARTERIOSCLEROSIS almost from birth, depending on the quality of your DIET, EXERCISE and general way of life. It gradually stiffens and narrows your arteries throughout your life, but chiefly in adulthood. The ANGINA which affects a minority in middle life is a direct result of the slow strangulation in this way of your heart's blood supply and is easy enough to understand.

It is more puzzling that you should have a sudden, devastating and irreversible blockage of a coronary[1] artery, perhaps without any warning. The underlying arterial disease has built up gradually over decades. Some parts of your coronary arteries must for several years have been as vulnerable to sudden blockage as they were when it actually happened: why now and not then?

The immediate answer relates to the clotting behaviour of your blood, whose 'mono'* mechanism is still largely mysterious but capable of great variations. It is clearly affected by a wide range of 'mono' factors, such as medication and nervous tone; it seems also to respond to changes in 'colour'* mood. Furthermore the muscles in your artery walls can tighten during periods of TENSION, narrowing the artery further. So you will discover the reason for your coronary in the circumstances which surrounded it.

Your DIET at the time and for several months before determined how clean or burdened your blood was, and pre-existing disease helped to determine what your heart could cope with. Thyroid deficiency causes COLDNESS and weakens your arteries long before it becomes obvious to your doctor. OVERWEIGHT, raised BLOOD PRESSURE, SMOKING and excessive fat in your blood are indicators your doctor can measure, but do not correlate closely enough with abnormal clotting to cause it directly.

ALCOHOL consumption relaxes the muscle of healthy arteries and opens up the circulation beyond them. This does not happen in stiff diseased arteries, which tend to be the ones nearest your heart. Consequently the warming effect of alcohol elsewhere in your body is at your heart's expense, and highly dangerous to it.

STRESS is not in itself a direct cause of coronaries, but exhaustion of your ability to cope with it seems to be (Chapter Two). Great weariness or hopelessness under pressure, coupled with a heavy meal with wine and several cigarettes the night before, could therefore determine a coronary at three the following morning.

Fundamental to the timing of this catastrophe is a critical breakdown in the integrity of your whole person, usually at a high 'colour' level. Either you are seriously disappointed or aggrieved by something that matters very much to you or you have simply reached the limit of what you can endure.

---

[1] 'Coronary' means 'crown-shaped' and was originally used to describe the architecture of the arteries which feed your heart. In modern usage it means 'of the heart'. 'Coronary heart disease' is a tautology; 'coronary artery disease' is accurate, and better English.

HELPING YOURSELF

If you survive the first two days after your coronary, your chances of full RECOVERY are good. They may be better at home than in hospital, and you should discuss with your doctor at an early stage whether there is any real point in your being in an intensive care unit or hospital ward at all.

Spend the first few days SLEEPING, literally to your heart's content. This is far the best way to heal the effects of exhaustion under STRESS.

Convalescence at home gives you plenty of time to reflect on your life up to now and identify why your coronary happened. Any pressure you could not throw off before is shed for you by your illness. Use it well to review what matters to you in life and what further purposes you wish to pursue. Identify the changes you mean to make and how you will implement them.

If you are OVERWEIGHT, adopt the DIET for healthy weight reduction. Include lots of fresh garlic, which favours your recovery and protects your heart in various harmless ways. SUPPLEMENT this diet with Zinc (15mg daily), Selenium (200microgm twice daily) and Dolomite (500mg three times daily). You should also have extra Vitamin B_6 (Pyridoxine 50mg twice daily) if you cannot remember your dreams each morning, Vitamin C (1000mg three times daily with Dolomite) and Vitamin E (400IU twice daily with Selenium).

Lecithin (600mg three times daily with meals) lowers your blood cholesterol* level and helps to mobilize fatty deposits from ARTERIOSCLER-OSIS, progressively reducing over several months your risk of a further coronary.

BREATHE efficiently, making sure to fill your lungs properly for at least ten breaths, twice each day.

As soon as your doctor advises, begin to EXERCISE gently but persistently to improve your fitness and hasten weight loss.

If inappropriate COLDNESS is a feature of your life, consider the advice on that topic.

If you are prone to worry or TENSION, see that topic for better ways of dealing with their cause.

Make some room in your life for being yourself. You have probably not had proper and adequate recreation* for decades; it is important now.

Your coronary is not the disaster it might have been, but a second chance to live life abundantly. How you heal depends on grasping your opportunity. If you feel finished, you will be; but if you are determined to live, you can. Do not be intimidated by any prognosis you are given; it is only an educated guess pleading to be defied.

Having set your course for recovery, cherish every one of the days you might so easily not have seen.

COT DEATH, sudden infant death, SIDS

'Is he all right?' is the first thing a new mother wants to know about her baby. A few in every hundred are not quite perfectly formed, though most of these will lead completely normal lives unhindered by their birthmark. A few in every thousand have more serious defects which will handicap them to some extent and may involve many visits to doctors and hospitals during their childhood. Apart from this tiny minority, the answer comes back 'He's fine!'

Occasionally, however, the defect is too subtle to be seen. An UNDERWEIGHT baby may have been retarded in his growth at all stages, so that although no one organ is actually malformed they are all too small and contain too few cells. That leaves most of them with reduced overall power for living, and perhaps a few with defective or unbalanced metabolism. This may weaken their *primal adaptive systems** right from the start, opening them up to serious mistakes in the early weeks and months of life which threaten their survival.

Unfortunately, the possibilities do not end there. Western culture has undermined the intimacy with his mother that should sustain and reassure a baby throughout his infancy. Despite the pleas of Leboyer, many babies are still born roughly into glaring lights and clashing noise, upended, slapped and probed vigorously with an unkind plastic tube. Most are taken away to be weighed, cleaned up and checked soon afterwards. Some are then 'cot nursed' in the mistaken belief that a *'mono'** trained nurse can care better for a weak or injured baby than his *'colour'**-attuned mother. A baby who is frightened and cries a lot is usually put away in a nursery to let the mother have some peace, rather than given to her in bed to suckle and comfort. All these habits undermine BREAST FEEDING and are easily taken home by parents anxious to bring up their baby loved but unspoiled.

The result is that your baby is removed from you just when he most needs your presence. An infant who cannot feel his mother's warmth and movement – nor hear, taste, smell or see her – has no means of knowing that she still exists. Nothing could undermine him more completely than this. Obviously that is not your intention; you accept in good faith the management you are taught by people you believe know better than you do. It is dreadfully upsetting to realize that well-intentioned caring may bring him to the edge of despair.

A few babies every year actually go past that point. Subtle birth defects or utter hopelessness break down their IMMUNITY completely, and without warning they are discovered dead in their cots. There is no illness to account for it. Many theories have been offered, none of which explains more than a minority of cases. Yet there are enormous variations between ethnic groups, and deliberate attempts to look after especially vulnerable babies and STRESSED parents dramatically reduce the number of these tragedies. It should not be difficult to prevent the vast majority of them; we have only to realize their connections with the worst in Western attitudes to baby care.

HELPING YOURSELF

Take FAMILY PLANNING seriously. Never produce a baby casually or resentfully.

Begin in PREGNANCY to be friends with your baby, knowing that his 'colour' communications are wide open. Talk to your medical attendants about your plans and fears for the delivery, and make very clear what you would prefer to happen. On the day, father can oversee the implementation of your plans – adapting them to medical advice but not letting that overwhelm your aspirations.

Avoid injected drugs during your labour if you can, so that both you and baby are alert to experience the moment of birth. Hold him then, and keep him with you unless one of you urgently needs medical attention. You are the one to vitalize, comfort and console a tired or shocked infant – not an incubator!

Suckle him as soon as he shows interest, and BREAST FEED exclusively. SUPPLEMENT your own diet with Vitamin C (200mg three times daily) throughout your lactation.

Get home from hospital as soon as you can.

Do not be afraid to have him in bed with you – all night if you would like to and have the room. Feeding him in the night is then much easier, and he is continuously reassured by your presence. Unless you are drunk or drugged, the risk that you will suffocate him during your sleep is tiny compared with the risk of cot death.

Even if you put him to sleep in a cot, keep that near your bedside until he is WEANED. Do not banish an infant to a separate room unless you are desperately TIRED yourselves – a dangerous state of affairs that needs lots of support from relatives and friends.

Get a sling or baby-carrier and make a habit of carrying your baby around with you for a lot of the time. All babies prefer movement and a changing scene, especially attached to mother. In shops and among crowds a sling is safer, virtually proof against cross-INFECTION, and much less frightening for him than the unfriendly sight of people's towering bodies from a pram. He will be much more alert, contented and confident for this kind of handling, and correspondingly more fun to be with.

Do not rush to WEAN him from your breast, not even with the occasional solids or bottle of cowsmilk when you are out. He will indicate clearly enough when he is ready for that step, usually around five to seven months of age. Since this moment marks the end of infancy it deserves to be waited for, then savoured and celebrated. Do not rush your baby into childhood.

COUGHING

Of all the parts of you that are exposed directly to the outside, the skin of your lungs is far the most delicate and vulnerable. Yet it devotes hardly any effort to self-defence, concentrating entirely on its highly specialized function of exchanging gases between the air and your blood. For its protection it relies as in COLDS on the efficiency of air conditioning in your nose, and other defences in your voice-box and *wind-pipe** through which the air must pass to reach your lungs in the first place.

Your nose and throat join in your *pharynx,** so that you can by-pass your nose when breathing hard. Just below that your wind-pipe begins, with two curtains of elastic skin drawn across it to act as *vocal cords** and sluice-gates. They can shut tight to keep out food and sea-water, but that stops you breathing too – not practical except in extreme emergencies. Routinely they protect your lungs in a more dynamic way. Your vocal cords close briefly when you swallow food, which does not even touch them, so that fragments do not drip through afterwards.

But you make mistakes sometimes, especially with drinks, and there is often a little mucus or moisture to be cleared out of your lungs. To deal with these you almost close your vocal cords, then blow out hard. For a split second air roars through the narrows at gale force, carrying all before it. That is coughing, a natural protective function quite healthy in itself. 'Clearing your throat' is normal, but you need to understand why you sometimes cough too much.

The usual problem is that uncomfortable air is still getting through, despite the best your nose can do. In cold weather it may simply be too chilly and dry, shocking your wind-pipe as well as your face. More often, irritant gases, airborne chemicals and SMOKE penetrate to your vocal cords from over-whelmingly polluted air; coughing is your reasonable but ineffectual protective response.

COLDS, ASTHMA, HAY FEVER and CATARRH can spread to your vocal cords and wind-pipe, making them touchy. Mucus from an INFLAMED wind-pipe needs clearing anyway, so some of the coughing is useful; most is not. Hoarseness and loss of voice often accompany the cough.

Least common is what you most expect, the cough that indicates BRON-CHITIS or lung CANCER. Any chest INFECTION is likely to make you very breathless, or produce lots of *sputum** or pus from your chest – tablespoons-ful each day. The vast majority of coughs at any age arise from above or around your vocal cords, not deep inside them.

The cough of PERTUSSIS (Whooping Cough) is highly characteristic and usually gives the disease away – a prolonged paroxysm of explosive coughing which exhausts all the air from your lungs and leaves you blue, followed by the long whooping sound as the air sighs gratefully back in; retching or actual SICKNESS commonly follow. It is caused by toxic infiltration of NERVES in the skin of your windpipe which may outlast the infection by months.

HELPING YOURSELF

Steer clear of smokers and SMOKING, still the largest avoidable cause of cough. Uphold smoking bans in public places if you see them defied. Never let anyone smoke near your children, and ventilate any smoking-place well.

Practise BREATHING deeply every day, in the freshest air you can find.

Muffle your face and throat in cold weather, to re-breathe some of your exhaled air. This saves you warming and moistening every breath from scratch. Ventilate your bedroom at night but cover your face well with warm bedding.

Mask your face effectively during any dusty DIY job. Choose muscle-power over chemicals every time, but ventilate any fumes thoroughly to the outside. Never run the car for long in an enclosed space.

Humidify insulated, draught-proofed and centrally heated places with flowers, pot plants, a fish-tank or radiator accessory. An air *ionizer** may be helpful in high-tech or smoky rooms.

The best first aid for cough is steam, inhaled slowly and deeply through your mouth and exhaled through your nose. Cover the jug with a cloth held across your upper lip and cheeks, to confine the steam but leave your eyes free. Five minutes' inhalation every hour is the highest useful dose. Menthol and Eucalyptus Inhalation, Karvol or Olbas Oil on a clean handkerchief in a warm pocket is almost as good for use away from home, and safer for small children.

A night light candle under a pan of hot water containing one teaspoon (5ml) of Menthol and Eucalyptus Inhalation makes a cheap, safe and effective vapourizer to run in the victim's bedroom. Keep it well out of harm's way.

Cough Drops (Weleda UK Ltd) are a useful and safe alternative to cough linctus, but are only available on private or NHS prescription. Your doctor may be prepared to let you try it.

*Homoeopathic** remedies vary widely according to your detailed symptoms, so get further advice from a competent practitioner.

The Honey Cider Vinegar RECIPE makes a wholesome substitute for cough syrup.

CYSTITIS

Your bladder is only required to transform a steady trickle into an occasional and manageable torrent, but must meet an exacting specification to accomplish this. Its lining must be capable of enormous stretching several times daily without tearing or discomfort, despite the sour and irritant nature of its contents. Its muscles must relax absolutely while your bladder fills passively with urine, yet generate and hold a steady voiding pressure until completely empty. Its outlet valve must give way widely to this flow, then remain tight but at ease until the next time you release it. The whole organ must combine the suppleness of your *heart** or GALL bladder with corrosion resistance and chemical tolerance far beyond that of your COLON.

It is small wonder that in some people that tolerance breaks down. This is seldom because of INFECTION, although a few doses of ANTIBIOTIC treatment are often dramatically effective in dealing with it. Even if it were, the repeated courses of treatment you may have to endure are highly undesirable and invite THRUSH to intervene. Most bladder symptoms arise instead from INFLAMMATION against the irritant *waste acids** which are concentrated in your urine, and may crystallize into kidney or bladder *stones.** The more flesh food you consume the more probable this is, whereas vegetables, fruit and cereals create a more comfortable reaction nearer neutrality, with plenty of buffering capacity to keep minerals dissolved, greatly reducing your risk of forming stones.

These waste acids not only irritate but support vagrant COLONIC *bacteria** that make a living by splitting them like firewood to release the energy they contain. Instead of ash this yields ammonia, which smells like rotten fish and means you have a genuine INFECTION. In babies this commonly takes place externally as NAPPY RASH, but in adults it more commonly tracks back up your urinary outlet to reach your bladder and lodge there. If the infection is eradicated with a single ANTIBIOTIC course the outcome may well be straightforwardly successful. But if you are prone to infection, repeated treatment again leaves you prone to THRUSH development.

As a woman you may have additional problems. Your bladder outlet valve may have been strained and weakened during successive PREGNANCIES. Your exit pipe is short and opens right by your VAGINA, where it is eternally damp with secretions, vulnerable to chafing and difficult to ventilate. Two layers of underwear inside tightly fitting jeans accentuate these adverse features, and make you much more prone to INFLAMMATORY or INFECTIVE cystitis and THRUSH than seems fair.

Sometimes structural anomalies in your kidneys or bladder make it possible for bacteria to migrate through the system and cause repeated infection. Otherwise cystitis in men or boys is hard to account for by penetration of bacteria from outside, since your outlet pipe is much longer – anything up to 15 centimetres. This strains the credibility of current theories of INFECTION, which is a topic discussed at length elsewhere.

HELPING YOURSELF

The DIET for health reduces waste acid formation, allowing your urine to remain only slightly sour and far less irritant. Avoid sugar, meat and alcohol in particular. Home-made lemon barley water RECIPE is very alkaline, and quickly eases the discomfort of cystitis by neutralizing urine acidity.

Wear cotton underclothing and avoid nylon tights especially inside jeans. Internal sanitary tampons are usually preferable to external towels, so long as they are introduced and removed carefully.

Firm massage to your lower spine for ten minutes and a brief *Sitz** bath can be repeated daily, or up to four times each day if need be. The aim of these measures is to tone up the NERVES supplying your bladder, making it sufficiently energetic and controlled to overcome irritability. The Sitz bath should be cold, and deep enough to immerse your bottom completely and wash over the crease of your groin. Drop yourself in it for 30–60 seconds after urinating or during your morning wash. The initial shock gives way quickly to numbness, then to a creeping tingly glow. The bath is then over, but its effects will stay with you for one or two hours. The benefit is not immediate but accumulates over several weeks. If the effect of the bath is disappointing, complete Sitz's original recommendations by bathing your feet in hot water at the same time.

If none of these simple measures improves your condition or you BLEED painlessly from your bladder, seek further medical examination and tests. Your doctor will look for evidence of recurrent INFECTION, and if he finds it will look for structural reasons why you cannot prevent them for yourself. This may involve ultrasound examination of your kidneys or perhaps some detailed X-ray procedures to reveal stones or ineffective valves in your urinary passages. If something is discovered that SURGERY cannot help, continuous ANTIBIOTIC treatment may be necessary to prevent chronic kidney infection.

More likely no cause will be found and you can confidently build up measures of your own. A SUPPLEMENT of Vitamin E for several months (200mg twice daily, emulsified if possible) will strengthen your bladder skin if your usual supplies are scanty; a little extra wheatgerm oil should maintain it adequately afterwards. Vitamin C (1000mg twice or three times daily) is a useful urinary antiseptic, but should be combined with Magnesium Orotate 500mg three times daily to prevent stone formation. Magnesium and Vitamin B$_6$ (50mg three times daily) help dissolve stones otherwise inaccessible to treatment.

Make sure THRUSH is not at the heart of your problem, and deal with it even if your suspicions cannot be fully substantiated.

*Homoeopathic** Apis mel 3x or Cantharis 3 are most commonly helpful; consult a homoeopathic practitioner (ADDRESS) before giving up.

A *medical herbalist** has many remedies for bladder symptoms, including some reputed to dissolve urinary stones gently over several months. Contact the ADDRESS for a qualified practitioner near you.

DANDRUFF, scurf

WHAT HAPPENS

Dandruff is one of the commonest complaints of all, a stubborn ITCHING scaly condition of your scalp and eyebrows that sometimes spreads to other parts of your body as *seborroeic dermatitis.** Many shampoos claim to be medicated to deal with it but none abolishes it completely. Doctors usually confine themselves to distinguishing it from PSORIASIS, seborroeic ECZEMA, NITS and other INFECTIONS, and prescribing a *steroid** lotion if the condition is a serious nuisance.

Scurf is the name that gives it away as a derangement of skin nutrition. It was formerly recognized as part of SCURVY, resulting from drastic deficiency of Vitamin C. However SUPPLEMENTS of that vitamin do not necessarily cure it, since many other food factors are likely to be deranged too. Minerals such as Zinc are particularly important, and commonly deficient nowadays in people whose food is mostly processed or refined, especially since household plumbing has been based on copper. Small quantities of copper dissolve in your WATER and compete with zinc for access to your body. Even more of it gets into your hot water from the copper tank and can soak through your skin if you spend too long immersed in a hot bath. As it happens, large supplements of organic acids such as Vitamin C enormously increase your absorption of all these minerals, helping to put right this modern difficulty.

Overconsumption of animal fats is another important factor in weakening the health of your skin. It neutralizes much of the benefit of the *essential fatty acids** in vegetable oils, however much of these you may also consume. Their purpose is quite different. They are essential ingredients in the skin structure of your body cells, which when cemented into a patchwork quilt form skin as you know it.

Essential fatty acids are also important raw materials for your *sebum,** which keeps your hair water-proof and conditions the climate of your skin – your scalp in particular. Its slightly acid and greasy character is essential for health whatever the advertisements may say. Whilst frequent washing with detergent shampoos certainly removes the scales and suppresses the itching for a time, it also destroys the climate without which your skin and hair cannot regain their resilience and health. Water that is too hot can do this too, without any help from soap or shampoo. Sebum only accumulates slowly, so you cannot afford to wash it out of your hair every few days.

Dandruff arises when there is too little sebum to protect your scalp from drying out. When this happens there is not enough oil to keep the *cells** in its surface layers stuck together. (Vitamin C plays an essential part in the cement substance which normally does this, which is how it comes to be implicated sometimes in dandruff.) Scales therefore flake away prematurely, exposing raw and immature layers underneath which are even more vulnerable to soap and heat than the mature outer cells. Far from curing dandruff, washing with hot water and shampoo keeps it going.

HELPING YOURSELF

Wash your hair in tepid water only, massaging your scalp thoroughly as you do so. Accept the fact that it will still feel greasy afterwards. Dry it patiently with air at a comfortable temperature; carefully avoid overheating your hair or scalp.

Meticulous brushing twice a day is the key to restoring your scalp to health. Obtain two good quality bristle brushes if your hair is short and fine, or a pair of well-made 'pin-cushion' brushes if your hair is thick and long. The bristles must penetrate to your scalp easily, but should not scratch it.

With one brush in each hand and using them alternately, groom your hair twice daily for three to five minutes. For half that time stroke systematically up towards your crown from the hair-line on each temple and at the nape of your neck. Then brush backwards from your forehead and follow through from your crown, backwards and downwards in all directions, respecting the natural lie of your hair. Finish with further strokes from each side up towards your crown against the lay of your hair, then settle it in place with gentle combing. Comb out the brushes carefully each time, and scrub one on the other with warm water and soap once or twice each week. This routine will keep your hair clean, manageable and in excellent condition.

Adopt the DIET for health, which will set your consumption of animal fats within reasonable bounds. Fresh oily sea fish (eg Mackerel) contribute to your intake of essential fatty acids; Egg Nog and Honey Cider Vinegar RECIPES augment your mineral supplies.

SUPPLEMENT this with Zinc (15mg) and Vitamin C (1000mg) daily, taken together. A good Multimineral (eg Nature's Own Ltd) and Essential Fatty Acid source (eg Lane's Glanolin, or Evening Primrose Oil) are worthwhile extras for a month or two, if the expense does not daunt you.

Many herbs are valuable adjuncts to good scalp hygiene and form the basis of several ranges of natural beauty products – Weleda, and Beauty Without Cruelty for example. Levy's BOOK gives details for home use of fourteen different herbs. Any medical herbalist or natural beautician (ADDRESS) would give you appropriate professional guidance.

DEPRESSION

Depression behaves like a cloud, covering the face of the sun and stealing the colour from your world. It threatens whenever severe and unremitting STRESS exhausts and breaks down your capacity to cope with it. You are not just winded and sick at heart, but incapable of any feeling at all except a very aggressive and painful kind of deflation and hopelessness. You awaken early each morning feeling particularly desperate, with plenty of time to savour it in solitude before the distractions of the day begin. You cannot even then raise the effort to do anything, however ordinary or essential the task may be. Everything seems pointless and dull, and decisions are particularly difficult. You consider your plight hopeless and beyond help, and are convinced everyone knows and is discussing behind your back how worthless a person you are.

Such a profound collapse of your NERVES and *primal adaptive system** comes about only after deep disappointment or grief, a prolonged and exhausting effort which has drawn heavily on your *'colour'** reserves. Environmental STRESSES such as chronic pollution with pesticides, lead or other chemicals are slowly becoming recognized as capable of this. So is severe and protracted nutritional imbalance or deprivation, especially in relation to trace mineral nutrients – which are essential in any case to help you keep lead out.

CONSTIPATION can cause or contribute to depression by creating a reservoir of toxic fermentation products in your large bowel, which are then reabsorbed to hinder your *metabolism** generally and chronically lower your spirits. The COLDNESS of marginal thyroid insufficiency not only contributes to constipation but dulls your mental function in its own right, thereby contributing to depression both directly and indirectly.

People vary greatly in their tolerance of STRESSES like these, so that some are much more prone to depression than others. But some circumstances hit particularly hard. When a new mother has spent the effort of her pregnancy and enters parenthood physically drained, hormonally confused and personally hurt, humiliated or disappointed by her experience of childbirth, the anticlimax may precipitate *post-natal depression** – the product of frustrated biological impulses and shattered dreams. Otherwise, exhaustion and grief from nursing your DYING life's partner, job redundancy and long-term unemployment, moving house, SHINGLES and PREMENSTRUAL TENSION are all powerfully depressing experiences.

RECOVERY is slow and cannot be safely cut short. It depends on *re-creation** of your bodily reserves and restoration of your damaged 'colour' spectrum – your emotional integrity, self-esteem and sense of purpose. Some of these may be deeply laid on vulnerable lines from way back in your life and can only be changed with a lot of patient hard work. And yet the breakthrough to recovery may then be quite sudden and unexpected – like the gleam of light as a cloud withdraws from the sun.

HELPING YOURSELF

Recognize your condition, and confide in a reliable friend, relative, priest, *Counsellor** (ADDRESS) or *Clinical Psychologist.**

Your doctor may not be in a position to give you the time you need, but can relieve the most debilitating symptoms with anti-depressant drugs that usually help more than they hinder your progress, are not addictive and can be stopped gradually after six months or so. That gives you time to get yourself sorted out personally and nutritionally.

Commence the DIET for health, making a particular effort to obtain raw live food from an *organic** source and commence each meal with it. SUPPLEMENT this with a good multimineral formula – Nature's Own Ltd manufacture a reliable one. Essential fatty acids such as Blackcurrant Seed Oil 500mg (Glanolin – Lane's), can be taken twice daily half an hour before food with plenty of water and a capsule of Vitamin E 100IU, preferably emulsified. Brewer's Yeast (9 tablets daily) and extra Vitamin B_6 (50mg three times daily) are prudent additions, especially if you cannot recall your dreams at all. Vitamin C 500mg three times daily completes the requirement for most people.

Stop relying on ALCOHOL or tranquillizers to obliterate your misery. It has to be faced and dealt with – that is where your confidant comes in. He can contest your hopelessness and lend you 'colour' encouragement to get moving instead.

Arouse yourself each morning by brushing your skin vigorously all over, or by following a hot shower with cold water for half a minute. BREATHE deeply and sing loudly in your car or any private place; run, dance or skip sometimes. Light-heartedness would make you feel like doing it: doing it can make you feel a little more light-hearted.

*Homoeopathic** treatment should be prescribed and supervised by an experienced practitioner, but you can try choosing the Bach Flower Remedy that best suits your need. Contact the ADDRESSES for advice on how to proceed.

A spiritual *healer** or practitioner of *Traditional Chinese Medicine** (ADDRESSES) will adopt a different approach to your case that safely complements your self-help measures.

When you recover, read Dorothy Rowe's BOOK which is written with good sense from a wealth of personal and clinical experience.

DIABETES Mellitus, sugar diabetes

You digest starchy food and sugars by breaking them down to their basic components and absorbing these into your intestinal bloodstream, which flows direct to your liver before going anywhere else. Some is stored and used there, but most of it passes on into your general CIRCULATION. The level in the blood to your pancreas regulates how much *insulin** is released from store by the special cells there that produce it. Insulin then circulates with the sugar to all the tissues that need it as fuel, and opens the gate to let it in.

This mechanism has some delay built into it, and works best when sugar is absorbed from your intestine in a steady trickle. This happens automatically with whole natural foods whose raw starches are large and complex, like felled trees; your enzymes have to saw the sugars off each branch, one log at a time. What is more, the plantation is dense with undergrowth (the indigestible cellulose fibre in the food), which slows down the work of removing the logs. Lorries (insulin) arriving one at a time can easily cope with a flexible daily routine for carrying them away.

Refined and processed foods present quite a different problem. Their simple *carbohydrates** behave like a deluge of ready-sawn logs falling on clear ground. During the shower you need every lorry you can get to stop the log-pile spilling all over the road. But no sooner have you mobilized your fleet and workforce than the shower stops, and the work ends as suddenly as it began – only to start up again whenever you next eat, several times each day.

This is very STRESSFUL for your pancreas, which cannot synchronize your response to such heavy and erratic demand. So your blood sugar level ranges above and below your ideal, more and more wildly as your pancreas fatigues. People vary a lot in how fast this happens. HYPOGLYCAEMIA may happen first, or diabetes may show only during PREGNANCY. But decades of abuse inevitably weaken any pancreas, making many people mildly diabetic by their forties. Tablet treatments only loot your insulin stores, exhausting them eventually. Injections replace your own insulin imperfectly, and do not seem to prevent degenerative complications like ARTERIOSCLEROSIS from eventually setting in.

Many other factors help to decide whether you will become diabetic or not. Being OVERWEIGHT or physically inactive considerably increase your risk. The COLDNESS of thyroid insufficiency aggravates both these conditions, and interferes directly with the work of your insulin as well. So if your reaction to cold weather is to huddle idly around a fire wrapped up warmly, the chances of your becoming diabetic are higher than if you are prepared to keep warm by EXERCISING actively.

Steroid* medication given for any other reason powerfully favours the development of diabetes, so you should assume that any hormone growth promoters you accidentally consume with your food may have the same effect. This is most likely to occur with meat, at least until the EEC ban on the use of growth promoters comes into effect – and in the past a black market has continued to circulate such items after they have been officially banned.

HELPING YOURSELF

Whether or not diabetes runs strongly in your family, protect everyone with a healthy DIET which excludes refined flour, sugar and all manufactured and refined foods containing it. Beware particularly of the food additives Sucrose, Sugar, Glucose (or Dried Glucose Syrup), Dextrose, Fructose, Hydrogenated Glucose Syrup, Hydrogenated High Maltose Glucose Syrup, Invert Sugar, Isomalt, Lactose, Maltose and Xylitol – all stressful refined sugars. Additives with 'Starch' in their names are best avoided until more is known about their effects on human digestion. See that you get whole wheat (or wheat germ and bran) regularly for the chromium and manganese they contain, both vital to the health of your pancreas. Regular helpings of raw carrot and onion, and lemon juice instead of milk in tea, all have worthwhile anti-diabetic properties.

If your family is susceptible to diabetes, SUPPLEMENT this diet with Chromium Orotate 1mg twice daily, and Manganese Orotate 50mg twice a week. Be sure to EXERCISE regularly to keep reasonably fit. Do not allow yourself to get appreciably OVERWEIGHT. Avoid using an oral CONTRACEPTIVE, to be on the safe side.

Once diabetes is discovered you need to adopt all these measures in full, doubling the chromium and manganese supplements for three months. Balance your total carbohydrate intake carefully against your physical activity, and confine it to naturally starchy foods, whole vegetables and fresh fruit. Eat plenty of dark green leaves fresh in season. Add Vitamin B_{15} (Pangamic Acid 50mg twice daily) and Folic Acid 2mg twice daily to your Brewer's Yeast (9 or more tablets daily). Take Vitamin B_6 (Pyridoxine) 50mg daily until you regularly recall pleasant dreams.

Numerous herbs and homoeopathic medicines are available if additional help is required, but you should contact a *Medical Herbalist** or *Homoeopathic Practitioner** for personal assistance, through the ADDRESSES given.

If tablets or insulin proves necessary despite your best efforts, persevere with them nonetheless. People who lean more heavily than necessary on their medication are more likely to suffer the complications of diabetes – high BLOOD PRESSURE, CORONARY, *stroke,** blindness and insufficient CIRCULATION to their legs.

Bring up your children to these habits, to prevent diabetes in their turn.

DIET, nutrition

Most people suppose that nutrition is now an exact science which we thoroughly understand. Do not believe it. What we have now is a rather dull technology designed to help us balance the nutrients in artificially refined, processed and preserved food. If your food were whole, natural and fresh your APPETITE could do the work without any help at all.

Real nutrition had its heyday fifty years ago, when biologists still studied whole diets in whole live animals and people: its degeneration began when biochemists began to focus their attention on our 'mono' parts. It is disturbing how quickly a tradition can be forgotten once it is eclipsed.

Sir Robert McCarrison was one of the great pioneers, still honoured by the society named after him, who publish a BOOK of lectures on nutrition he gave in 1936 that still sound radical today. He based these on experiments in which healthy animals chose their food according to APPETITE from the usual fare of a particular group of people; their progress was compared with control animals on a perfectly constituted fresh diet. Whilst the latter continued in excellent health, the test animals faithfully reproduced the pattern of diseases characteristic of the human group whose diet they were eating! McCarrison concluded that 'the greatest single factor in the acquisition and maintenance of good health is perfectly constituted food', and said what he meant by that.

His contemporary Dr Max Bircher-Benner established in Zürich a revolutionary healing centre that is now world famous. He first visualized how your *'colour'** pattern, energized by sunlight consumed with your food, shapes the growth, form and function of your *'mono'** body. He demonstrated in practice the healing power of this principle over a wide range of serious diseases and established the principles of biological treatment.

These ideas have been opposed with irrational hostility by the professions, for unpublished reasons of their own. It is certainly not innocence that motivates them. Many have had the opportunity of trying nutritional treatments on their patients, or seeing the results in patients they have shared. A Royal Free Hospital trial of dietary treatment for RHEUMATOID ARTHRITIS was spectacularly successful as long ago as 1937 (see p. 40). I have not found reference to it in any medical literature since then, and it certainly made no impact on the direction of subsequent medical research into this disease.

In the absence of any other explanation for this from doctors themselves, we may suppose that ideas like these are too cheap, too successful and too little dependent on professional help to win medical approval. They completely undermine the time-honoured basis of medicine in classification of disease, which diminishes in significance like a punctured balloon when the same diet will prevent and even cure most if not all of them! Doctors who deny or mock this claim have never tried it, have no training for it and are not competent to give opinions or advise you. But you can quite safely try it for yourself.

HELPING YOURSELF: THE DIET FOR HEALTH

Realize first that doctors do not in general understand nutrition, having been taught very little about it. Do not expect them to advise you well.

Then restore your natural APPETITE, using the freshest foods you can get, whole from nature and unadulterated with chemicals. Some food grown without chemicals to 'organic'* or 'biodynamic' standards is now available in supermarkets and wholefood shops; this gives far better value for money.

Take advantage of vegetables and fruit in season locally, and grow them organically in your own garden. Eat them as fresh as possible, and have a portion raw as the first course of every meal.

Cook everything else as little as possible, avoiding unnecessarily high temperatures. Eat it fresh from the cooker; do not habitually save food, frozen or otherwise, for eating later.

Use the sprouting RECIPE for seedlings to supplement your raw food. Stored raw carrots, potatoes and onions are good winter reserves of live food.

Chew everything carefully and well, to get all its 'colour' and give digestion time to work properly. Postpone a meal rather than eat in haste.

Most people thrive best on a wide variety of vegetables, cereals and fruit garnished with smaller quantities of eggs, fish and dairy products. Animal food of any kind is inessential, and meat in particular presents digestive difficulties and hazards for some. As the quality and range of your plant food increases, your craving for animal foods will decline. Vegetables contain plenty of protein and enough of everything else.

Be careful to eat sparingly of foods scarce in nature but plentiful in Europe – butter, oils, honey and all animal products. Animal fats from modern farms are particularly hazardous and reduce the benefit of vegetable oils. Nevertheless a little butter from healthy cows is still preferable to lots of vegetable margarine, if you work hard enough to burn it off.

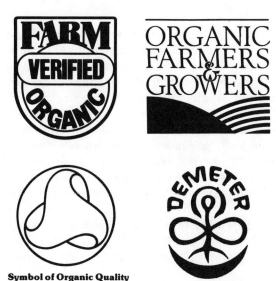

Symbol of Organic Quality

WEIGHT CORRECTION, CONVALESCENCE

The same diet will correct OVERWEIGHT and UNDERWEIGHT conditions, provided their fundamental causes can be put right. Even if you cannot solve your basic problem, keep to these principles and accept the result.

Give yourself plenty of time to eat and get properly in the mood for it. Make the meal a social event whenever you can.

Begin every meal with a course of live fresh salad – fruit in season, grated root vegetables or onion, fresh coleslaw or seed-sprouts.

Chew every mouthful thoroughly before you swallow it.

Avoid drinking during and just after the meal since this makes digestion less efficient. Drinking before the meal is fine, but avoid coffee and strong Indian tea if you are nervy and underweight.

Breakfast: Your main energy meal, based on cereals. Use the muesli RECIPE, including the condensed milk or fresh cream if you are undernourished. Moisten with live yoghurt if you are convalescent, skimmed milk or water if you want to lose weight, whole fresh milk or fruit juice otherwise.

Midday Meal: Small fresh salad or fresh fruit in season, then wholemeal bread, whole-rye crackers or baked potato with light garnishes – yeast paté or spread, boiled free-range egg. Spread your bread with cottage or cream cheese, nut butter, tahini or good dairy butter if you are underweight. Otherwise go for a low fat spread, live yoghurt or a little fresh mayonnaise, and limit yourself to one slice or two crackers – spread on the *smooth* side!

Evening Meal: Fresh coleslaw or salad, then any rich protein you may wish – meat, beans, fish or cheese – with a suitable light garnish. A wholemeal pasta sauce or baked potato is a good and easy companion for vegetables if you do not want meat. Add some anyway if you are underweight, and have cream with fresh or stewed fruit to follow, but sweeten them with raisins only.

FOR CLEANSING

If you really mean business, begin with a two-day fast on barley water RECIPE; you may prefer freshly squeezed fruit juices diluted with mineral water or filtered tap-water. Do not be put off if it makes you feel ill, but take time off work if necessary; you have ''FLU'. Illness as soon as you fast calls for urgent cleansing and does not usually take more than a week or ten days. This may need nerve; the support of your doctor or a friend is very valuable.

After two days start eating one or two pieces of fresh fruit at mealtimes. You can add or substitute any raw vegetable for variety.

When you feel well and hungry, commence two meals a day – a late breakfast or lunch and an evening meal. Drink juice or barley water between meals as desired, but not during or for an hour after eating. There is no need to go hungry.

Breakfast: Start if you wish with a cup of juniper berry tea prepared overnight, or freshly brewed broom or parsley piert. Proceed to a generous fresh fruit course, as many pieces as you wish in any variety; try some exotic ones.

Pause, and if you remain hungry eat dry wholemeal toast, or nuts and raisins, until you are satisfied.

Main Meal: After herb tea again if you want it, start with a generous fresh coleslaw. Pause, then have one baked vegetable of your choice: potatoes, a root variety, beans (not from a tin), broccoli or cauliflower. Cook them gently and slowly in a closed dish, in their own juice.

After three weeks you should be ready for a more normal diet, avoiding routinely the items you now realize are unwholesome. You can then afford to take part in occasional celebrations and restaurant outings without expecting mishap.

In ARTHRITIS your cure will take several months longer. Continue to avoid *all* meat, fish, shellfish, tinned food, eggs, salt, spices, coffee, Indian tea, alcohol and tobacco. You may have a little butter and cottage cheese, otherwise avoid all dairy products too.

See also SUPPLEMENTS.

PREGNANCY

Eat normally, but pay special attention to foods derived from the reproductive parts of plants and animals. Cauliflower, grains, beans, nuts, fruit, roe, eggs and whole fresh milk are obvious examples. If you can find genuinely free-range hens managed naturally, their eggs will be better value. The same applies to 'green top' unpasteurized milk sold at the farm gate by a local dairyman. Fresh goat's milk is another option, but should not taste at all 'goaty'; a good producer will be proud to show you his herd and tell you how he feeds them.

Consider SUPPLEMENTS at least during the six months leading up to your pregnancy, especially if you have been on the CONTRACEPTIVE pill; get your husband to take them as well. Persevere after conceiving for another three months. Thereafter take only what you normally use to support your general health.

ALLERGY TESTING

To discover whether foods or chemicals are responsible for chronic symptoms you may have, you need to convert your blurred everyday reaction to them into a brisk rejection response. This can be accomplished by eating none of the suspect food for just four days, then reintroducing it. The weekdays from Monday morning until Friday afternoon are convenient, reintroducing the test food at teatime on Friday. Any reaction will be over in time to test something else on the same days of the next week.

But to be sure of a clear result you must eat nothing in those four days that could deputize for the food you are testing. This means in practice that you must exclude all members of the same biological family at the same time.

The fullest published list can be found in Mansfield and Monro's BOOK, but here are the families most commonly troublesome:

Beef, suet, beef stock cubes, Oxo, Bovril, milk chocolate; items including dried skimmed milk, casein, whey powder, milk solids, cow's milk, butter, cream, yoghurt, cheese.

Wheat, wheat flour of all kinds, wheat bran, semolina; packaged items including wheat, gluten or flour.

Potato, tomato, aubergine, pepper (cayenne, chillies, paprika, pimento), ground cherry, physalis, tobacco.

Chicken, hen's egg, chicken stock cubes.

Coffee, tea (Indian and Sri Lankan), chocolate, cocoa, cola.

Aspirin and the following which contain natural *salicylates*:* many permitted food additives (colourings, benzoates, hydroxybenzoates, gallates, trihydroxybenzoates); almonds, apple, apricot, blackberry, blackcurrant, cherry, cider vinegar, cucumber, currant, gooseberry, grape, lemon, marrow, peach, pepper, plum, prune, orange, raisin, raspberry, rosehip, strawberry, sultana, tomato, tangerine, wine vinegar.

Cereals containing *gluten*:* wheat (including that advertised as 'gluten free', which may still contain up to 2% of gluten), barley, oats, rye.

CANCER

Anyone setting out to use diet as a means of getting well from cancer must read BOOKS by Brenda Kidman and Dr Alec Forbes; nothing less can prepare them adequately for the changes that will be called for.

In principle you will be using the diet for cleansing given above for at least six months, probably a year. After that you will be able to relax onto something like the diet for health. But in both phases you should note the following points which specifically relate to cancer.

Eat lots of live raw salad, amounting to at least half of all you eat. This should include fresh grated carrot or carrot juice daily, agitating the juice with a little oil in a liquidizer to dissolve some of the Vitamin A it contains. That portion will pass straight into your CIRCULATION and act directly against the remnants of your cancer, without first being stored in your liver.

If you wish to eat meat or other food from animals, fresh cod is the safest. Otherwise only meat, chicken and eggs that are fully 'Organic'* can even be contemplated with safety.

Avoid dairy produce of all kinds, or consume it only on rare occasions.

Bruised, unhealthy or stale samples of parsnips, parsley and celery are the only fresh salad vegetables you should be wary of. They contain in appreciable quantity members of a group of substances known as psoralens which are rather toxic and encourage cancer. Of these celery is no great loss, being a fibrous stem and containing little else of value. On the other hand parsley is weight for weight one of the most nourishing of all green vegetables, and its strong flavour prevents most people from being able to eat more than garnishings of it in any case. If these sprigs are selected for their health, freshness and perfection of form, you gain something and risk little by eating such small quantities.

See also DIABETES MELLITUS. For Wind see GAS.

WHAT HAPPENS

When you are living every moment of your life to the full, you are not concerned to know in advance where it may lead you, and the ultimate certainty that you will die some day holds no fears. As a child you are fascinated by the world of physical things, though you may be made very aware how powerfully your mind can alter them. As you get older you gradually realize that 'mono'* objects and events are not as concrete as they appear to be, and that they sometimes behave in defiance of science. If you are fortunate enough to grow old gracefully and with a clear mind, this transient and fluid quality in the *'colour'** substance of things becomes increasingly real for you, exposing physical strength and durability as less solid and more vulnerable than they pretend. It is a natural extension of this process that you should eventually grow right out of physical existence, and embrace wholeheartedly that rarified 'colour' world, a fragment of which was always the real you.

I cannot yet from personal experience say more about death and what may follow it; Dowding and Kübler-Ross both go further in their BOOKS than I intend to. But I am certain that the prevailing attitude towards the process of dying is mistaken, and grossly unhealthy. It saps the honesty of your last communications with dying relatives, poisons your grief with regret and sadness and makes an anxious nightmare of your own last days.

Crude remnants of dead religious dogma are in our culture overlaid with shallow materialism to suggest a world of polarized opposites – Heaven or Hell, success or failure, life or death. This makes death seem profoundly disturbing, particularly for doctors repeatedly confronted with it. It challenges them to review their 'mono' attitudes and technology, and rebukes them when they do not.

Other scientists, however – Bentov, Bohm, Capra, Lovelock and Sheldrake among them – have in their BOOKS explored a version of the truth in which many levels of meaning may attach to commonplace things and events. This 'colour' version of the world may not be reassuringly solid or clear cut, but penetrates life more profoundly than materialism or dogmatic religion, and is replacing them. Dying becomes a transition from one level of meaning and existence in which your 'colour' self navigates a 'mono' world to another where 'mono' considerations play no part. Your 'colour' substance – identity and purpose, consciousness and love, insight and experience – survives to live by timeless rules; only your body rejoins the common 'mono' pool.

Such an insight dignifies your dying when that becomes inevitable, and sets you a purpose in it. You have some 'colour' relationships to anticipate and others to confirm – none near to you will lose your intimacy. Your 'mono' affairs are easier to settle. Above all you are free to relinquish your body gracefully, instead of hanging on to the last shreds of your material identity in self-deluded panic. Others are free to be unguarded in your company and so enjoy it to the full. Your wake is a celebration, with no funereal misery on your account. Your love continues as a present intimacy, not a memory.

HELPING YOURSELF

Think regularly through your attitudes to fundamental things, revising them as your experience requires. Face up to prospects you are afraid of and discuss them with the others they concern. Read the BOOKS already mentioned. You cannot really live without some notion of what dying is, and how to die.

Try to live each day as if it were your last, postponing only what you can bear to leave undone. This teaches you to rank deliberately the priorities of your life and to recognize the trivial. Above all, 'let not the sun go down upon your wrath'.

Share your views with others, particularly your children. Never discuss death with them in morbid or sepulchral tones. Work with them through the deaths of their pets, their grandparents and the plight of those victims of famine or disaster who are so regularly world news.

Treat a corpse of any kind with respect, in honour of the life that has just left it. Bury it naked, or wrapped in a bio-degradable fabric, in fertile shallow soil where it will compost naturally.

Discuss with your intimate relatives how you wish to be disposed of, and what relationship you hope to maintain with them when you have died.

Talk over the issues you consider important enough to die for, if need be.

Suicide* is the ultimate abuse of however much personal IMMUNITY you have left; life only ends wholesomely when all of that is spent. Your consciousness will survive to regret it. By deliberately ending life you deny yourself the possibility that something new may turn up: if things are that bad, anything new has got to be better.

When illness such as CANCER or a CORONARY brings the real prospect of death, maintain your honesty and live out your preparations like you do everything else, without melodrama. Engage your doctor in this; he will be visibly relieved. Do not jump to the conclusion of death; simply relish each day without fear of dying, indifferent to when that may come.

Deep burial* in sterile subsoil is a fairly recent and most unhealthy custom; cremation* is wasteful and seldom well done, though more practical. We need the option of shallow burial in bio-degradable wrappings, within small, well-tended and protected orchards or gardens of remembrance that our bodies can enrich. This is contrary neither to hygiene nor any British statute, and was customary in Mediterranean countries well into this century. There is no prospect of such a garden becoming offensive or overburdened. Clean, dry bones can after two years be disinterred and preserved in a casket or ground and scattered. The land devoted to burial can be contained at a manageable level and need never become derelict or require redevelopment. Once we have become civilized enough to do this, our culture can claim to have healed itself back into Nature.

WHAT HAPPENS

Each ear occupies a cave in the side bone of your head, with a long narrow inside entrance leading from a valve at the back of your nose. There would be a large entrance from the ear-hole on the outside of your head, but this is covered by your ear-drum. Vibration of this double thickness of skin enables you to hear.

When the two valves in your nose are working well, the air in the caves (your middle ears) stays around the same pressure as outside so the ear-drums are relaxed and fully sensitive to sound. But the ear cave is also a crude lung, slowly absorbing air into your CIRCULATION; the valves open regularly to make up for this. You can feel them easing when you swallow or yawn, sometimes with improvement in your hearing. This is most marked as the pressure outside increases when you descend in a lift or plane. Air leaks out easily past the valves on the way up, but they must be opened actively on the way down to let it back in.

During a COLD the skin of your nose tends to swell, and it is up to you to keep that as local as possible. If the valve gets involved it becomes sticky and requires a greater pressure to open it, which may stretch your ear-drum PAINFULLY. This kind of fleeting earache lasts up to half an hour at a time and is not too severe; but worse may follow.

The lining of your ear tube does not have to swell much before it blocks the air passage completely where it passes through the bone of your skull. That blockage can last for days. The air goes on dissolving into blood vessels in the cave, making a vacuum which sucks your ear-drum in. Or the lining of the cave runs like the skin of your nose, and CATARRHAL mucus trapped there presses your ear-drum outwards. Either way the PAIN is miserable, weakening and protracted, and your hearing may be quite markedly reduced.

There are only two ways this situation can resolve itself naturally. Either the catarrh accumulates enough to burst your ear-drum and let itself out, or your COLD clears up and the mucus escapes through the reopened drainage tube to your nose. Provided your CATARRHAL tendency is over by then your ear-drum will heal perfectly, and you will be none the worse for the episode.

Doctors are rather inclined to assume that every swollen pink ear-drum is automatically INFECTED and prescribe ANTIBIOTICS on the false assumption that *bacteria** are involved. This is rarely the case, unless they get in through your ear-drum after it has perforated. In that case treatment is well justified to stop pus trickling through the hole, which prevents its two skin layers from healing across as they should. The frustrated energy is diverted into healing the outside and inside skins together around the margin of the tear like a button-hole, making it much more long-lasting. It may not be permanent even so, but gradually get smaller and vanish. But this is the way chronic ear infection used to get established in the past.

HELPING YOURSELF

Work on preventing COLDS and other VIRUS INFECTIONS and on limiting their extent. Earache is much less likely if colds are well contained.

Children need to chew hard and long on unrefined cereals, raw vegetables, dried fruit, liquorice root and the like from an early age. This challenges the jaws and their muscles to become strong and bulky. That broadens the whole face; a wide nose leaves the ear-tube valves unobstructed. Pap-fed children grow up with fine jaws and narrow noses which block far too easily.

Learn how to 'blow' your ear-valves, and make sure they do it regularly. Pinch your nostrils firmly, then pressurize your nose and swallow. Get a child to try blowing up a new balloon while you pinch his nose for him. It may still work if he laughs instead!

When earache happens give plenty of pain relief. Warm oil sometimes soothes, or a very cold ice pack may work better – you will have to try each in turn. *Bach Rescue Remedy** in the outside ear passage may help, so long as your ear is not already running. A hot water bottle to lie on is usually soothing.

Homoeopathic* Arnica tincture or tablets often reduce panic if not the pain. If you use paracetamol or aspirin, take an adequate dose: you can safely repeat an ineffective dose after half an hour.

Accept decongestant medicine to shrink the ear lining, but decline an ANTIBIOTIC unless the ear is running or you are terribly ill. *Mastoiditis** – a high-pressure infection of your middle-ear cave that gets into all its deepest crevices – is now rare, but infected discharge makes a permanent hole more likely. It is well worth a course of Penicillin to avoid that.

If the drum does not burst the catarrh may persist, with prolonged deafness. Decongestants are no good long-term: take them in full dosage for three days of each week, persevere with ear-valve exercises and take homoeopathic Merc. sol 30 three times daily for the remainder of the week.

Work on preventing chronic CATARRH.

If the doctor suggests a grommet operation to restore your hearing after prolonged catarrhal deafness, consider it. It is an elegant and safe application of SURGERY which nicely complements measures you can take yourself. A tiny plastic tube keeps open a surgical incision of your ear-drum for long enough to ventilate your middle-ear cave and restore it to normal function. It is gradually extruded in the course of the next six to eighteen months, as the skin of your ear-drum rejects it and seals over, leaving a soundly healed scar. You should manage to shed the grommets, and any need for them, within a year or so. You will still need to use the measures already discussed to correct anything in your constitution which would make similar incidents likely, but you do not have to wait months for your hearing to be restored.

EAR WAX

Your ear-drum lies three centimetres inside your skull, at the bottom of a passage that takes a rather twisted course, slightly upwards and forwards from your ear-hole. The skin which lines this passage is constructed in just the same way as your skin elsewhere, with one exception. Everywhere else, spent scales from the surface of your skin are rubbed away by friction of some kind. This is not possible in your ear passage; without some means for clearing out old scales your ears would quickly become blocked with them. Your ear-drums would become distorted and PAINFUL, and you would be tormented with NOISES in your head which are worse than hearing nothing at all.

Wax is the answer. It is formed by *sebaceous glands** in the skin in the outer half of your ear passage, and transforms the scaly debris into a cylindrical glacier. This very slowly creeps outwards, rotating like a cork-screw. At its edge near your ear-hole, pieces of overhanging wax break off and tickle so that your finger tip finds and removes them every few weeks or so. In this way not only scales but dust, and the remains of any insect that gets in there, are efficiently parcelled up and removed.

This arrangement can be unsettled in three ways. If you grope inside your ears with twists of cloth, cotton buds or hair-pins you can easily turn back the edge of the glacier to coil in on itself, and will eventually ram it down against your eardrum like the charge in a cannon. If so it gradually dries out and shrinks into a hard core, for a time making space for more wax to collect. Eventually the hard pebble fills the canal, and symptoms begin. This only takes six to twelve months, if no wax escapes at all.

Alternatively the shape of your ear passage may frustrate the movement of your wax glacier, so that it accumulates even without your help. If its shape is markedly oval instead of circular, wax cannot easily follow its corkscrew course and its outward flow grinds to a halt. Some people's ear tubes narrow at some point, which is just as difficult for wax to negotiate; the shoulder of an abruptly narrowing tube may even reflect the wax back on itself, to form a ball just as if you had tampered with it. Although they may not be constitu-tionally inevitable, you cannot control these misfortunes once they have taken shape.

Your DIET is one factor you can control. The character and amount of wax is influenced by your food, being more profuse and irritant the more fat, waste acids and chemicals you unload into it from your over-burdened CIRCULATION.

Syringing is the time-honoured treatment in all cases of wax accumulation, usually after softening with warm oil. It is surprising that doctors have never given any thought to preventing it, since they stand to reduce their work-load considerably by doing so. Perhaps they are glad to have problems like these that are gratifying and easy to solve. I doubt if their patients agree, and am sure that the first scientists who bother to take prevention seriously will be gratefully patronized by tens of thousands.

HELPING YOURSELF

Never reach for ear wax with anything sharper than your finger end. To have waxy ears is not dirty, but evidence that your glacial cleansing mechanism is working properly. If you succeed in keeping the passage clear, you are removing its accustomed protection and making INFLAMMATION or INFEC- TION much more likely. If you fail, wax will accumulate helplessly in the normally waxless part of your passages, where there is no mechanism for getting rid of it.

A healthy DIET, in which flesh floods, fats and chemicals are consumed as exceptions, makes no demands on your ear wax as a medium of excretion. Consequently it remains non-irritant, soft and flexible, and manageable in quantity.

If your ears do require clearance of wax, use Glycerine BP (Glycerol) or Almond Oil to soften it for four or five days first. Olive Oil is quite good if you already have some, to save a special purchase; but a large wax plug will swell with olive oil and may give you EARACHE. Tackle your ears one at a time, the worst affected first, to keep some useful hearing throughout. Warm the oil in a cup of hot water for a few minutes, then lie your head on the good side and drip oil slowly into the bad ear until it fills. Maintain that position for a few minutes, then grease a twist of cotton wool with vaseline and carefully plug the ear with it. One thorough daily application at bed-time is ample.

The syringing will be quick and easy after this preparation, and you can repeat the process for the other ear if necessary. Ask your doctor if the anatomy of your ear passage is awkward in any way (slit-shaped, unusually narrowed or tortuous) that might account for the wax blockage. If so, persevere with at least one application weekly of Glycerine or Almond Oil to each ear in turn (ie each ear twice a month), to keep the wax as fluent as possible. A special purchase would in this case be worthwhile since glycerine does not cause the wax to swell, and almond oil is the least irritant of those available.

If your ears are not unusual, put into each just two drops of the softener you now have once each week. This dose moistens your ear drums then gradually flows outwards, which may help to establish a new glacial flow in the right direction so breaking at source your dependence on the ear syringe, and even on the drops.

ECZEMA, (atopic) dermatitis

Your skin is not just a container but a remarkably sophisticated organ which regulates losses of heat and moisture from your body, can store and excrete surpluses from metabolism and receives sensory impressions. Despite its permeability it is a very effective barrier against *microbes** and moisture and can regulate the penetration of sunlight to the tissues inside. It wears tirelessly and will grow into a form appropriate to the physical work expected of it. Its elasticity enables it to cope with changes over the years in your shape and size.

Its thin surface sheet grows from a foundation layer one cell thick. Successive sheets of cells created there mount up in layers, each flattening and hardening as it ages. The oldest layer forms your outside surface, with its cells arranged like slates on a roof. Wear scrapes off these oldest cells as flakes of dry scale, which are larger and greasier where your HAIR is thickest and *sebaceous glands** most active. The DANDRUFF in your scalp arises in this way; some degree of it is inevitable, since even in health your surface skin must flake off eventually.

Habitual friction arouses your skin to thicken up, especially on your palms and soles; some long-distance runners prefer this natural foot-leather to shoes. Small areas of contact with rough seams in ill-fitting shoes can produce the same effect, especially around a WART; but being localized and lumpy these *corns** are uncomfortable. Sudden unaccustomed wear raises *blisters** instead, the only adaptation you can make in the time available.

All this sophisticated life is thrown off balance if your skin is required to excrete or store poisons your blood cannot cope with. These are dissolved in your sweat or incorporated in your skin cells to be worn away six weeks later. They combine to poison your skin metabolism, which deranges drastically its evolution. It INFLAMES, grows faster and sheds its disordered surface faster still as it attempts to right itself; this leaves vulnerable immature skin exposed, still chronically poisoned.

This is eczema, or dermatitis. It takes many forms and is distributed variously on your body according to the precise *'colour'** imbalances associated with the underlying cause of your problem. Doctors have for a century fascinated themselves with distinguishing these different manifestations, naming and describing them, and researching their biochemical and micro-anatomical nature. Yet when it comes down to treatment, all that can be done for the non-INFECTIOUS conditions is to suppress their appearance. *Steroid** creams and ointments are the mainstay of this approach. But after a year or two their effect weakens. And after years of continued use your skin gets thin and delicate, all its vitality spent – almost as if you had borrowed from its future to clean it up today and had nothing left with which to redeem the debt.

Unless your rash clearly arises from ALLERGY due to surface contact, look deeper for its cause from the beginning. You will not then be let down.

HELPING YOURSELF

Avoid using soap when you do not need to; cold water is sufficient for ordinary washing, with cold cream (Aqueous Cream BP) as a lubricant if necessary. Soap removes fat from your skin and makes it much more vulnerable to irritants, FUNGI and bacteria on its surface. Prolonged soaking in a hot bath does the same. Emulsifying Ointment, much favoured by eczema sufferers, only puts back in what the soap and hot water take out!

Try a modified version of the *Priessnitz pack.** After a short hot shower or bath wrap your body tightly from armpits to hips in a cold damp sheet; if the sheet oozes water when tightened, it is too wet. Wear a long warm woollen sweater over this, under a house-coat, for two hours; at night, just get into bed. After the initial chill you should quickly relax, glowing with warmth under the sheet. When you take it off (or waken in the morning) it will be dry, and may be stained with what your skin has excreted. Repeat this several times a week. It does not matter if your eczema is not covered by the sheet.

Practise deep BREATHING several times daily, one of which can coincide with ten minutes' brisk EXERCISE in the open air. Shower afterwards while still perspiring, and finish with cold water for 20–30 seconds, especially on your eczematous patches. Pat yourself dry.

If your skin is chronically bad commence a cleansing DIET, with raw food only for the first week and avoiding salt. Check whether you are ALLERGIC to food from the cow in the early stages of this diet, and if so avoid it absolutely for several months.

If your problem is intermittent or reasonably limited, a normal healthy DIET should be fine; but check yourself for ALLERGY to each family of foods you wish to eat regularly. After a rest from them for a few weeks, you will get away with occasional portions of almost anything.

SUPPLEMENTS of Zinc, Vitamin C and Essential Fatty Acids, with Honey Cider Vinegar or Egg Nog RECIPE for other minerals, are well worth while for three months, especially in DANDRUFF; your diet should be sufficient thereafter.

*Homoeopathic** treatment is often helpful, but you will need to stop using *steroids** first. If Sulphur fails, take expert advice about alternatives.

Steroids creams and ointments are the mainstay of medical treatment. They only suppress the effects of the condition, though even that can be an immense relief at times. Get your doctor in the first place to help you off the more powerful fluorinated ones and back to plain hydrocortisone ointment; covered with polythene gloves or food bags this is quite effective, and much safer. Urea is good for soothing irritation, and is combined with cortisone in some preparations. Your cure will in time get you off even this, except perhaps for accidental relapses.

ELECTRICITY DISEASE

You need electricity to function. Appliances and furnishings which drain the electricity from your room may give you HEADACHE or make you drowsy, congested and confused; your body is likely to work much better when the charge is put back.

But everyone nowadays, no matter how you live, is exposed to much more electricity than has ever been possible before. Since we began to explore it, less than a century ago, it has become the dominant '*mono*'* medium of civilization. Whatever we may do about chemical pollution and energy conservation can only reinforce our dependence on electronic energy.

It has various manifestations. The flow of electrical current is the least important of these, though it can cause the most troublesome kind of BURN. The magnetic field that is generated around any electrical current has more biological significance, but is not new; birds and large sea creatures have for millions of years navigated during their seasonal migrations by the earth's magnetic field. Static electrical charge is familiar in nature too, most dramatically as electrical storms; but any flowing or agitated water generates static in the air above it which has a tonic effect on the creatures BREATHING it – hence the appeal of mountains and seaside for *convalescence*.*

The invention of alternating current is what made oscillating high-energy magnetic fields and electro-magnetic radiation possible, at intensities far beyond what animals and people have been used to. Since living things of all kinds have electrical field activity too, we are beginning to realize that electro-magnetic pollution must be taken seriously. Your body fields extend well outside your skin and interact with a full spectrum of magnetic, electrical and radio fields generated for all kinds of purposes by a wide range of authorities and businesses. The interaction inevitably distorts the shape and energy of your own output, which must alter your WELLBEING in some way, however subtly. Little by little we are discovering how.

High-tension power cables, for instance, distort the electromagnetic fields in the nearby landscape. People in various parts of the country seem to have been made irritable and unwell by these, in ways it has been impossible to substantiate by conventional medical means. But Dr Jean Monro, in collaboration with electrical engineers from Salford University, has been able to show that some of her very allergic patients are affected badly by electricity, with typical ALLERGY symptoms in response to fields from ordinary domestic electronic appliances, turned on without the subject's knowledge.

Accidents with radar during the Second World War showed how *microwaves** can heat flesh enough to burn it. Parts of your brain may be especially susceptible, since HYPERACTIVITY, muscle weakness and marked TIREDNESS have been observed in people who work with micro-waves. Many other studies detailed in Jane Clarke's BOOK suggest they are capable of affecting all major systems of your body and may trigger MULTIPLE SCLEROSIS attacks.

154

Ventilate your rooms naturally from the freshest outside air available. Use natural furnishing fabrics and carpets. Avoid aerosol spray-cans and smoke; extract kitchen fumes efficiently to the outside. These measures maintain the natural charge of the air for as long as possible. House-plants and indoor fountains positively reinforce it.

Radiant and fan heaters, air conditioners, tube lighting, televisions and VDUs all leak the charge near them away to the earth. Unplug them when they are not in use, and look for substitutes.

Ionizers can recharge and clean the air in rooms deprived of good natural ventilation. Clear your bedroom of electrical equipment and artificial fabric furnishings, then run an ionizer in it continuously, night and day. This may refresh you sufficiently to cope much better with HEADACHE, MIGRAINE, or other STRESS symptoms you cannot otherwise avoid.

If you use a microwave cooker be sure that its door seals effectively, and get any damage to the door or its seating attended to before you use the appliance again. A leaky door will allow micro-waves to circulate in your kitchen, which may affect its occupants. We do not yet know enough about the biological effects of these particular micro-wave frequencies to be sure they are safe, whatever their advocates may say; but an undamaged and well-made appliance of approved design is likely to be quite safe when used in accordance with the manufacturer's instructions.

Ionizers Currently Available

Medion Ltd (ADDRESS) have for many years manufactured a range of models for various uses from the car or desk top to the full scale concourse, open plan office or board-room.

This is however a technology that lends itself to small-scale industrial development, and a number of firms have appeared in various parts of the country. They can often compete effectively on price terms, but the quality and power of their equipment varies enormously. They are also more difficult to keep track of, and some of them have probably ceased trading.

When answering an advertisement by a lesser known manufacturer it is as well to explore these matters as much as you can before agreeing a purchase. If at all possible, obtain the use of equipment on approval before committing yourself. Even if it functions perfectly, it may not provide the answer to your problem.

EPILEPSY, seizures, fits, convulsions

WHAT HAPPENS

Anything that over-excites your NERVOUS system or interferes with its control can cause a riot somewhere in your brain, resulting in abnormal movements or sensations corresponding to the normal function of that part. You may only ever have one such fit in your life, or repeat them only in particular circumstances – after FAINTING or HEAD INJURY perhaps. Children between six months and six years old are susceptible to fits during any high FEVER; some toddlers have a *breath-holding attack** that can end in a fit whenever they are really furious. None of these has serious implications, and they are only harmful if they interfere with BREATHING or result in INJURY.

That covers the vast majority of all fits, but they get a bad name from two much more serious causes that mercifully turn up rather seldom – CANCER or ARTERIOSCLEROSIS affecting the brain. Besides these, however, quite a few TEENAGERS begin to suffer from epilepsy for which no cause can be found, but which may pester them to a greater or lesser extent for the rest of their lives.

Doctors take all these matters very seriously, and will investigate the cause of any fits they cannot easily explain. This usually rules out the serious conditions everyone fears, and a decision is taken as to whether medical treatment is likely to help. Most doctors do not give daily drugs to prevent fits that happen seldom in case side-effects turn out to be more troublesome than the disease. This leaves you simply putting up with your complaint under occasional medical supervision, unable by law to drive a car and with a number of occupations and *recreational** pursuits closed to you. Even if treatment is offered and succeeds, it only ever suppresses the riots without removing their cause, and must continue indefinitely. *Temporal lobe epilepsy** is particularly difficult to deal with, because it occurs in a part of your brain sometimes concerned with behaviour. Violent and unreasonable outbursts get blamed on it when HYPERACTIVITY could be causing both.

Research into epilepsy is far too preoccupied with brain chemistry and ignores the obvious. Irritant chemicals are used increasingly in urban societies, and are accumulating in your body as well as your environment. Lead continues to pollute car exhaust fumes, cadmium gets into canned food and chemically fertilized soils, and mercury continues to fill our TEETH when fluoride has failed to protect them. Insecticides based on nerve gas are sprayed regularly on farm land and gardens. All these increase your liability to fits, can be detected if we decide to look for them and respond safely to active measures for their removal. In addition we could be much more energetic in legislation and regulation of these problems as a community, once interests vested in the present state of affairs have been overcome. Meanwhile you should not accept the excuse that insufficient scientific evidence exists to link epilepsy with these environmental factors. The work necessary to establish those links has simply not been done, because policymakers and directors of research show insufficient interest in them. The Conservation Society's BOOK shows what comes to light when the subject is taken seriously by a reputable scientist.

HELPING YOURSELF

Start by adopting a positive, confident, campaigning attitude. Anything that helps to integrate your outlook also steadies the temper of your NERVOUS system as a whole, and of its irritable part in particular.

Once your doctors have investigated your fits and you know the effect of any treatment they have prescribed, arrange for yourself a cleansing DIET SUPPLEMENTED for cleansing. This will require many months to complete its work but you can relax onto the DIET for health after a month or so. Avoid coffee, SMOKING, ALCOHOL and strong tea indefinitely; cocoa, chocolate and cola drinks are also best avoided. On the other hand eat fresh onions, garlic and asparagus whenever they are available, raw if you can.

Have no canned food or any processed items labelled as containing Aspartame ('Nutrasweet', 'Canderil'), Patent Blue V (E131), Thiabendazol (E233) or Ammonium salts (380, 381, E402-404, 503, 510, 527).

SUPPLEMENTS of Vitamin C (3000mg daily), Zinc (15–30mg daily), Manganese Orotate (50mg daily), Dolomite (500mg three times daily) and Vitamin B_6 (Pyridoxine, 50mg daily) for the first three months will top up your reserves of nutrients known to soothe your nervous system and help coax copper, lead, mercury and cadmium out of you. After that your diet should maintain the nutrients adequately, but you would be wise to carry on taking the Vitamin C.

A *Medical Herbalist** can offer many appropriate remedies, such as elder bark and valerian root. Consult one (ADDRESS), or follow Juliette de Baïracle Levi's instructions, given in her BOOK.

A practitioner of *Homoeopathy** or *Traditional Chinese Medicine** or a reputable *Hypnotherapist** may be able to help you when others cannot. Consult the ADDRESSES for possibilities nearby.

None of these measures need interfere with your medication, but once you are established in them you will want to try cautiously reducing the drugs. Be candid with your doctor about this and try to win his cooperation; this is always easier if you frame your approach as a request for advice. If he can see that you are prepared to venture on your own responsibility, he will carry his obligations to you more easily. Once you have a bargain keep him informed of progress, preferably including an honest diary of all your fits.

It is mistaken to associate physical fitness too closely with health, which it can at best only garnish and may just as easily undermine – as the rapid increase in sports INJURY clinic facilities makes only too plain.

The confusion in most people's minds arises from supposing that health and physical efficiency are one and the same. This is patently not so. It is possible to be perfectly beastly to your family and aggressive towards your neighbours yet physically very fit. A man capable of a heavy sustained effort may not so much be healthy for choosing to make it, as stupid for avoiding a more sensible alternative. Another may make the pursuit of fitness his excuse for avoiding family relationships or work he dislikes but should not neglect, in favour of the adult equivalent of play. Aerobic fitness, the rate at which your body can make use of oxygen, is merely the easiest kind of efficiency for 'mono'* enthusiasts to measure and understand.

There is obviously some point in being reasonably efficient at anything that enables you to use your wits and faculties acutely, energetically and without TIREDNESS. It is nice to be supple, strong, nimble and quick for its own sake, just for fun. Sometimes you need to be exceptionally fit just to survive your job or the circumstances you live in; you do not need to make any special effort, just keep going. Others need to offset the effects of too sedentary an occupation, and whole communities may need a substitute for tribal warfare by which to settle scores and rivalries. For no-one else is there any point in exercising to maintain your fitness at a level you are never really going to use, unless you actually enjoy doing it.

Even then, get your general constitution in order first. No body improves for exercise if it is cluttered with rubbish, fatigued, ill-fed or badly worn. Rest, a good cleansing DIET and sound healing for dilapidated parts must in this case take priority over yet more work. A reflective kind of recreation, like painting or fishing, will then do you much more good than anything based on physical exertion.

Once your diet is nourishing and you have got over the worst of your wear and tear, an appetite for activity will arise quite naturally. You will feel more spring in your step and walk more vigorously because you enjoy it. That is the time to look at other forms of active recreation that will give you a chance to extend this enjoyment.

Some people run because they like it, but a lot more simply follow fashion. Think for yourself. Sustained brisk walking about town is just as valuable, and a steady lope up stairs is far more hygienic than crowding into the lift. Bikes beat public transport and traffic hands down, are a lot easier to park than any car and give you the means to burn off TENSION and exasperation in harmless bursts of acceleration.

You may prefer to organize a vigorous pastime into your way of life. The clubbable sports – golf, court and pitch games – are obvious choices if you enjoy the *après jeu* routine but waste time and money if you don't. Many loners like swimming, which makes a convenient lunchtime habit. If straight exercise bores you, try more adventurous water sports like wind-surfing, sailing, sub-aqua or water-skiing, where fun or competence is the chief object and exercise is incidental. Horse-riding can work this way too, provided you avoid the more equitation-oriented stables.

If all-round health is all you are interested in, avoid exercising for its own sake. Take it in your stride, as part of living. That way you keep invigorated with the minimum of wear and tear, and actually contribute to your overall vitality instead of draining it. There is no need to feel foolish, bored or exhausted.

It takes remarkably little effort to keep your body acceptably efficient. Ten minutes three times a week of sustained moderate exertion will save your CIRCULATION and BREATHING from stagnation. Activity brisk enough to make your simultaneous conversation difficult is quite sufficient, whatever your condition; the fitter you are, the harder you will be working to achieve this effect.

From this state of readiness, a well-fed and clean body leaps into condition very fast whenever you ask it. Your first holiday swim may tire you a bit, but in two days you are back on reasonable form. Games in the garden with energetic children need hold no fears. You can take a heavy gardening spell or three sets of tennis in your stride any time you want.

You can extend this exercise routine as a useful aid to weight reduction. Once you have sustained your effort steadily at this level for twenty minutes you begin to burn deep-seated stores of energy and to make less economical use of them than you would at a slower or more intermittent pace. Your *metabolism** takes on an active tone which mobilizes fat, conserves muscle, heats you and reduces your APPETITE. What is more, these effects persist for up to twenty-four hours. So thirty minutes' vigorous exercise daily ensures that you shed OVERWEIGHT without reducing your vigour – especially if your exercise replaces a meal.

Whatever your interest, it is dangerous to use a sport to get fit, or fitness training to get well. Clean up your constitution, first and foremost. Then train it, by all means, into good enough condition to enjoy your chosen sport. If you want to excel, a good coach can take over your training from there.

FAINTING

WHAT HAPPENS

All your blood vessels are capable of expanding widely when they need to, by relaxation of the muscles that are wrapped round them like crepe bandages. If they all chose to open up at once their total capacity would exceed the volume of your CIRCULATING blood many times over; your BLOOD PRESSURE would collapse, because no blood would get back to your heart to keep it primed.

That does not usually happen because your NERVOUS system keeps the emphasis of your circulation on the tissues where the work is. That varies smoothly throughout the day, from restfully digesting your last meal to vigorous muscular exertion. The only part of you that always needs blood is your brain, whose ground floor houses the control centre which regulates the distribution of your blood everywhere else.

This arrangement is not proof against upset. Any *shock** or STRESS severe enough to disrupt your brain routine will leave your circulation unattended for a few seconds, which is quite enough for valves along your blood vessels to relax indiscriminately. When this happens a large fraction of your blood can quickly gravitate to your legs, leaving you with insufficient to pump uphill to your head or elsewhere. So the blood drains from your face, your vision goes grey, and all the control functions of your brain go haywire – you sweat, feel giddy and may be SICK. Finally you lose consciousness altogether and slump to the ground. You may have a brief *fit** while you are unconscious, if other parts of your brain are similarly affected. But unless you INJURE yourself in falling, no permanent or serious harm is likely to be done.

This whole fainting sequence may only take a few seconds, but it does usually give you some warning. If you are prone to faints you may recognize circumstances that generally bring one on. If they are inclined to follow a meal by several hours and come on gradually, you may be HYPOGLYCAEMIC and should explore that possibility.

But the underlying cause is usually far more prosaic. Standing still for a long time, especially in the heat or in stuffy and airless atmospheres, will eventually wear most people down. Any PAIN will cause fainting if severe enough. Painful PERIODS are particularly liable to affect you if your loss is heavy so that you have to cope with *anaemia** as well. Prolonged TIREDNESS, excessive exposure to the cold or going without meals often cause people to faint under more immediate STRESSES that would not normally affect them. TEENAGERS during their adolescent growth spurt have less stable circulation, and PREGNANT women are in some POSTURES liable to trap a large part of their blood supply in their legs, if their babies weigh heavily on the veins from there.

Medical investigation usually reveals nothing abnormal, and suggests no useful preventative action. But there are several valuable clues you can follow through for yourself. In particular, since sluggish nervous reflexes account for the mechanism of fainting, anything that improves these will reduce your liability to faint.

HELPING YOURSELF

'Eat breakfast for yourself, share your lunch with a friend, give your supper to an enemy.' If your bigger meals come early in the day you have ready fuel for all your activities. Missing out breakfast is a great mistake, for TEENAGERS especially; TIREDNESS from SLEEPING too little and too late heightens any apprehension you feel about the forthcoming day and destroys your APPETITE. In adults this more often goes with eating and drinking too large and too late at night, which you may be using as a way to relax after a long TENSE day.

Besides sufficient unrefined energy food in a generally healthy DIET, you need plenty of the Vitamin B group, Vitamin C (at least 200mg daily) and nutrient minerals. Nine Brewer's Yeast tablets daily are enough if you are reasonably well, but a Strong Vitamin B Complex is better for the first month if you are not. Egg nog or Honey Cider Vinegar RECIPE provides the minerals cheaply, reinforced for a few weeks with a good multimineral formula (eg Nature's Own).

Tone yourself up generally by brushing your skin vigorously all over first thing each morning, or finish a hot shower with thirty seconds of cool or cold water and rub yourself dry vigorously instead.

Practise good BREATHING several times each day, preferably in fresh air out of doors. EXERCISE regularly to become reasonably fit. Get enough SLEEP, starting well before midnight.

Meanwhile three *homoeopathic** remedies for fainting are worth trying: Arsenicum album 3 while you remain debilitated, Moschus 3 or Ignatia 3 if you are well but are the NERVOUS or excitable type, inclined to worry. All can be taken every four hours for a few days at a time, when you feel the need.

A *pot pourri* of Lavender, or massage with its essential oil, helps to reduce a fainting tendency and is a useful restorative after attacks. Peppermint tea reinforces this, especially if used instead of your customary stimulants.

*Traditional Chinese Medicine** and *Reflexology** understand instability of your nerves and circulation better than conventional doctors do. Consultation with a local practitioner of either (ADDRESSES) may prove very rewarding.

When you feel faint loosen clothing round your neck, suck hard against your closed throat to get blood into your chest, and lean well forward. If necessary lie down flat in good time, with your legs up on a chair. When the moment is past get upright again in gradual stages, so as not to risk a recurrence.

FAMILY PLANNING, pre-conception

It is comparatively easy to avoid PREGNANCY by CONTRACEPTION, and many people still think conceiving a baby is merely a matter of removing this precaution. This may work out for you in practice, if you are healthy and ready for parenthood. But remember that you are embarking on the most creative thing you will probably ever do. Do not undertake this lightly, but get into the right frame of mind and prepare your bodies for the task. Every livestock farmer nurses the health of his breeding stock before mating them, making sure that they have the best of everything available at this important time. Yet most of the offspring of these matings will be dead and eaten within two years! You are laying down the foundation of a life that may last fifty times longer. Treat yourself at least as well as a farmer treats his animals.

Every baby starts as an egg and a sperm which have to be grown by you, his parents. Your eggs were made before you were born, but mature gradually for at least three months before one of them is chosen for release at *ovulation** to be ripe for fertilization. Meanwhile sperms are formed in a continuous supply, maturing over a period of at least two months. During this period both egg and sperm are vulnerable to damage by chemicals (including tobacco SMOKE and ALCOHOL), RADIATION and INFECTION. If these coincide with the critical *cell** divisions that are part of the process of ripening for both eggs and sperms, non-conception, MISCARRIAGE or a damaged baby become much more likely.

Perfectly formed germ cells have then to unite in the right place and conditions and continue to develop in the womb you have meanwhile prepared for it. Major errors cause MISCARRIAGE. Minor delays place your *placenta** too low for comfort, which makes the *umbilical cord** more liable to coil round your baby's neck and tighten during birth. Lower still a pregnancy rarely survives, and only with SURGICAL help. Without it your *placenta praevia** is torn before your baby can be born and BLEEDS profusely, creating a SURGICAL emergency.

None of this can work unless your life maintains a reasonably prosperous *'colour'** tone. Your fertility is reduced if you are unsettled, TENSE, under STRESS, EXERCISING strenuously, UNDERWEIGHT, extremely OVERWEIGHT or suffer from COLDNESS all the time. But failure to BLEED menstrually every month does not rule out pregnancy, since highly 'coloured' passions may arouse you to *ovulate** directly, just when you need to.

Your general health helps determine how much of the slippery fertile womb mucus you produce for a few days before you ovulate; it will string out between your fingers, like egg-white. Sperms only survive at all if they can reach this mucus, and can collect from successive intercourses while it lasts. This gives you a harmless means of influencing the sex of your child. Intercourse once only in that time, as soon as you feel the mucus, is more likely to give you a girl. A single intercourse just before the mucus disappears is more likely to produce a boy.

HELPING YOURSELF

Pregnancies are not conceived by taking thought but by indulging your instincts. You need a comfortable nest to get broody in. Otherwise you may fail, and seek unnecessary medical investigation, which only weakens your nesting behaviour even more. So leave the rat-race, relax self-indulgently into your home and enjoy your present prosperity without any sense of guilt.

Delay conception for a minimum of nine months following a previous pregnancy, though gaps of two to three years between birthdays give you more time to rally your resources for each one, especially if you BREAST FEED for a year or so. After illness or your last oral CONTRACEPTIVE pills, postpone pregnancy for at least six months. If your general health is good and has not recently been drained, a minimum of three months' preparation is sufficient. This is your pre-conception interval. Keep careful track of your PERIODS during this time, and of the mucus days in between.

Both of you need to adopt the DIET and SUPPLEMENTS for pregnancy. If you are UNDERWEIGHT or very OVERWEIGHT, bias it accordingly. Do not slim drastically – you will manage pregnancy much better plump than lean, and your baby is much less likely to develop abnormally.

Give up SMOKING, and ban it in your living rooms. Avoid ALCOHOL; not even small quantities are completely safe. If you take regular medication, ask your doctor if you can safely reduce or stop it during your pre-conception interval and until your pregnancy is three months old. At the same time be checked for *rubella**** IMMUNIZATION and sort out any VAGINAL DISCHARGE.

Avoid medical X-rays and ultrasound scans during your pre-conception interval. Do not sit close to television and computer screens, especially colour ones. If the door of your *microwave** oven should be damaged, do not use it until it has been competently repaired.

If your work involves you with hazardous chemicals, anaesthetics, radio-isotopes, X-rays, radar or ultra-sound equipment, oscilloscopes or colour-screen computer monitors, arrange if you can to keep out of the most active areas during your pre-conception interval.

The only leisure pursuit known to threaten pregnancy is skin-diving. Otherwise keep up your EXERCISE and *recreational** pursuits throughout pregnancy and pre-conception, but keep comfortably within your capabilities. Deal with SLEEPLESSNESS if it persists or recurs more than occasionally.

Notwithstanding all this *'mono'** advice, pre-conception is a 'colour' event. Relax and enjoy every minute of it. Cultivate your sense of wonder with the BOOKS by Nilsson and Templegarth Trust (ADDRESS). This calm interlude is soon eclipsed by busy family life, for up to twenty years. Each wait between children is a private lull amid that turbulence, something very special that only you two share.

After repeated MISCARRIAGES or if pre-conception lasts eighteen months or more, see your doctor to discover why, and contact Foresight (ADDRESS).

FEET

WHAT HAPPENS

Your feet are not at first much use to you. They kick and POSTURE automatically while you gradually take over control of your NERVOUS system from above downwards. Your hands and mouth may actually discover them first, before you are otherwise aware that they belong to you. They are soft and smooth, simply shaped with no arch or any other obvious functional bias; you take some time to work out what to use them for. As long as you sit or lie they are in view, and serve as extra hands; but when you get interested in crawling and walking you lose sight of them, and they begin to develop as shock-absorbers and springs, specialized for balancing and moving over all sorts of ground surface.

When fully functional, each of your feet forms a springy arch between your heel and the bases of your toes, braced by the muscles within your foot and on your shin. This sets up your *ankle** perfectly level, making SPRAIN unlikely and providing the foundation for your upright POSTURE. Your legs rise at a comfortable angle with your *knees** poised for smooth function and minimum wear, able to lock properly when fully straightened. Your thighs are therefore comfortably aligned, and your *hips** too can rest in their most economical position. The posture of your pelvis then provides the ideal platform for a well-balanced *spine.**

Walking must be a precarious skill for human beings, because a lot of us develop poorly in this respect. Footwear cannot be entirely to blame for this, since the errors seem to be present from birth in many cases and may be to do with the posture imposed on your feet in the last months of PREGNANCY. You may consequently have failed from the beginning to brace up your foot arches adequately, which splayed your feet and ankle tendons outwards, destroying their springiness and making you very flat-footed. Your legs twisted inwards to compensate, which made your kneecaps 'squint'. The *ligaments** on the inside of your knees are over-strained, and may begin to hurt. Meanwhile your thigh and pelvic postures are distorted, making you prey to *osteoarthritis** in your hips and lower spine. All these errors get built into your bones as they grow.

Mass-produced shoes and elastic socks certainly do not help. They cannot usually be expected to improve on the function of your naked feet. The best you can expect is that they do no harm; but if you wear shoes too young they are almost bound to. They splint your feet and mould them into an unnatural and inefficient shape. This considerably cramps their style, so that you are forced to use them in a different way. The shape they adopt as they grow corresponds therefore to a function that is less than ideal.

If they were built and fitted properly, shoes could correct early postural errors and enable your bones and JOINTS to grow into the best shape for ideal life-long function. But designers are a long way from realizing that, and will respond best to commercial pressure from a much more discriminating shoe-buying public.

HELPING YOURSELF

Avoid substantial footwear for your children up to about two years of age. For outdoor trips in winter dress them in loose-fitting socks or leggings only. Let them learn and practise walking barefoot. This is safe even on gravel, and will properly toughen the soles of their feet.

If when they walk their ankle tendons seem to be splayed outwards when viewed from behind, consult a *Podiatrist** (ADDRESS). He is able to correct this error inexpensively and permanently in a toddler; older people may need expensive tailored insoles for the rest of their lives. Since this will probably prove to be a major cause of osteoarthritis, treatment is worthwhile at any age. Lobby for it to be properly investigated, and incorporated into the National Health Service if the results justify this.

By the time they are ready for shoes their feet will be strongly formed. Choose the right shape as well as an adequate size of shoe, very supple and light. Do not accept shoes which distort their toes, setting them up for *bunions** – the prominent knuckles that develop at the roots of their big toes under STRESS. There must be room for big toes to point straight forward.

Beware of elastic socks in artificial fabrics, which usually offer a very limited range of sizes. When stretched they squeeze your toes quite powerfully, distorting them almost as surely as badly shaped shoes.

Review the size of your families footwear every few months. It may get too small before it wears out.

Do not permit young TEENAGERS to wear high heels (above 3cm) all day. These pitch their body weight forward, ramming their feet into the front of the shoes and deforming them, however well styled the shoes may be. Low heels and a generous style are essential for day-long wear at school and work, at least until their foot bones solidify permanently, usually by 18 years. Leisure outings for a few hours two or three times a week wearing something more modish do little harm and make room for compromise.

Choose leather or canvas uppers always, for good ventilation. Cool, well-aired feet are proof against *athlete's foot** and resist *verrucas** better.

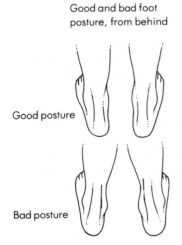

Good and bad foot posture, from behind

Good posture

Bad posture

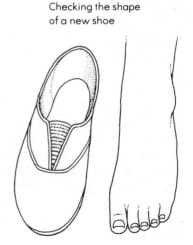

Checking the shape of a new shoe

FEVER

Your temperature is usually controlled very accurately at around 36.8°C (98.4°F) by a thermostat in the base of your brain. This is the setting at which your *metabolism** works best. But you sometimes need to go into overdrive to outrun a disease process such as INFECTION of some kind and regain your health more quickly. Raising your temperature is the easiest way.

You start by re-setting your thermostat a few degrees higher. That makes your body behave as if it were too cold; you save heat by cutting down the CIRCULATION to your limbs and skin and feel you want to curl up in a ball wrapped up warmly. If the need is urgent you may shiver, which is a trembling movement of your muscles that burns fuel to make extra heat quickly.

In a few hours you reach the new thermostat level and relax again. You may now feel comfortable but your skin is hot and dry, and your pulse is faster. Because your body is concentrating on RECOVERY you do not want to do anything or eat, and may only manage to sip a little fluid at a time.

Eventually the fever 'breaks'. The thermostat goes back to normal, so your body now feels too hot. Your skin flushes and perspires, you throw off clothing and appreciate cool draughts. When you have cooled to your usual temperature you become comfortable once more.

A feverish illness usually has a definite daily rhythm. You wake up feeling normal, but become feverish and unwell late in the morning when your temperature has begun to rise. It runs high all afternoon and evening, breaking naturally in the early hours of the next morning. So your nightwear and bedding are damp and need thorough airing.

This routine continues as long as you need it, and usually stops within a few days without any other symptoms arising to indicate why. Children, who use fever more than adults, often shrug it off overnight. Your body has healed itself without snags or complications, so pat yourself on the back.

Remember however that your fever mechanism evolved vigorous enough to cope with prehistoric conditions, in which you needed to raise your temperature in much colder and draughtier circumstances. That would justify your instinct to wrap up warmly. But wrapped in an efficient quilt in a centrally heated draught-proofed house you can easily over-reach your target – usually around 39°C (102°F). Over-heating is the result, reaching as high as two or three degrees above the optimum for healing. This causes HEADACHE, *vomiting** restlessness or *delirium*.* Children between six months and five years overheat easily and may then *convulse** alarmingly.

Fever can accompany some diseases which will eventually require treatment from the doctor. Consult him after two days, or sooner if you have PAIN, severe HEADACHE or any other localizing symptoms such as a very SORE THROAT. But brief uncomplicated feverish episodes at intervals during childhood are not unhealthy in themselves. It is not irresponsible to manage these yourself once you are familiar with them.

HELPING YOURSELF

Manage fever: do not attempt to abolish it. Medicines and food tend to get in the way, but frequent small sips of tepid watered fruit-juice or home-made barley water RECIPE are very refreshing.

Cover up just enough to avoid shivering – one layer of light billowy clothing, plus a sheet or one blanket. Avoid quilts of any kind. Ventilate the room for a through draught. Turn the heating down. These precautions make over-heating much less likely. Leave a feverish child to sleep like this. If he gets too cold he will wake you, or cover up more. Do not risk his overheating in the night; you will get far less warning and may have to work for several hours to get his temperature back within bounds.

If over-heated but not delirious, use a bath even hotter still to get warm and pink. Get out and dry, then wrap up tightly from armpits to hips in a cold damp strip of cotton or linen. If it drips when you tighten it, the wrap is too wet. Pin it every few inches to keep it tight, and get into bed. The fever drops as the towel dries. At the same time blood is drawn away from your head, relieving headache and irritability.

Delirium or convulsion needs urgent cooling. Strip the child and wipe him all over frequently with a hot damp sponge. Play warm air over him with a hair-drier or fan heater. Support him face downwards in a kneeling or crawling position and make sure he can breathe freely. Speak to the doctor for advice.

Try *homoeopathic* * Belladonna 6, as drops or a tablet held on the tongue for a few minutes, half hourly until your symptoms are relieved. Persevere for two or three doses.

If this fails or you prefer conventional remedies, stick to Paracetamol Dispersible BP. Aspirin is even better, if you know it does not upset you. Only medicate a child when you cannot watch him and manage the fever by nursing. Half to one tablet, creamed to froth in a few drops of water or milk, treats a small child safely. If it makes him sick, cool him down for half an hour and try again.

'FLU, chill, influenza

After SICKNESS, diarrhoea and perhaps BACKACHE, 'flu must be the commonest reason given by usually healthy people for being off work. It means a bad COLD with FEVER, HEADACHE, muscle PAINS and terrible weakness which strikes very hard, gives four or five days' symptoms and leaves you weak and grey for another week after that.

Influenza is probably not the usual cause. Any generalized VIRUS INFECTION which enters by your breathing passages will mimic true influenza, and ''flu-like illness' is probably much more common than the real thing. In practice it does not matter very much which exact virus is responsible, except that *influenza vaccination** may not protect you against all the others.

Sometimes, however, a 'flu-like illness or bad COLD does not arise from infection at all. Identical symptoms can occur whenever your body refuses to tolerate any more contamination with *waste acids** from your *metabolism,** or irritant chemicals from your food. This INFLAMMATORY rejection of chemical contaminants can be precipitated by any STRESSFUL turn of events, from overwork to chilling by exposure – exactly the same circumstances as would favour INFECTION and in which many people 'catch cold'. The situation produced by non-infectious 'flu is very similar to that in MIGRAINE or RHEUMATISM, two diseases in which a 'cleansing illness' or 'healing crisis' of this kind was familiar to the naturalistic physicians of half a century ago.

Some of the causes of a cleansing illness are quite modern, however. In particular, residues of the *pesticides** used routinely in agriculture persist in many samples of fresh vegetables and fruit. We know these accumulate in your body fat, but whether they cause disease is regarded as controversial. Research data from various sources, published in reputable scientific journals throughout the world over at least a decade, strongly suggest that they do. Chronic ALLERGY, mental confusion, swollen lymph GLANDS and *glandular fever** may all be associated with pesticide contamination at levels well within the range now found in Europeans and Americans.

Acute 'flu may seem to occur whenever weight loss, infection or any other sudden STRESS flushes accumulated pesticides and other fat-soluble chemicals out of your fat stores into your circulation. The symptoms arise from INFLAMMATION of the *tissues** irritated internally by these chemicals, and from your attempts to excrete them externally through CATARRH, diarrhoea, urine and sweat.

Modern allopathic medicine does not understand or believe in this problem, to the extent that no routine laboratory tests can be arranged to check whether an individual patient may be suffering from pesticide contamination. Indeed, pesticides are now in use for which no laboratory test yet exists! Doctors simply diagnose VIRUS INFECTION and recommend Aspirin, Paracetamol or Caffeine – which merely herds the chemical back into your fat and frustrates your attempt to get rid of their cause. This undoubtedly contributes to chronic degenerative diseases later in your life.

HELPING YOURSELF

Regard 'flu symptoms as evidence of your body's self-healing efforts. If you can possibly tolerate them, do not interfere. Avoid in particular all the pain-killing medicines, coffee, strong tea, chocolate, cola and tobacco.

Home-made Barley Water RECIPE is your best drink, whether the cause is chemical irritation or infection. Decline cordials and squashes; unsweetened fruit juice is preferable, diluted at least half-and-half with water.

You will not want to eat, and there is no need to. Leave food of any kind alone until your APPETITE returns. Then start with fresh fruit on the first day, add cooked vegetables on the second; wait until the third day before trusting your digestion on richer food.

Try to manage a shower each day; this will help ease FEVER and pain, and wash away dried perspiration.

Good BREATHING promotes excretion of volatile chemicals, many of which are difficult to excrete in any other way. It also helps prevent complications arising in your chest from CATARRHAL congestion there. Ventilate the room well, to keep the air fresh.

Infludo (Weleda UK Ltd) is an *anthroposophic** medicine based on herbs and low-potency homoeopathic dilutions, and specifically designed to relieve 'flu symptoms harmlessly. It can only be supplied on a doctor's prescription, privately or under the NHS.

Rest during the acute illness, and do not rush back to work when the obvious symptoms subside. Your stamina after VIRUS INFECTION will at first be very poor and needs time for convalescence. As a rule, allow two days of RECOVERY for every day of obvious illness. You may feel a fraud, but any attempted short-cut will prove that you are not.

*Influenza** IMMUNIZATION every autumn has some value against genuine infection with influenza or closely similar viruses and may stimulate your immune system generally. I should be happier if a more natural route than injection were developed. If you seem to get 'flu often, reinforcing your IMMUNITY by DIET and appropriate SUPPLEMENTS would be safer and more comprehensive.

If chronic accumulation of chemical residues seems the most likely fundamental cause of repeated 'flu bouts, use the special DIET and SUP-PLEMENTS recommended for cleansing elsewhere.

FOOD POISONING (adults), gastro-enteritis

WHAT HAPPENS

Your intestine forms part of your outside skin, folded through you like the hole in a cotton reel and sufficiently protected to be able to specialize in digestion and absorption. Large parts of its length become elaborately corrugated and pitted with crypts, all lined with fine fronds of delicate tissue – excellent for its purpose but very vulnerable.

Any foods synthesized artificially from refined ingredients, or contaminated with residues of agricultural, processing or preservative chemicals, unsettle this delicate situation. Damage is not gross or severe at first and is easily overlooked in the kind of laboratory safety tests applied to foods. But it nags away at you, spoiling the efficiency your digestion is capable of. If you eat these foods regularly their deleterious effects spread through your system, seriously eroding your overall health, which will eventually let you down badly. Quite a few people suffer irritable symptoms for years without realizing that their food is the cause.

Your gut obviously cannot tolerate anything grossly corrosive, irritant or INFLAMMATORY and takes uncompromising steps to get rid of it. Vomiting forcibly expels it by the way it came in, and rapid violent contractions hurry it along in the normal direction to be excreted as soon as possible; diarrhoea is watery because you have no time to reabsorb digestive juices from your bowel contents. This calls for exceptional activity in the wandering nerve that controls your intestine; its energy reverberates in the base of your brain, making you feel faint and shocked as well as nauseated.

This wretched condition occurs most suddenly and violently in chemical poisoning, and is then over fairly soon unless serious structural damage has been done, when continued pain and vomiting are less useful and may extend the damage. The diarrhoea may then be bloody, and a constant ache may underlie the rests between spasms of colic.

*Microbes** may need time to multiply into a colony large enough to cause symptoms, which are delayed and more gradual. They are usually prolonged as well since the microbes continue to multiply, undermining your efforts to expel them. That gives pus time to form as slime in the diarrhoea. Structural damage is less likely but significant losses of fluid, protein and minerals often occur. So long as these are replaced, RECOVERY coincides with the formation of specific antibody defences, which may take up to ten days in the more exotic INFECTIONS. These are still contracted sometimes, not only on holiday. At least two dysentery-type illnesses occur regularly in Britain, and resistance to ANTIBIOTICS is making their treatment increasingly unreliable.

Chemical contamination of your intestine affects your susceptibility to gastro-enteritis of this kind. By killing some of the *bacteria** that normally inhabit your intestine and play a part in digestion, chemicals can radically change the normal balance of microbial life in there. This means you have less to fight back with if more hostile microbes threaten to colonize you; they then have a better chance to get established, and are harder to throw off.

See also SICKNESS AND DIARRHOEA in children, and TRAVEL SICKNESS.

HELPING YOURSELF

Grow, buy and eat *'organic'** and *'biodynamic'** food in preference to anything else, because they are declared to be chemical-free. Be wary of processed and convenience foods, most of which list at least some of the chemical additives they contain; consult Felicity Lawrence's BOOK for details.

Wash fresh vegetables and fruit as thoroughly as you can, scrubbing skins that will be cooked or eaten. Soak leafy vegetables for some time, agitating them occasionally. A handful of salt in a basin of washing water helps to detach insects and slugs but must be rinsed off well afterwards.

Keep utensils free of non-nutrient chemical residues and bacterially contaminated food. Do not tolerate chipped, grubby or smeared cutlery and crockery on which microbes can easily persist. Even dampness gives them hope.

Rinse washing-up liquid off dishes very thoroughly, as residues get into your next meal and may erode your intestine.

Carefully scrub your finger-nails first thing every morning and after dirty work of any kind, and wash your hands fairly thoroughly with soap and water before handling or eating food. That keeps accidental doses of germs, THREAD-WORMS and chemicals small enough to cope with.

Avoid heavy consumption of anything rich or highly manufactured; spend the same on less of the good quality authentic food. A party that makes you sick is a pathetic way to have fun.

Control sudden violent *vomiting** by keeping warm and still between bouts. Try holding drops or a tablet of *homoeopathic** Ipecacuana 6 or 30 in your mouth whenever you can. A few drops of undiluted *Bach Rescue Remedy** can be used in the same way. If not relieved within half an hour, sip a wet slurry of arrowroot or three teaspoons of Kaolin Mixture in a little hot water.

Intractable vomiting cannot be allowed to continue for longer than four to six hours. It is then worth your doctor's attention.

Be slower to control *diarrhoea** in an adult. Use a long soak in a hot bath, followed by a tight wrap of cold damp cotton around your belly, to reduce the pain and violence. Homoeopathic Arsenicum album 6 often moderates it. Gentle slow clockwise massage of the stomach is comforting. After 6 hours take three teaspoons of Kaolin and Morphine Mixture in a little water, and repeat after four hours if the symptoms persist or return. Consult the doctor after three doses or in any case if blood or pus appears.

FUNGUS INFECTIONS

Fungi are quite different in their behaviour from *bacteria*,* VIRUSES and other one-cell organisms. They are very primitive microscopic plants, but are unable to make food for themselves by photosynthesis in the way most plants do. All fungi are therefore obliged to scrounge their nourishment from the better equipped creatures they live on, which is why moulds are so consistently associated with decay. But they are by no means always parasitic in their habits. Many lodge with their hosts rather than living at their expense, and some even pay for their keep.

Their usual pattern of growth is to form a *mycelium*,* a network of root-like fibres which cling to and feed on the surface of their host. From this foundation grows a microscopic forest of stems which may support *spores** – very tough and heavily coated seeds that will resist drought, time and many chemicals without losing their viability. From this exposed position the spores are easily scattered on a puff of air or brushed onto the coat of a passing animal. A wide selection can always be found in the dust of even the cleanest houses. Out of doors they live on the skins of practically all fruit varieties and play an important part in their ALCOHOLIC fermentation to wines.

Mycelia of various fungus species can grow in your skin, as a spreading ECZEMATOUS ring in *ringworm** or producing a rash of deathly-coloured soggy scales and crusts in warm damp places, such as your groin or armpit or between your toes; *athlete's foot** is probably the commonest infection in the developed world. It or its relatives can infiltrate your finger tips and nails, cracking and deforming them. In AIDS or other IMMUNO-deficient states mycelium may invade your lungs but otherwise are never permitted so far.

The spores of some fungi do not necessarily form a mycelium but are able to adopt a cellular habit more like bacteria. Fungi that can rely on shelter and abundant provisions from their hosts may spend most of their lives in this cellular form. Yeasts are the most familiar examples, many of which have lost or else rarely use their mycelial habit. Some however retain the possibility of transforming from cells to mycelium and back again, according to the conditions they find themselves in.

*Candida albicans** is one of these. It depends on people for its livelihood, and inhabits your intestine shortly after birth in small cellular colonies that digest remnants of sugar and starch, make a certain amount of GAS but do no real harm.

However, if your IMMUNITY is temporarily deficient for any reason, these colonies may spread and transform to mycelia, which are much more troublesome. THRUSH is the commonest cause of VAGINAL DISCHARGE, which may be very tame or stubbornly aggressive. Internally THRUSH mycelium has no respect for the natural barriers of your body and can penetrate almost anywhere. It can then run down your IMMUNITY much further by conveying from your intestine to unauthorized places partly digested food not yet stamped with your *'colour'.** But it remains well camouflaged and takes a very long time to eradicate.

HELPING YOURSELF

Keep your skin well aired and cool. Do not over-dress and keep to natural fabrics – cotton and wool – for the clothing next to your skin. Stockings and suspenders are usually better than tights.

Choose shoes with leather uppers at least, as these will ventilate your FEET; they also return good value for money if you look after them, by packing them with dry newspaper immediately you take them off to absorb their moisture. Wear sandals without socks or go barefoot at every opportunity.

Sun bathing is sometimes hazardous, but air-bathing never is. Simply wear the minimum clothing and let the air get to your body. This restores it to the climate which most naturally resists significant fungus infection. Ten minutes spent naked each day makes a significant difference, even indoors in winter.

Make a habit of brushing your skin all over with a soft brush or dry loofa every morning during your dressing routine. When you bang the loofa afterwards against the palm of your hand, clouds of spent skin scales billow out. These are meat and drink to fungi, which cannot thrive on you without them. What is more this habit hardens your skin appreciably over several weeks, so that spores are less likely to lodge there and germinate.

Take the precautions against internal THRUSH given elsewhere; they also help to prevent CONSTIPATION and GAS.

GALLSTONES'

Your *liver** is a highly organized *metabolic** factory with five different trees of branching pipework to cope with its complex functions. One of these is to make *bile,** which is a bit like golden washing-up liquid. It trickles into its own pipe system and collects between meals in a small balloon called your gall bladder. This is the nearest thing you have to a squeezy-bottle, but much cleverer. It concentrates and acidifies the bile by reabsorbing three-quarters of its water and some of its solids, leaving behind a liquid loaded with emulsifying salts made from *cholesterol.** You squirt this liquid into your intestine whenever there is fat in it, to emulsify that into droplets fine enough to be absorbed from there and carried back to your liver for digestion.

Fats are not easy to dispose of and you take advantage of bile to get rid of several, including a little cholesterol. The amount in your bile is very small, considering the trouble it can give you. It depends on a careful balance with the emulsifying salts also present to stay harmlessly dissolved.

This is drastically upset if you become accustomed to eating sugar, as most people in all economically developed countries have done. In coping with an increase in annual sugar consumption over the last century from one to twenty-five kilograms we Westerners have considerably increased our cholesterol production. Some research workers believe that the corresponding reduction in fibre intake has interfered with conversion of this cholesterol to emulsifying salts, so that the amount entering your bile is proportionately less than the cholesterol there and cannot cope with it.

These disturbances precipitate small solid particles of cholesterol out of solution, usually mixed with chalk (calcium carbonate). Unless you change your DIET enough to tip the balance decisively in your favour, these particles grow very gradually into dust, then grains and finally small pebbles.

At some stage in this progression you are likely to experience PAIN as one of the stones blocks the exit tube. INFLAMMATION and INFECTION provoked by such episodes eventually wear out your gall bladder, which becomes leaky and unable to maintain the necessary balance of acidity and salts in your bile. Stones then enlarge out of all control, to the size of sugar lumps. You can easily have twenty or thirty of these, after a few decades of gradual development. But occasionally, by a slightly different process, you form just one or two much larger stones of pure crystalline cholesterol. The only treatment doctors ever consider is SURGICAL removal.

Gallstones form in around ten women and two men out of every hundred industrialized people. They do not always produce disease, and only after about forty years; but when they do it is costly and dangerous. There is a respectable scientific basis for classifying it with the *saccharine diseases** described in Cleave's BOOK, all of which would be decimated by a drastic reduction in the sale and consumption of refined sugar and starches. No profession or government that fails to tackle this clear-cut and simple issue can seriously claim to be interested in promoting public health.

HELPING YOURSELF

Start on the DIET for health as a matter of urgency if stones are discovered or suspected in your gall bladder, whether or not they are already causing you disease. Reduce drastically your consumption of animal fats and meat, and cut out all sugar and refined flour. Emphasize instead apples, citrus fruits, tomatoes and berries in season, whole-grain cereals, the cabbage family and parsley. These keep your cholesterol intake low, and the types of fibre they contain help you to get rid of cholesterol from your intestine instead of recycling it.

SUPPLEMENT this with lots of Vitamin C (1000mg three times daily) to make fat deposits easier to handle. Lecithin (500mg daily), or Choline and Inositol (500mg each twice daily), from which you can make it, strongly reinforces this effect but adds to the expense. Vitamin E (200IU twice daily) would be an additional advantage. Continue all these for six months, then depend on your diet and the Vitamin C alone.

Mineral supplement foods are rather important. Egg nog and Honey Cider Vinegar RECIPES provide them inexpensively, but additional Zinc 10–20mg daily for 3–6 months would be wise. If money is no object take two Nature's Own Multimineral tablets daily, obtainable through the mail order ADDRESS.

Check that COLDNESS is not part of the reason for your cholesterol problem.

Angelica herb tea or Liver Herb extract (Nature's Own Ltd), has a useful tonic effect on your liver function.

If PAIN from stones in a reasonably healthy gall bladder is getting troublesome, consult a *Naturopath*,* spiritual *Healer** or Practitioner of *Traditional Chinese Medicine** (ADDRESSES). The first can guide you through a two-day fast followed by a pint of olive oil emulsified with orange juice, taken as quickly as you can manage. This strongly promotes gall bladder action, which can extrude the stones into your bowel. Do *not* try this one on your own! The other practitioners may be able to help you achieve the same by less strenuous means.

If it looks as if you may need SURGERY, delay it as long as possible by excluding fats from your diet and help your surgeon by getting rid of OVERWEIGHT. Alter your diet anyway to prevent the basic disease continuing.

Once your gall bladder has been removed you will not be able to digest fats so efficiently, so continue to avoid large quantities indefinitely.

GAS, wind, flatulence

From childhood, nearly every Westerner makes wind that smells unpleasant. You were taught to hold it in company, and let it out quietly in the toilet or out of doors. Learn now to avoid making it in the first place and you can give your children a valuable legacy.

Healthy digestion makes no gas, and the little you swallow accidentally with your food makes up most of what you have to contend with. The small colonies of THRUSH that survive in your bowel digest sugar residues into carbon dioxide, which is inoffensive and never in health amounts to much.

If your food contains too little fibrous vegetable matter, however, the *coliform bacteria** which normally thrive peacefully on that take to living on meat instead. As a result they make more complex nitrogenous gases that are both obnoxious and toxic. These gases, together with other chemicals the bacteria produce, change the climate of your COLON from acid to alkaline. That very much favours THRUSH which, like many other FUNGI, can live peacefully alongside you in small colonies throughout your life but quickly takes advantage of any opportunity to multiply. That adds increasing quantities of carbon dioxide to your gas problem.

If you eat lots of sugar some gets through to your colon, actively feeding your thrush. They soon outgrow their usual limited quarters and are not easily confined. Furthermore the kind of diet that lacks fibre and contains lots of sugar is also likely to lack B Vitamins; in the absence of one of them, Biotin, THRUSH is apt to transform from its cellular form into a *mycelium.** This enables the colony to break bounds and spread up into your small intestine, where the alkaline climate still favours them. Yeasts you swallow with your food can grow in the upper part of your stomach, and spores may survive its acid bath to reach your intestines from above. Once there they can feed sumptuously on any sugar you eat, making lots of gas and spreading more complex effects elsewhere.

All this is very insidious, and is not yet recognized at all by most doctors though they have useful remedies at their disposal. Most of them regard wind as inevitable and harmless, and their patients give up consulting them for it. This throws away an excellent opportunity to prevent more serious trouble many years later in your life, when continuing chronic irritation from these noxious chemicals has begun to produce COLITIS or chronic CONSTIPATION, perhaps ultimately bowel CANCER.

Unfortunately some of the remedies put forward by alternative schools of thought are unreliable, depend on expensive supplement programmes and may have to be continued for many months or even a few years to produce satisfactory results. As is usual whenever professional groups disagree but will not debate the issues sensibly together, real progress stagnates and their patients lose out. Even if you understand and can cope with this, you must add to your medical problem a tactical one you could do without.

HELPING YOURSELF

Your doctor or chemist can supply medicinal charcoal tablets or sachets, which will soak up the gas like blotting paper; but do not depend on these as a remedy, merely as temporary relief. Homoeopathic Carbo Veg (vegetable charcoal) in low potency may be just as effective and more economical.

Then recondition the climate in your bowel. Eat lots of fresh root and leaf vegetables, as in the cleansing DIET. Avoid absolutely all sugars and starchy foods such as cereals, especially bread; candida mycelium can feed on intact starch grains (CATARRH). To begin with you will also need to be wary of starchy roots and fruit such as potatoes and bananas. Broken nuts and citrus fruit are unsafe because they are usually teeming with fungi. Avoidance of meat, coupled with this increase in fibrous vegetable food, will coax Coliforms back onto their cellulose diet, which tames them dramatically.

Stewed apple purée is a first class intestinal cleanser; cook and store it in steel or glass as it cleans aluminium too! Eat it exclusively for two days and watch your tongue become clean and pink – a sign of similar improvements further down.

Once your tongue is clean and you have a hearty APPETITE again, make raw fresh vegetables or fruit your first course; these will pass easily through your stomach* and get your intestinal* digestion going, ready to greet any cooked food that follows. Next eat the rich protein food – meat, fish, eggs, hard cheese, nuts or unsprouted beans – which can sit alone in the acid bath of your stomach and get the attention it needs. Finally eat the starchy vegetables or bread, which can sit in your stomach hopper digesting in your saliva. This way you are far less likely to make gas by mistakenly mixing up these separate processes.

Make live yoghurt RECIPE and add this to your first course. The Lactobacillus used to make it is of the Acidophilus kind, and a proportion will get through your stomach in small vegetable or fruit meals to thrive in your large bowel. Less will survive as the dessert to a heavy meal.

Beware of expensive 'Acidophilus' cultures, because most of them die before they are consumed. A SUPPLEMENT of Biotin (50–250mcg with three meals daily) is wise, however, because it helps to prevent mycelial transformation. Other items may be necessary if you appear to be ALLERGIC to lots of things; your IMMUNE system may need boosting.

Explain your problem to your doctor, and see if he would be willing to prescribe Nystatin tablets for six months or even a year, on NHS prescriptions; the charge is good value, even if you have to pay it monthly. Even one month will be useful; most of the real work is done by your diet anyway. You need one or two tablets four times daily, at least one hour before meals and as regularly spaced as possible. Wash the colouring off the tablets and crush them thoroughly in water before taking them.

A Homoeopathic practitioner can offer an alternative remedy, a high potency of Candida Albicans; you should consult his advice.

Raw fresh garlic deters Candida very strongly.

Lymph GLANDS

Most people think of the arteries, capillaries and veins which contain their blood as a closed CIRCULATION around their bodies. This is anatomically accurate, but does not adequately portray what is involved in nourishing and cleansing each *cell** in every *tissue** your capillaries pass through. To manage this, nourishing and aerated blood liquid – *plasma** – must ooze out of the capillaries at their high-pressure ends where they enter the tissue as the final branches of the artery to that *organ.** This fluid then disperses around the tissue and bathes every cell, exchanging its fresh contents for stale residues the cell no longer wants. Most of this fluid is then gradually sucked towards the capillaries again – but this time at their low-pressure ends where they are really tiny veins. Your body fluids actually spend most of their time adrift in your tissues in this way.

A small proportion of this fluid does not return to a blood vessel directly after its wanderings but is drawn into a secondary system of blind-headed drainage gulleys called *lymphatics,** which pick up the spilt fluid and take it back to your circulation by another route. Lymphatics are very numerous everywhere in your body but are less obvious than veins and arteries because they are small and transparent and consequently rarely thought about. The tiniest contribute their contents into larger and larger trunk vessels in just the same way as veins, although they are never anything like as large. The largest eventually meet in the centre of your body and empty into a main vein on the left side of your neck.

This secondary circulation provides your IMMUNE system with an opportunity to sample what is going into the core of your body from the periphery, and intervene if you come under any kind of threat. The lymphatic system washes your tissues clean of any *microbes** that penetrate the skin of your mouth or nose, and any pieces of dirt that get into your body through any INJURY. Most of these are fortunately too large to soak into blood vessels in any case, but must not get any chance to do so. Material like this can clog the capillaries in your lungs or else quickly INFECT the whole of your body.

So whenever injury or infection riddles a local area of your body with microbes or debris, your lymphatics take on greater importance and drain away a greater proportion of the tissue fluid – especially if tension in the area flattens some of the venous capillaries, effectively shutting them down. But this would convey no advantage if the lymphatic system did not include some means for filtering out all this unwanted material and making it harmless.

Your lymph glands provide this. They are small soft rounded swellings stationed at intervals along your lymphatics, often at junctions. They vary in size from a lentil to a broad bean according to their importance and activity. They swell most when dealing with living microbes, since these actively resist destruction and arouse a full INFLAMMATORY response. This includes making a permanent stock of IMMUNE antibody tailored to that microbe, so that in future you can deal with it quickly and without fuss, wherever in your body it gains entry.

HELPING YOURSELF

Swollen glands can often be felt on each side of your windpipe during a SORE THROAT or COLD. Usually they subside within a day or two, except in children who meet new microbes more often than adults and may go on making antibodies for several weeks. If they are thriving despite their enlarged glands, you need not worry for at least a month. Otherwise see your doctor.

Glands at the back of your neck are smaller, and drain your neck, scalp and ears. Swelling of these glands is a feature of *rubella (German Measles)*,* but more usually follows infected ear-piercings, insect BITES and scratches. In these cases antiseptic on the sore place settles the gland quickly as a rule.

Glands in an arm-pit or groin drain the corresponding limb and nearby skin structures on your body, such as your BREASTS. Minor shaving wounds, *sebaceous cysts*,* scratches and insect bites are still common causes of swelling, but see your doctor if you cannot find an obvious cause.

*Glandular Fever** is a generalized, prolonged and weakening illness with swellings everywhere. It is supposed to be a particularly aggressive VIRUS INFECTION, but it can happen with any generalized virus if your resistance is poor. Vitamin and mineral SUPPLEMENTS to enhance your IMMUNITY help most people recover more quickly but are better used to prevent it in the first place.

Lymph glands are an important line of defence when spreading tissue damage occurs for other reasons, such as CANCER. In that case they demonstrate your body's readiness to tidy things up and regain command of the disordered part: do not panic, help it! But see the doctor too. You can be healed, and maybe you can be cured. You just have to find out why things went wrong and set that right. There are many groups and treatment agencies available to help you, and you have the time you need. Remember – panic only spreads dismay, whereas wholesome action gives you fresh heart and a completely different outlook. Even at the very worst, you have nothing to fear but fear itself.

HAIR LOSS, baldness, alopecia

Your scalp, the skin on the dome of your head, is rather special. It is firmly stitched to a fibrous layer underneath it called the *galea*,* which moves freely over the surface of your skull. It is anchored to the back of your head by a sheet of muscle that extends almost to your crown, with which you can twitch your galea back and forth. Its front edge is also muscular but unattached, able only to wrinkle your forehead and raise your eyebrows. Its breadth extends on either side of your crown almost to your ears. This unusual arrangement means that the CIRCULATION to your scalp can only get in at its edges. Several arteries terminate there in a web of connections under your scalp, from which capillaries feed the hair roots all over it.

Men have an additional factor to contend with. From your late TEENS to your mid fifties, when male hormone production is at its strongest, its influence makes your galea gradually thicken and get tougher. Dense unyielding fibrous undergrowth becomes its dominant feature, and exactly underlies the area of typical male baldness. This fibrous tissue is liable to shrink gradually, corrugating your forehead, tightening around your capillaries and starving your hair roots of blood. Only the onset of middle age checks this development, and by RETIREMENT the fibres are weakening again.

Your inherent virility influences the outcome of this very much, because having lots of male hormone makes the process more aggressive. Consequently baldness tends to run in families, on the men's side. But many other factors help to determine how well your CIRCULATION copes with it. Your DIET and scalp hygiene are foremost among them. Virile men on processed Western diets who shampoo their scalp regularly are on balance very susceptible to hair loss over the galea.

This is the commonest form of hair loss, but not the only one. Any deterioration in the health of your scalp, such as DANDRUFF, may thin out the hair all over your scalp and shorten the life of each strand. COLDNESS attributable to thyroid insufficiency has the same effect. Sometimes a small patch of your scalp goes bald for a time, when its CIRCULATION is badly hit; in this case hair usually grows again as the blood vessels RECOVER.

The most common cause of widespread hair loss is medical treatment with certain anti-CANCER or *immunosuppressive** drugs, which interfere sufficiently with hair growth to shut it down temporarily. Hair usually re-grows normally when you have recovered from the course of treatment. Rarer than this is the dramatic generalized *alopecia** that affects a very few people quite suddenly, often in your TEENS, in which you may in quite a short period lose every strand of hair from all over your body. This can affect either sex, often after a serious STRESS or shock, and does not usually recover. Its cause is a mystery.

None of the common forms of alopecia seem to interest doctors much, for very few have taken the trouble to explore them. No drugs work so they assume there is no treatment, and give complacent advice or none at all.

HELPING YOURSELF

Look after your skin and CIRCULATION to prevent baldness of any type, whatever your inherited tendencies may be. Give them plenty of air and a fair share of sunlight.

Never bunch a pony-tail or bun tightly, or use curlers or rollers overnight. These habits stretch your hair root capillaries, narrowing their blood flow; this not only weakens the hairs you have now but can starve their roots to death.

Beware of wearing hats that fit tightly; these spoil the CIRCULATION to your scalp unnecessarily.

Brush your hair thoroughly for three to five minutes twice each day. Use a fine natural bristle brush, and vary the direction of your strokes – from the crown downwards in all four directions, then from every direction up towards your crown, for half a minute each. This massages and cleans your scalp and hair very thoroughly without disturbing its natural chemical climate, and prevents DANDRUFF far better than shampoo. Shampoo your hairbrush often, by all means – not your hair.

Make your DIET healthier, cutting down especially on meat and animal fats, refined starchy foods and salt – all of which clutter your blood and crowd out the necessities. Abundant fresh fruit and vegetables, supported by wholegrain cereals, supply most of what your hair needs. Honey Cider Vinegar or Egg Nog RECIPE, SUPPLEMENTED with a tablet of kelp and a teaspoon of cod or halibut liver oil each day, augment your supply of the relevant minerals, Vitamins (A and D) and Essential Fatty Acids.

Stop SMOKING.

You can reinforce all this with massage for five minutes twice daily if you have the time. Plant the tips of all your fingers and thumbs firmly in a close pattern on one area of your scalp; stretch it in every direction, wriggling it as vigorously as you can, for a few seconds; then move on to another area. If you find this tiresome, use a simple vibro-massager instead.

If your hair is thinning or you are recently bald, intensify your efforts. Pad an old door with foam rubber for use as a slant-board, and arrange to support it at one end 18–20" (45–50cm) off the floor. Lie on this for fifteen minutes twice a day, on your back with your head downwards. Massaging and brushing your scalp in this position powerfully restores its circulation. Additional SUPPLEMENTS of Brewer's Yeast (six tablets daily), Vitamins A (as Halibut Liver Oil), C (1000mg twice daily) and E (100IU twice daily), Lecithin (500mg twice daily) and Essential Fatty Acids (eg Blackcurrant Seed Oil 500mg twice daily with your Vitamin E) are worthwhile for three months.

So is trial of a local stimulant such as Aloe Vera gel, castor oil or cayenne in spirit; look up BOOKS by Airola, Levy and Mellor for details.

HAY FEVER, chronic rhinitis

The predominant vegetation throughout Europe and most temperate regions of the world was originally forest. Human beings have since medieval times gradually cleared the trees to make way for agricultural pastures and crops, including cereals bred from many wild grass varieties. Grasses are now the predominant greenery of the developed world, and yield an unnaturally intensive harvest of grass pollens during the months of May, June and July.

Your IMMUNE system can cope much better with a wide diversity of small STRESSES than large doses of a few. Consequently you can tolerate almost anything you inhale or eat as one of many small challenges in a rich and seasonally variable cocktail. But anything that looms large or persistently in your environment begins to irritate, and can provoke you into ALLERGY or an over-reaction resembling it.

*Atopic** people are as a result often ALLERGIC to grass pollen, with all the constitutional changes doctors expect to find in such cases. The proportion has never been high, and is probably not rising. In addition to features such as ECZEMA and ASTHMA, these people commonly endure hay fever from May to July, during which time any exposure to grass provokes sneezing, ITCHING and profuse clear nasal CATARRH.

But many others are becoming *intolerant** of the non-nutrient chemicals which increasingly contaminate your food, water and air. Something like thirty thousand different chemicals are now in use. About four thousand are deliberately added to manufactured foods, and many more get there by accident. Ten new chemicals are coming into use each week. It seems you simply cannot cope with the novelty of all this, and develop intolerance symptoms much more easily than a few years ago. Perpetual chemical irritation has in turn reduced your IMMUNE tolerance of the foods themselves – especially those that are now unnaturally plentiful throughout the year.

Wheat and other cereals are in this category, so that many people only just manage to tolerate them without symptoms. A heavy seasonal barrage of closely related pollens finally breaks you down, with violent expulsive efforts in your nose, eyes and throat. Sneezing, ITCHING, congestion and copious watery discharge may give way to more chronic INFLAMMATORY changes, perhaps including stubborn COUGHING or even ASTHMA.

Unfortunately the season may never seem to end. Once your immune tolerance has been breached, intensive effort will be needed to restore it to its former strength. Otherwise your nose remains chronically irritable, provoked as easily by substances inside your blood as from the outside by irritants you inhale. Unaccountable bouts of *chronic** or *allergic rhinitis** are the result, which you probably mistake for repeated COLDS. No VIRUS INFECTION would last as long as these bouts can – up to months at a time. Explore instead what is irritating you; otherwise your symptoms will get more stubborn and more disabling as your IMMUNE system progressively loses its grip.

HELPING YOURSELF

Try to identify exactly what you are reacting to, by the method described in Mansfield and Monro's BOOK. The special DIET for ALLERGY is a simplified version of their recommendations.

If your problem is still mainly seasonal, obtain nine pounds of honey collected from local hives just afterwards, and eat a tablespoonful of it daily throughout the three months preceding your next hay fever season. This will acclimatize you to the pollens you have to tolerate then, and may enable you to do so without symptoms. The British Beekeepers' Association (ADDRESS) can put you in touch with members in your area, but a local wholefood shop may stock their produce anyway – look for the characteristic label, over-printed with the bee-keeper's name and address.

You cannot help what you breathe, but have control of what you eat. Throughout the hay fever season and for two months beforehand eat the DIET for health, leaving out all cereal foods to reduce your overall exposure to grasses. Do not then rely too much on something else, in case you break down your tolerance of that as well. Rotate your foods, sampling each family for three consecutive days and avoiding it for the rest of the week, as detailed in Mansfield and Monro's BOOK. By staggering your use of each food family through the week you can still have a diverse and interesting diet.

If necessary SUPPLEMENT this diet for IMMUNITY. Large doses of Vitamin C, from 2000mg daily upwards, are particularly helpful and inexpensive.

Keep fresh cultivated flowers in your home throughout the winter, and sniff them hard several times each day. Flowers are bred for their blooms at the expense of their pollen, so this habit keeps you accustomed to inhaling it regularly in small amounts. The pollen season therefore comes as less of a shock, and you may cope without symptoms.

Cold water showered directly on your face for several minutes helps control an attack of allergic rhinitis, if only for an hour or two. *Homoeopathic** Mixed Pollen (Weleda UK Ltd) abolishes the symptoms of about half the people that try it. If it fails at first, try raising the potency.

Decongestants are less sedative than the antihistamines most doctors prescribe. Try not to use either for more than four days in each week, to retain their full effect and avoid dependence on them.

*Yoga** teaches a method of breathing which gradually reduces the sen-sitivity of your nose over a period of years, and has on occasion cured hay fever outright. Contact a local teacher through the ADDRESS.

Beards and moustaches are a liability to rhinitis sufferers. Try the effect of shaving them off.

HEADACHE

Headache is probably the commonest symptom of all, suffered by almost everyone at some time or another. It rarely signifies any serious *'mono'** disorder that your doctor is at home with – very high BLOOD PRESSURE, or something pressing on your brain. After that his expertise is less precise; your hunch can easily be as good as his or better.

It cannot be comprehensively explained in 'mono' terms. Generalized congestive and INFLAMMATORY problems may cause headaches, and arise in turn from accumulation of waste acids in your blood-stream; these require the same treatment as MIGRAINE. SINUSITIS, EARACHE, SORE THROAT and TONSILITIS are all inflammatory diseases localized in your head, so that the PAIN which always results from inflammation in confined spaces may seem like headache. A FEVER that is too high dilates blood vessels in your head and makes it feel as if it will burst. *Meningitis** or *encephalitis** headache is very severe, and makes you want to hold your head back to relieve it a little. These require urgent medical attention.

Structural disorders of your *neck,** and CONCUSSION or other INJURIES to your head or spine, even many years ago, are much more chronic than inflammatory conditions and often relate predictably to POSTURE or TIRED- NESS; they are described in more detail elsewhere, and can usually be dealt with. The headache of ELECTRICITY DISEASE can be remedied by modifying the electrical quality of your surroundings. HYPOGLYCAEMIA headache goes with mental confusion, and tends to occur during long gaps between meals, whether you are aware of hunger or not. Brain ALLERGY, such as can occur in severe generalized THRUSH, may cause headaches that coincide with ALCO- HOLIC bouts and are wrongly attributed to drunkenness.

Quite a few headaches coincide with CRAMP or muscle TENSION in your neck, scalp or face; even your jaw muscles get involved if the set of your TEETH is wrong. You can spot all these by the tenderness and rigid feel of the muscles affected, especially when compared with someone else's.

When all have been explained this way that can, many headaches remain to be accounted for. They cannot be precisely located in your brain as 'mono' sensations are, and seem to be a purely *'colour'** disease in which energy around your head is excessive.

Yogic philosophers understand this from the way 'colour' moves into your body – entering from above your head, flowing down your spine, and spreading forward into your softer parts through seven energy centres cor- responding to important nerve plexuses in your 'mono' anatomy. That flow is frequently blocked in modern Westerners, by unhealthy 'colour' will or by inadequately treated INJURY in or near your spine. Frustrated energy is not only confined in your head but reverberates there, like an oceanic swell breaking in a sheer-walled cove. It is little wonder that you feel so ill at ease and out of balance, with little APPETITE or energy for action.

Relax and massage your face, neck and scalp. Stretch, and take a quick break of routine, in fresh air if you can. Take ten deep BREATHS with your diaphragm, giving each all your attention; sigh and relax as you exhale. Close your eyes if they feel tired or heavy. Splash your face freely with cold water or apply *Eau de Cologne* to refresh you before resuming work.

If headache persists into your leisure time, recline comfortably while someone wriggles the skin of your scalp and brow with gentle, quick circular motions of their finger-tips, moving them to a new site every few seconds. Ten minutes of this is very soothing and almost hypnotic.

Or take a hot relaxing bath with sprigs or oil of lavender. After drying wrap a cold damp (spun-dry) cotton or linen cloth tightly around your body from armpits to hips, fastening it with safety-pins at close intervals. Cover it with a warm woollen garment, or get into bed. This draws frustrated energy down your body and decongests your head.

A simple foot bath may have the same effect, with less fuss. Note whether your feet feel cold or hot during the headache, and immerse them in water of the opposite temperature for several minutes.

A tea of fresh or dried mint or rosemary often relieves headache. It is usually helpful to drink something but avoid coffee and strong Indian tea.

If you regularly have sick headaches in the morning or during leisure time, a process similar to that in MIGRAINE is probably responsible; a special DIET for cleansing is the most direct route to a dependable cure.

*Homoeopathic** books devote pages to distinguishing headache remedies, according to their precise location and character. You will need to take professional advice for a chronic problem. Meanwhile try Bidor 5% tablets (Weleda UK Ltd), an *anthroposophic** headache remedy with wide application.

An *Osteopath** can often cure minor dislocations in your spine which frustrate energy flow and give you repeated headaches. Cranial osteopathy can tackle old injuries to your head. Find a practitioner near you from the Register of Osteopaths' ADDRESS.

All this may fail to abolish the headaches that arise easily in responsible, reliable people under pressure. The 'colour' of the situations in which they arise is probably familiar; that may tell you how it started, and gives you some clue about what to do. How severe it becomes is some guide to urgency: step aside from your obligations if necessary to get right. Try to see the common denominator in headache situations which will explain why they recur, so that you can learn to handle their cause more wholesomely. *Counselling**, *Relaxation for Living** or *meditation** (ADDRESSES) may help you succeed at all these levels.

HYPERACTIVITY, difficult children, hyperkinetic syndrome

Twentieth-century industry has introduced to the world many chemical substances that can never have existed before, because the conditions to create them do not occur naturally. Their commercial potential has been exploited long before their full effects on people could possibly have been discovered, and they have inevitably leaked accidentally into parts of your environment where they have no place. Many of them are accumulating there and in your body because neither you nor the rest of nature have yet worked out how to exploit them, make them harmless or dispose of them permanently. Almost without exception they are individually irritant or poisonous, sometimes in very small concentrations. Their possible inter-actions with each other are almost infinite, and virtually unexplored; nonetheless we can be sure that together they profoundly disturb the balance of natural things.

The coincident exploitation of *electro-magnetic radiations** is exploding even faster and more boldly, if that is possible. Their quality is not new to us, but the spectrum and intensities of human exposure have altered beyond recognition. A new ELECTRICITY DISEASE consequently affects some people, which only unbalances their IMMUNE mechanisms further.

Children are especially vulnerable to all these disturbances, receptive as they are to new impressions of every kind. Their brains mature slowly, and are wide open to chemical and electromagnetic contamination which may distort the *'colour'** blueprint for their development, with lifelong consequences.

So by no means all the irritability and awkwardness children display nowadays results from bad parenting or weak social control, but it has been hard to convince doctors of this. The symptoms are only obvious in 'colour', and have evaded *'mono'* detection until recently. But acceptable measures of environmentally disturbed behaviour are now in use in Germany and the USA, and reveal effects from chemicals and common foods in about two children per hundred. I believe the true proportion is now nearer 5%, and rising steeply.

The behaviour is fully described in BOOKS by Barnes and Colquhoun, and Mansfield and Monro. Its severity and persistence vary widely, and is likely to coincide with ALLERGIES such as nasal ITCHING and CATARRH, ECZEMA, seasonal HAY FEVER and ASTHMA. A normally likeable child is seized by spells completely out of character, when he is unaccountable, unpredictable, impulsive, very clumsy and inept, often violent, intolerant and easily frustrated. His energy seems inexhaustible, on very little sleep. He is not in control, but at odds with himself. All this begins twenty minutes to two days after the beginning of a new exposure, and rumbles on continually if the irritant is not withdrawn.

If they grow up undetected, affected children are likely to become violent and vandalous, and will sooner or later come into conflict with the law. Evidence is accumulating that many young people in remand homes, prisons and Borstal institutions are hyperactive, and respond dramatically to improvement in their DIET and withdrawal of common chemical irritants.

HELPING YOURSELF

Commence a cleansing DIET straight away, scrupulously eliminating sugar, refined flour, artificial food colourings and preservatives, and fluoride toothpaste or supplements. Put up with the tantrums withdrawal of favourite foods may precipitate; you must at all costs get the victim's APPETITE on your side.

SUPPLEMENT this diet for IMMUNITY and CLEANSING alternately, six weeks each way. Vitamin B$_{15}$ (Pangamic Acid 50mg twice daily) and Siberian Ginseng (600mg three times daily) are particularly useful additions.

If he does not improve dramatically check for food ALLERGIES using the special DIET, starting with the food families he craves most passionately. Food from the cow, wheat, chicken produce, citrus fruit, fish and the potato family (which includes tomatoes, peppers and aubergines) cover most of these. Consult Mansfield and Monro's BOOK for full details.

If you draw a blank try the salicylate-free DIET for at least three weeks, keeping otherwise to the basic exclusions listed at the beginning of this section.

If you are still in trouble you need help. Write to the ADDRESS for the Hyperactive Children's Support Group, who have the most reliable self-help experience and advice to share with you.

Occasionally people fail because sensitivities are too numerous, and include chemicals it is difficult to exclude. In that case use the ADDRESS of the Environmental Medicine Foundation, who can help you identify the sensitivities and prepare vaccines or drops to neutralize them. If your doctor is willing, on-going treatment can be covered by the National Health Service.

Although the problems are daunting at first, success rapidly simplifies them. Intolerances get fewer, general health improves, mistakes become easier to spot and rectify, and normal life becomes possible again. So persevere!

HYPOGLYCAEMIA, low blood sugar

WHAT HAPPENS

This is a topic most doctors simply refuse to believe in, mainly because they are not prepared to prolong the test for DIABETES sufficiently to spot it, or else make no attempt to reproduce the STRESSFUL tone of ordinary life as a background to the test. Yet experienced physicians who look for it claim that it affects up to one American in ten during some part of their day; Europeans are unlikely to be far behind. Fredericks' BOOK sets out the details.

When your healthy body is deluged with refined sugar, it is forced to respond with a huge pulse of *insulin** wrenched urgently from storage in your *pancreas.** This synchronizes imperfectly with the arrival of the sugar in your blood, so that spare insulin is still around when all the sugar is dealt with: the level of sugar in your blood goes on dropping, which provokes release of *steroid** hormones from your *adrenal** gland to offset the insulin effect.

This exactly corresponds to fast acceleration in your car followed by savage braking, and is just as wasteful and wearing. Before too long your pancreas and adrenal tire and begin to respond more sluggishly to these relentless mealtime challenges. Even more insulin needs mopping up, and it takes longer to work up enough steroid to do it. Consequently your blood gets very short of sugar for a time, around three or four hours after the meal.

This makes you giddy, confused, FAINT, inattentive, irritable, NERVOUS or TIRED, and may produce severe HEADACHE. You are much more likely at these times to behave unreasonably or violently, to make stupid and serious mistakes, to be involved in accidents or to take decisions you later regret and may not even remember.

Every time it happens you crave for a sugary snack – ALCOHOL, sweet bakery or confectionery. Any of these works in the short run, but only brings on another hypoglycaemic bout a few hours later. Over a period of months or years this habit progressively unbalances your general nutrition, and may lead to serious dependence on alcohol or manufactured counterfeit foods.

STRESS, NERVOUSNESS or PREMENSTRUAL TENSION are all made much more difficult to bear by hypoglycaemia. On the other hand they conspire to exhaust your adrenal sooner and more precipitately, thereby bringing hypo-glycaemia into the open. However, since the symptoms are vague and apparently neurotic, they tend to be discounted even by sympathetic medical advisers, especially after painstaking routine biochemical investigations have failed to reveal any well established disorder. You are then discredited in your doctor's eyes, and left to suffer; any return visits you may make only reinforce and harden his attitude. For the lack of simple advice your pancreas follows your adrenal into feebleness over the next decade or so. By then you are DIABETIC, but unlikely to be discovered early because you have 'cried wolf once too often'.

Hypoglycaemia is easily and inexpensively treated, and gives ample warning of a serious preventable condition that now spoils RETIREMENT for many people. It is scandalous to neglect it so complacently.

HELPING YOURSELF

If your symptoms appear to fit this description, consult your doctor and say so. Receive his reaction, and follow his advice if you reasonably can – it may involve referral to a hospital clinic for tests. If this gets you nowhere try the following, but keep a note of your progress and summarize it briefly and clearly in writing for your doctor's interest if you succeed. Send or deliver it to him after an interval, with thanks for his advice. This may be tedious, but is how doctors will learn to take the problem seriously. A decline in your use of his time will convince him more than anything else.

Without an Extended Glucose Tolerance Test, lasting six hours after three days of preparation, hypoglycaemia cannot be proven – and it may not show clearly even then. If a hospital doctor declines to do this, the next best thing is to try the diet which follows for yourself. If it does not quickly abolish your symptoms, you are unlikely to have hypoglycaemia.

Commence the DIET for health, avoiding every scrap of sugar (whether refined or not), glucose, malt, and honey; all refined flour, pasta, rice, confectionery and bakery; all coffee, tea, chocolate and cola; all ALCOHOL; all soft drinks and packaged snack foods. To begin with avoid dates, bananas, grapes and oranges too. You are allowed whole milk, butter and soft cheese, eggs, peas and lentils, peanut butter, oils and Mayonnaise RECIPE (no sugar) and fresh fish to your heart's content. You can have moderate amounts of all other sweet whole fruits, fresh or dried, any unsweetened whole-grain cereal product and black strap molasses (the residue of whole cane syrup *after* the sugar has been removed).

Have smaller meals frequently, or add legitimate snacks to fill the gaps in your present routine. In either case, breakfast well and sup lightly.

If this seems to help, continue and SUPPLEMENT it for three months with a Dolomite or Bonemeal tablet, three Brewer's Yeast tablets, 500mg Vitamin C and 15mg Zinc with each of three meals daily. Chromium Orotate 1mg three times daily would insure you against deficiencies in the yeast.

You should by then be able to reduce your SUPPLEMENTS to the Brewer's Yeast and Vitamin C alone, and broaden your DIET a little. Never take your RECOVERY for granted or you still risk a slow slide into DIABETES.

WHAT HAPPENS

Very few medical subjects have received more intensive research than this one, so that a great deal is now known about the *'mono'** basis of self-defence.

Your Lymph GLANDS are packed with blood cells called *lymphocytes,** which are made in your bone marrow and continually circulate between these glands, your lymph and your blood. When challenged by substances foreign to your body (*antigens*),* which usually penetrate your body via lymph passages, these lymphocytes begin to multiply and become *plasma cells,** which make antibody tailored to bind on to the antigen. Some microbes are directly neutralized this way, others are then swallowed by blood *phagocytes** (eater-cells) and dismantled inside them. This mechanism evolved from a much more ancient 'cellular' defence in which antibody is not involved. You still use this for some viruses and bacteria like *Tuberculosis.**

These facts cannot answer questions of *'colour',** such as how you recognize what is foreign to you. Your *primal adaptive system** evidently uses your *thymus** gland to train lymphocytes as agents for this purpose. A proportion of them spend time there before rejoining in your Lymph GLANDS their fellows that came direct from your bone marrow. By deciding when it should switch on and off, these thymus-trained *T-lymphocytes** provide your immune system with the 'colour' judgement it needs to function sensibly.

But your immunity is much more positive than even that suggests. Your thymus is invested with a vital life-long integrating function, known to the ancients but eclipsed by the anatomists of the past century. It is the seat of your vitality and WELLBEING, waxing and waning as they do. It rallies to caresses and to beautiful sights, sounds and smells; it shrivels rapidly with TIREDNESS and illness. By maintaining your sense of purpose it gives all your actions personal meaning, however menial they may be. It upholds your self-respect, which enables you to maintain relationships of positive mutual regard with all other independent beings, not just people. It regulates your instincts and passions, by which you can resist disturbances imposed on your life by others. Only when all these positive functions break down need any question of self-defence arise.

If external STRESS or inadequate DIET cause your primal adaptive system to lose its grip, your 'mono' defensive responses get clumsy. They are still appropriate but exaggerated, so that you mobilize far too much effort to overcome small challenges. *Intolerance** symptoms are of this kind, and becoming very much more common because chemical challenges and subtle errors of nutrition are now more easily come by, even than a decade ago.

If things get bad enough, your immune system starts to make errors of 'colour' judgement. By then you are reacting inappropriately against foods and other familiar natural substances that you should be able to tolerate perfectly well. The list may include your relatives, even your own flesh, and rapidly gets absurdly long. This ALLERGIC emergency affects a tiny but increasing minority of Westerners, and is only just being tackled adequately.

HELPING YOURSELF

Keep all your habits positive. Do not make gestures of negation – arms folded, legs crossed, face covered. Relish the beauty in the sights and sounds of life around you. Keep a light heart, and smile a good deal. Give yourself regular doses of song, poetry, pictures and music. All these maintain your spirits and sustain your thymus.

However heavy your responsibilities, keep space in each day when you are your uninhibited self.

Consciously cultivate a personal sense of purpose large enough to comprehend all your talents, energies and wildest dreams. Then act from it and maintain it in everything you do, and review it regularly.

Accept your passions as a legitimate part of you, even the shameful ones. Express them honestly, and wholesomely requite them all. 'Let not the sun go down upon your wrath.'

BREATHE in by lifting your breastbone, and hold it briefly while you thump your upper chest two or three times with your fist – exactly like an exhibitionist ape, but less conspicuously! This arouses your thymus. Do it whenever you feel down-hearted, instead of complaining or wringing your hands.

Always hold your POSTURE erect, with pride. Move boldly and gracefully. Learn how through *Alexander Technique,* * *dance,* * *yoga* * or *drama.* * Look up local ADDRESSES for options nearby.

Keep your DIET simple and healthy, with generous daily portions of live fresh vegetables and fruit. Rawness is not enough on its own; you may be eating raw cabbage that has been preserved by chilling for months and is long dead. Grated carrot, chopped onion and seed-sprouts RECIPE are easy and ideal.

Having prepared your food carefully in this way, treat it with respect and relish eating it.

SUPPLEMENT it for immunity during protracted or recurrent illness, and throughout RECOVERY. Vitamins B_3 (Niacin), B_5 (Pantothenic Acid) and B_6 (Pyridoxine), C and E are especially relevant, together with Essential Fatty Acids and Siberian Ginseng. Thymus Glandular Concentrate is available, and has value for anyone whose illness indicates feeble immunity. It cannot replace your own primal adaptive system, but offers it second-hand tools to replace your worn-out ones.

Traditional Chinese Medicine * has a more comprehensive approach to immunity than most others. Try a local practitioner when you have drawn a blank with your accustomed advisers and exhausted all these means of helping yourself back to buoyant and irrepressible vitality.

IMMUNIZATION

See also PERTUSSIS

WHAT HAPPENS

Active protection against particular diseases, by arousing your body to produce sufficient *antibody** before you risk natural INFECTION, is one of the successes which helped to establish the good name of modern medicine. But it cannot be offered until at least a few months of age, and only applies to a few diseases which once caused many premature deaths. The principal problem with infection nowadays is repeated or chronic incapacity for full living from a multitude of common causes which seldom kill. Immunization could never be a realistic protection against these.

Nevertheless public policy for preventing infectious disease now relies almost entirely on immunization because it can be packaged conveniently, evaluated scientifically and handled by community health services organized as they are now. You are not limited in these ways and can make up your own mind on the issue. Probably your chief concern is how to protect your children as comprehensively and harmlessly as possible.

GENERAL MEASURES

Babies fed exclusively at their own mother's BREAST are much better protected against infectious ailments of all causes, right from the start. Not only is your breast-milk alive with protective *cells** and loaded with antibodies and natural antiseptics, but it nourishes your babies IMMUNE system much better than any alternative. What is more, it makes an unambiguous distinction between food and non-food, so that your baby can confidently defend himself against the latter. Supplementation with even quite small amounts of other foods drastically undermines this confidence, and he begins to make mistakes. So stick with the breast alone if you can, despite doubting friends and advisers. Nevertheless, if you really cannot feed your child adequately, do not feel badly about giving up. To love and care for him generally is still the main thing.

Be sensible about outings to crowded places, especially in winter and during epidemics. Carry your baby in a sling on your chest, which stops people getting close to his face unless you let them. Do not put him down to roll around amongst CATARRHAL coughing children.

Avoid shopping at the busiest times, and use that sling. People much more often touch babies parked in push-chairs or on trolleys, and sometimes even give them things. The increased cross-infection risk is obvious.

Go out only on bright, breezy days – even in the pouring rain if necessary; you can stand within conversational distance and never BREATHE an atom of your neighbour's air. In contrast, on stagnant foggy days you risk *microbes** coughed out by others minutes before, hanging around for passers-by to inhale.

Get your older children immunized at entry to play-group or school, if not before then. Otherwise they may bring infections home to the baby.

Eat as for IMMUNITY and add some Vitamin C SUPPLEMENT for yourself if you are BREAST FEEDING: otherwise, put a few crystals of Vitamin C in a small daily bottle of watered juice or unsalted vegetable water RECIPE (*not* cordial or squash). You cannot easily overdo Vitamin C.

IMMUNIZING DOSES

WEANING is a good sign of readiness for active immunization, because babies do not begin to wean themselves until they are well able to face the outside world. That is unusual before five months. Three months is recommended officially to keep acceptance high and avoid risking convulsions, which start later; the injections are less effective that early, and more of a shock.

Some scientists have reservations about vaccines which enter your body unnaturally. They suggest that injections may work at the expense of general immunity, which is an objection that makes good sense to me. Oral or nasal vaccines against inhaled microbes would be welcome options, but so far there is little commercial incentive to develop them. But injection mimics exactly the kind of injury that lets in tetanus spores, and is therefore the natural route for immunization against tetanus.

Oral *Polio:** You swallow this live vaccine for a mild natural infection, but 15 people a year (1 per million courses) get polio from it. Otherwise protection is almost complete, although 7 Britons still get 'wild' polio each year. You still risk catching it abroad.

Diphtheria:* This injection is 100% effective; reactions and hypersensitivity are rare. Three Britons get the disease annually; most survive.

Tetanus:* Another 100%-effective injection. Temporary local reactions are common, lasting effects rare. Twenty Britons get tetanus each year; four die.

Measles: The first live injection, reserved until your second year. Often produces a mild 48-hour disease 5–10 days later, but protects 95% of people for 16 years or more. The balance of risks against benefits is rather finely poised here, since measles is rarely a serious illness in healthy children. If you are confident of your child's general resistance to infection, you could reasonably forego it. Community medicine specialists still emphatically recommend it because it prevents *meningitis** effectively and they have no means of offering it selectively to feebler children. The natural infection still kills 20 of them annually in Britain.

German Measles* – *Rubella:* Another live injection, preventing infection in 95% of girls right through their twenties at very little risk.

Tuberculosis* – BCG: A very safe skin reaction protecting most young people for 15 years; but a sore ulcer can form that lasts two or three months. Have the preliminary Mantoux skin test at least; you may be strongly positive already. If so check yourself for COLDNESS, even if you are passed free of tuberculosis infection.

Influenza:* A fairly safe injection of dead material, lasting only six months and of variable effectiveness. Worthwhile in chronic diseases and large households.

Boosters:Go for tetanus and polio when you leave school, and renew them every 5–10 years, especially if you travel abroad.

INDIGESTION, peptic ulcer, heartburn, dyspepsia

WHAT HAPPENS

Your intestines are fundamentally designed to cope with shoots, leaves, fruit and roots, the staple food of human beings from the beginning. You can digest these economically and at very low risk, using *enzymes** and *alkalis** which do not threaten your own flesh. People who stick to vegetable food make practically no acid in their *stomachs,** where they simply condition each meal for digestion by letting its fibre moisten and swell to a jelly pulp.

To cope with food from animals your evolution has equipped your stomach for an extra function. Its lower half is adapted to house an acid bath and extra enzymes which specialize in digesting flesh flood. But the meat in your meals has essentially the same quality as your own flesh; this acid bath is quite capable of digesting you!

To prevent this you depend on a delicately poised system of self-defence. Your stomach wall makes CATARRH, which acts as a barrier to acid attack. If your food contains plenty of vegetable fibre and you have chewed it enough, this swells to a stiff gel which takes up the sour gastric juice and prevents it from trickling too easily into contact with your stomach lining. And the massaging action of your stomach maintains its contents as a laminated whole, as if kneading flaky pastry; the acid and enzymes are kept inside, and the catarrh barrier is seldom overwhelmed.

If you abuse this system it easily breaks down. White flour and cereals provide too little fibre to gel and buffer your stomach contents, so that they slop about mischievously. Indigestible starch grains from white bread irritate your stomach like sand in your shoe. A quick bite chewed in haste will not moisten enough for proper handling in any case, however much fibre it contains. Eating hastily or in the wrong mood makes your stomach nervy and dry, too. It produces too little catarrh to defend itself, and acid irritation provokes clumsy spasmodic contractions instead of a smooth massage. These fragment its contents indiscriminately, increasing yet further their contact with its lining.

Your stomach skin cannot cope with this kind of challenge. At first it just gets rough and INFLAMED, feeling vaguely uncomfortable. You probably experience this at times, and know that it goes away once you have rested your stomach a while. For SMOKERS and ALCOHOLICS, however, *gastritis** can easily become a regular morning occurrence.

If this stage is neglected it gets worse, boring deeper into your stomach lining. So long as it can keep intact, the formation of new lining cells can hope to match the loss of damaged ones. But if once the lining is BURNT right through, repair of the hole slows down drastically.

This full thickness acid burn is an *ulcer.** It is much more vulnerable to acid and enzyme attack, so that the PAIN gets much sharper. Further neglect may lead to a hole right through your stomach or heavy BLEEDING from its veins; both are SURGICAL emergencies.

HELPING YOURSELF

Relax properly before a meal, and devote enough time to it. If you cannot, postpone the meal; but review your routine if this becomes a habit.

Chew every mouthful thoroughly and well, to gratify your APPETITE and get your digestion at work on it. Get everything liquid before you swallow it.

Do not neglect discomfort at the top of your stomach, just under your ribs, whether it occurs before or during your meals. Take dietary steps at the very least, every time. Cut out beer and spirits, coffee and strong tea. Mint teas make soothing substitutes.

Eat the DIET for health, avoiding sugar, white flour products, meat, fish, eggs and hard cheese for at least three weeks. Thereafter never hasten a meat meal, not even a sandwich; use only wholemeal and continue to avoid sugar totally.

You would be well advised to follow the advice on food combination given by Grant and Joice in their BOOK. The principle is to separate into different meals foods that require only alkaline digestion from those which need acid, so that the digestive climate in your stomach is unambiguous. The benefit of this approach to many people is undeniable. It may not require any change in what you eat at all, only when and with what you eat it.

Angelica and comfrey stems contain a mucilage which soothes your stomach; chew either when your stomach is empty. It may ease pain until your next meal relieves it. Liquorice root – *not* sweets – can be chewed regularly to promote ulcer healing. Witch Hazel (Hamamelis) tea is another useful remedy for gastritis and stomach ulcers.

SUPPLEMENTS of Vitamin E, 200IU twice or three times daily, will help you to heal up an ulcer and complement any other therapy.

If your pain persists, consult your doctor. He may arrange for tests to prove its origin, and give you medicines to neutralize the acid or tablets to stop it being formed. These allow the ulcer to heal, but make it hard for you to digest meat comfortably; follow the DIETARY advice as well. To get off the tablets and stay healed you will need to keep the diet going.

If TENSION unsettles you at mealtimes and produces too much acid, seek fundamental help to correct that. A *'Relaxation for Living'** course would be very suitable, next time one is organized in your area (ADDRESS).

*Homoeopathic** treatment works on your vulnerability, and depends on the details of your symptoms. You will need professional advice (ADDRESS) and must still attend to your diet.

INFECTION

It is a matter of scientific record, summarized in BOOKS by Odent and Hume, that *microbes** were first recognized 120 years ago by the French chemist Antoine Béchamp, whom Pasteur copied but misunderstood. An inferior scientist, but Napoleon's protégé and much the better publicist, Pasteur was celebrated for his interpretation and applications of work he did not really understand.

Our present science of microbiology therefore rises from false foundations which do not include the wider truths revealed by Béchamp. We have yet to rediscover how both microbes and larger organisms can arise from more fundamental living particles that Béchamp called *microzymas.** These roughly correspond with the *microsomes** that play an important part in the architecture and function of every *cell.** They are capable of surviving for remarkable periods of time – in limestone from deep caves, for instance.

These microsomes can assemble themselves into larger organisms or transform into *bacteria** according to circumstances. Dead or diseased cells can decay into bacteria, originating 'infections' deep inside a previously sterile tissue. Quite large organisms may interchange their basic particles in this way. Microbes are therefore by no means the invariable antagonists of human life that Pasteur gave us to believe. Had Béchamp's work received the attention it deserved, medical scientists might not have come to regard nature as our implacable adversary.

Germs* are not something to be killed. They do not cause infections but result from them. If your IMMUNITY is feeble or your home environment unhealthy, microbes prosper according to the ordinary laws of nature. They only reclaim resources your identity does not 'colour'* adequately. Otherwise they settle down alongside you in stable and prosperous cohabitation of your shared environment, contributing positively to your mutual health.

In this condition you are much less susceptible to COLDS, 'FLU and other common VIRUS INFECTIONS; FUNGUS INFECTIONS are never more than a nuisance in unhealthy skin, and THRUSH is not inclined to adopt its invasive *mycelial** form. More aggressive *epidemics** like HIV,* CHICKENPOX, MEASLES, MUMPS and PERTUSSIS are unlikely to originate in you; once begun elsewhere they will infect you only slightly or even pass you by.

It is suicidal to rely on substitutes for this healthy familiarity with the world of microbes. Active IMMUNIZATION is only available against a handful of them, and may prejudice your IMMUNITY to all the others. *Antiseptics** and ANTIBIOTICS are weapons of warfare which make no constructive contribution to your condition, but destabilize it. If ever they appear to cure you, it is really the effort your IMMUNITY has been able to rally with their support that you have to thank for your recovery.

Distrust of nature is what makes us warlike. Peace starts when you rediscover for yourself how false to life this distrust is, and what you lose by subscribing to it.

HELPING YOURSELF

Reassess your attitudes to woodworm, mould stains, weeds, caterpillars, rodents, wasps and flies. There may not always be realistic alternatives to killing them, but consider well your motives, and how you do it. Then apply the same principles in reconsidering your beliefs about infectious disease.

Do not use insecticidal aerosols or fly-papers; some of the chemicals in them are likely to accumulate harmfully in your tissues. Herbs like larkspur, rosemary, rue, sage and summer savory repel insects harmlessly and very effectively. Consult Juliette de Baïracli Levy's BOOK for details of how to use them.

Neither bring up your children to live in fear of germs nor do so yourself. You cannot sterilize your surroundings even if you try; be content with reasonably hygienic habits and water-tight, free-flowing drains. WORMS cannot trouble you if you scrub your fingernails after sleep and wash with soap and water after defaecating; the few you encounter will maintain your resistance to them. The same principle applies to every other disease-related organism.

Ventilate your home thoroughly, and throw open its windows to the elements on every day you can. If necessary, redesign its insulation to make this easier during the winter, when frequent airing is especially important.

Never use medicated or disinfectant toiletries without good reason, and then only briefly. If BOILS or infected skin is regularly troublesome, work on getting it healthier. This usually calls for adequate ventilation and cooling, and a regular rub with a rough towel or dry loofa, against the background of a healthy DIET. Bathing in fresh air always helps. So does splashing with cold water, especially after a hot bath.

Do not dress wounds with antiseptics unless and until they need it. Usually they do better without any dressing at all. If your doctor offers you a preventative course of ANTIBIOTIC treatment, ask him if there is any harm in waiting until the need arises, and indicate firmly that you would prefer this.

Whenever you feel the urge to kill anything, stop yourself and ask why. The more you think about life, the less inclined you will ever be to snuff it out. There is a living way of dealing with every problem; make it your purpose to find and pursue it.

INFLAMMATION

INJURY only occurs when wear or damage happen fast enough to overwhelm your body's capacity for continuous self-maintenance, so that a backlog of repair work is created. Inflammation is how that work gets done. It starts with engorgement of your CIRCULATION near the wound, from which a fluid swelling forms. This creates workspace, into which your blood cells flock to fulfil their healing functions: they are able to get out of your capillaries through enlarged pores which would normally retain them.

You commit precious reserves of energy and nutrients in an all-out effort to seal up the breach as quickly as possible. This makes it throb with heat, and swell if there is room; the pressure of this in confined spaces can make it PAINFUL. Even so inflammation is not part of the INJURY, but your means of RECOVERY from it. It deals comprehensively with any short, sharp injury – provided you survive it in the first place.

Your tissues vary in their readiness to inflame in this way, according to how often they need to. Skin is particularly vulnerable, so is equipped to cope especially well; inflammation starts in a wound within an hour, and has healed it five days later. NERVES and JOINTS, on the other hand, may take two days to get their healing effort going, and sometimes weeks to complete the task; they are too specialized to be versatile healers as well.

None of this works at all against damage that goes on continuously, day after day. If your daily healing effort cannot match it, your backlog of outstanding repair work simply mounts up. Unfortunately many modern hazards are not only relentless, but penetrate unhindered to your most vulnerable parts and baffle your defences utterly. For a time you do not even recognize the threat, and simply let it go on happening.

Eventually your damaged tissues provoke a futile response, a reaction against yourself. Inflammatory cells multiply wastefully, exhausting your resources and making the effects of your problem much worse. Inflammation intended to heal you may actually end up damaging you faster still.

This futile damage is mistaken for the problem itself, so that most medical effort is spent on distinguishing the inflammatory patterns of ALLERGY, ARTHRITIS, CANCER, ECZEMA, INFECTION, MULTIPLE SCLEROSIS, RHEUMATISM and so forth, and on devising treatments to suppress them. This may stop you suffering in vain, but leaves the underlying cause of your disease completely unaffected, and more effectively concealed now that your inflammatory smoke screen has been abolished. But there is no drug treatment that can do this indefinitely. The causative pollution merely accumulates eventually to the level that will overwhelm your treatment. Provided you escape or survive the side-effects and complications of the drug for long enough, you will sooner or later be brought face to face with your disease once more.

Removing its cause at any stage allows your inflammatory effort to achieve its objective, and turns your disease back into the short-term form your body can understand and heal – given sufficient time and resources.

HELPING YOURSELF

Work with inflammation in wounds, do not try to suppress it. *Contrast bathing** or a hot poultice will encourage your CIRCULATION, and cold water afterwards eases the throbbing or PAIN. Rest the part concerned, so that its effort is concentrated on recovery. If it is a hand or leg, try to keep it higher than your heart for good periods of time to prevent unnecessary swelling. Support a wounded limb with an elastic tubular bandage.

Only use anti-inflammatory pain-killers (with ingredients such as Aspirin, Paracetamol or Codein) to relieve intolerable discomfort that would prevent you from SLEEPING. Never consume them as a matter of routine. If you decide you need to, make the dose worthwhile but take it seldom, and only in response to great need. Routine repetition of a dose too weak to be effective gives you all the disadvantages of medication and none of its benefits.

Arnica ointment externally (if the skin is unbroken), or homoeopathic tablets internally, aid inflammatory healing wholesomely. Comfrey ointment speeds up the work of your white blood cells, and Vitamin C 200mg daily keeps them adequately supplied. SUPPLEMENTS of Pangamic Acid (Vitamin B_{15}), 50mg with three tablets of Brewer's Yeast twice daily, reinforces your inflammatory effort.

If you are still young and suffer from a chronic inflammatory condition such as rheumatoid ARTHRITIS or ulcerative COLITIS, you need to think seriously about your long-term outlook. *Steroids,** anti-inflammatory and immunosuppressive drugs neither arrest the progress of the disease nor remove its cause. Ask your doctor and specialist about this, and see what they think about your exploring these issues for yourself. Then consult an experienced *naturopath,** medically qualified *clinical ecologist** or *homoeopath** (ADDRESSES). Although most of what you need to do is within your scope, it may be hard work over a long period. Meanwhile continue to take what you need to cope for the time being, substituting wholesome treatment methods where you can. Keep your doctors informed, whether or not they are interested.

Whatever else you do, you will need the special DIET for cleansing for at least the first three weeks and intermittently thereafter; at all other times stick carefully to the DIET for health.

Good BREATHING, and the bathing routine given for PSORIASIS, are important aids to your excretion and tissue respiration without which your rate of healing will be impaired.

Use the DIET for ALLERGY to check whether particular foods or environmental irritants may be especially harmful to you, and avoid them.

Look out for a *healing crisis** within the first three weeks, which looks like 'FLU and may call for time off work. Expect steady progress thereafter over several months.

Full RECOVERY is often possible, especially when attempted at an early stage. It may take six months to become visible and two years to complete.

INJURY

Wear and tear constantly threaten to disintegrate your body, and it is marvellous how despite this your healthy self-maintenance effort manages to keep you whole and operational with scarcely any time off for maintenance or repair. Only when wear is sudden or overwhelming does it become an injury.

It need not necessarily become conspicuous and disabling, at least for a time. Injuries encountered during an important effort may be surmounted and even ignored, only to be discovered much later when the event is over. Soldiers have sometimes carried on normally after a wound which has severed a limb, only noticing their loss when they attempt to use it. What is more, sometimes the pain and BLEEDING only begin when the victim becomes aware of his injury. Conversely, Macmanaway reports, as a battlefield *healer*,* the extraordinary effect that a surge of willpower, or the determination to get well, can have in stopping haemorrhage and pain (BOOK).

On the other hand, the anticipation of injury may at times make it worse. When a drunkard falls off the platform of a moving bus he is often very little hurt, because he is so relaxed. Most sober people stiffen so much during their fall that they break several bones and bruise extensively.

Medical care for injuries is long established, and has not been improved by the drug age. There are however many things doctors can do to hinder complications, and because their confidence in your health is less nowadays they tend to give these routinely on a preventative basis. Many unnecessary anti-*tetanus** IMMUNIZATION injections and courses of ANTIBIOTIC treatment are given this way.

Few medical treatments actually promote healing. SURGICAL wound cleansing and setting of broken bones are the most constructive of these, and have scarcely changed in a hundred years. In view of this it is illogical that doctors show so little interest in much older healing traditions, particularly those based on *herbal* additions to your DIET which were the original basis of most drug therapy. And they have nothing to lose by exploring newer inventions such as *homoeopathy*,* *osteopathy** and *massage*,* which offer economical aids to healing that would complement admirably their established methods.

Whatever treatment you are offered, sound healing of any injury depends on vigorous self-maintenance, which is an aspect of your general IMMUNITY. If you are poorly nourished and over-STRESSED, you will be more susceptible to injury and take longer to recover from it. Even if you maintain your body well, your personal temperament and *action-pattern** may make you unusually *accident-prone*. This very real attribute may be hard to recognize unless you can compare yourself with other people. It is unhealthy in most ordinary circumstances, and deserves your attention.

Several specific injuries are topics in their own right: look for BACKACHE, BITES, BURNS, CONCUSSION, CORONARY, FOOD POISONING, JOINTS and SPRAINS. BLEEDING, INFLAMMATION, PAIN, RECOVERY and SURGERY are closely related general topics.

HELPING YOURSELF

Deal immediately with the inevitable *shock.* * To straightforward quiet, rest and warmth add Bach Rescue Remedy, two drops in half a tumbler of water sipped slowly; or homoeopathic Arnica 6 or 30, one dose every fifteen minutes until recovery. Make some fresh lemon barley water RECIPE, and serve it hot.

Simplify your DIET for a few days, as if for cleansing. The object is to avoid rich or sophisticated food which preoccupies your *metabolism* and distracts it from healing.

SUPPLEMENT this with Vitamin C, 1000mg in tablets or a quarter level teaspoon of powder in juice or barley water RECIPE, two or three times daily with meals. This scavenges *free radicals* * and feeds the blood cells involved in healing. Take additional Vitamin B_{15} (Pangamic Acid, or Calcium Pangamate), 50mg twice daily with six Brewer's Yeast tablets, to aid prolonged healing of complicated injuries.

Comfrey accelerates the work of the white blood cells that are involved in healing without loss of their efficiency. Its use can shorten the time it takes to heal a wound by as much as 30%. Use six 400mg tablets daily of the dessicated root for four to six weeks, or throughout the two or three months it takes a bone fracture to heal. If you want to take it for longer than that, stick to the above-ground parts of the plant which can be used fresh in wholemeal sandwiches or salads, or dried as tea.

Disabling PAIN that interferes with your SLEEP is worth attention. Contrast bathing is always helpful but not convenient in every case. Hot water for three minutes is followed by cold for thirty seconds, the cycle repeated three times finishing with cold. Infra-red heat for ten minutes is an alternative, followed by rinsing with a cold wet flannel. Arnica ointment 5–10% eases any closed wound, and support with an elastic bandage is worthwhile.

Massage eases muscle TENSION, which often causes most of the pain of bruising or blunt injuries. A physiotherapist or osteopath can treat you, and teach your companion how to follow on.

Accept any pain-relieving or muscle-relaxing prescription your doctor recommends to cope with whatever these measures do not help. Short-term use at the minimum effective dose is unlikely to harm you, but intolerable discomfort hinders your rest and recovery. Some medicines are best as a course, some can be used intermittently; make sure which type you have.

Full RECOVERY obviously takes time. Using your injured part again too early can undo weeks of healing effort. When you are doing all you can to help yourself, abide by professional advice and wait patiently for results.

A booster IMMUNIZATION against *tetanus* * is sensible if your last was more than five years ago. It is rarely essential to have a complete course of three doses. *Rabies* * protection is urgent if you are bitten abroad by an animal that may be infected; you should contact a local doctor or hospital immediately.

ITCHING, pruritus, urticaria

Everyone feels the urge to scratch or rub their skin sometimes, which is what itching does for you. Though rather disreputable, it is one of your basic and most familiar sensations, and plays some part in many normal functions and disease conditions.

But this has not made it any easier for 'mono'* physiologists to discover how itching works. There are no separate itching NERVES in your skin, as there are for pain and temperature. The sensation seems to start with the release of histamine* from storage in special cells in your skin or fine nerve endings; zinc is involved in the store-keeping. Messages then travel to your central NERVOUS system along the nerves normally reserved for PAIN, and can only be felt as itching once they have reached your brain. Either the nerve messages are very subtly coded or some 'colour' interpretation is necessary to make sense of them. Either way, the right amount of scratching sometimes abolishes the sensation – but just as often converts it to pain, or soreness, which is a mixture of the two. To confuse the situation further, scratching will sometimes start the itching off!

Its more useful varieties occur when a large insect is crawling on you, when a BOIL is ripe, in DANDRUFF, when EAR WAX loosens and under a spent scab in the final stages of wound healing. To scratch in these cases makes reasonable sense, though it may still at times be counterproductive. Insect BITES do not cause itching fast enough to help you prevent them, and the scabs of CHICKENPOX itch long before they can safely be scratched off.

In most other conditions the itching is useless or out of control. ALLERGY, ECZEMA and intolerance are getting much commoner, and frequently implicate food additives or common staple foods. Urticaria* (or hives*) is the most acute form of allergic skin reaction, and can appear very quickly and dramatically. Sometimes, particularly near VARICOISE VEINS on your legs, your skin itches because your CIRCULATION is weak at that point, so that the skin is inadequately refreshed by stagnant blood. PILES and itching of your anus without piles, probably originate in a similar fashion; the engorgement of veins in the area is then sometimes obvious and uncomfortable.

Most infestations with creatures larger than bacteria* are strongly associated with itching of an equally useless kind. LICE and scabies* are worth watching for as capable of causing the most intense and frantic scratching. THREADWORMS actually make use of the itching they cause to ensure that you consume their eggs from your finger-nails and maintain the cycle of INFECTION. VAGINAL THRUSH can itch so intensely as to constitute a medical emergency.

Antihistamine drugs often give good relief by simply neutralizing the histamine that originates itching. They are the mainstay of medical treatment for almost all non-infectious causes, but must be taken whenever it occurs and do nothing to solve your problem. Once your doctor has found no serious cause for it, you have everything to gain by probing this for yourself.

Make sure your skin is getting looked after. If DANDRUFF is part of your problem, deal with that. Otherwise air your skin thoroughly for five minutes every day, during your getting-up or bathing routine. Before you dress brush it all over firmly with a loofa or fine bristle brush stiff enough to make it blush but not to scratch it. Never use soap when you wash or bathe, and after any hot bathing rinse the part thoroughly with cold water for 15–30 seconds before rubbing dry vigorously. An all-over massage with oil for ten minutes once or twice a week is another pleasant aid to skin health.

Move towards a healthy DIET, first cutting out sugar, refined flour and the food additives listed in the special DIET for allergy.

Dry skin, with nails coarsely ridged or speckled with white patches, needs more Zinc; so do many women taking the oral CONTRACEPTIVE pill. Take 15mg daily, with Vitamin C (500mg or more) and Vitamin B_6 (Pyridoxine, 50mg daily) to enable you to use it. With time this increases the security of your histamine stores so that itching spells are triggered less easily.

If itching is due to ECZEMA or *urticaria** – great weals of raised red skin which come and go all over your body in a matter of hours – or is localized in your nose or eyes, look for ALLERGY or intolerance.

Sick skin that itches chronically may be INFLAMING against some irritant being excreted through it. As well as following the bathing routine already suggested, try a *Priessnitz pack.** After a hot bath wrap a cold damp sheet tightly once round your body from your armpits to your hips, pinning it at frequent intervals to make it hug you. Put on a warm woollen sweater over this, or go to bed in cotton nightwear. You should glow comfortably within a minute of putting this on; if water oozes from the sheet as you tighten it, take it off and wring or spin it drier. If after two hours (or overnight) the sheet is stained, repeat the pack three times a week until the staining fades. A special DIET and SUPPLEMENTS for cleansing will speed up your progress.

Wear natural fibres next to your skin, light and loose enough to be cool and airy. Adjust your clothing to the conditions, so as never to sweat into it; if you do, shower and change at the first opportunity.

Severe, protracted and generalized itching that is difficult to treat may originate in DIABETES, *jaundice** (build-up of a waste chemical from spent blood cells) and some forms of CANCER. If simple measures do not help your itching much and its cause is not obvious, you should see your doctor to explore matters further. He is more likely to rule out serious causes than to discover them, but it is worth taking some trouble to achieve even that.

JOINTS, elbow, hip, knee, neck, ribs, shoulder   See also ARTHRITIS

WHAT HAPPENS

Wherever two of your bones meet, a joint occurs. There are four kinds which matter: the cushion joints between the bones of your neck and BACK; the rolling joints between long bones, as in your legs and arms; the sutures – elaborately jig-sawn piano hinges between the separate bones of your head; and the *cartilage** joints between the fronts of your ribs and your breast bone.

Where you have a joint, it is intended to move; any that stiffen or are never used will eventually seize up for good. The only kind which can do that easily are your rib joints, which gradually lose their suppleness in the process of *ageing.** The others only fuse if they are badly INJURED or destroyed by ARTHRITIS.

Injuries arise in various ways. They may simply be damaged or worn very heavily by vigorous use. Intensive or professional athletes, such as hurdlers and footballers, are prone to exceptional joint wear that becomes obvious later in their lives because of the punishment their sport hands out. But anyone with an inefficient walking mechanism can wear the joints of their legs and lower spines more heavily than they can bear; this is probably the fundamental cause of most *osteoarthritis.**

The second main form of injury is *dislocation,** in which the normal relationship of the bones in the joint is disturbed. Usually this involves one bone slipping right out of the socket intended for it in the other bone. In a hip or shoulder this is a drastic and obvious change; but the small joints around your spinal bones may move too little to show clearly on X-rays yet still give rise to disabling symptoms.

Finally joints may become *impacted** or jammed as a result of either of these events. In this case its movement is restricted or abolished. The most important examples of this are the joints in your head. They move very little anyway, but quite enough to permit important rhythmic pulsations to reverberate freely through your nervous system and from there to your limbs. These pulsations arise every ten seconds or so, as a tick-over rhythm in the 'colour' mechanism that controls the movements of your BACK and limbs. If CONCUSSION, head or spinal injury impacts part of that joint system this 'colour' mechanism breaks down, spoiling your ease of movement and causing symptoms like HEADACHES for years, until the jammed joints are freed.

If you consult your doctor about a painful joint and he cannot find anything wrong with it on an X-ray, he may tell you that your cartilage is bruised. This applies particularly to knees and wrists, in which the cartilage is especially elaborate. He means you to understand that you have not got ARTHRITIS but have roughened the slippery elastic pads over the ends of your bones that enable them to rub together smoothly. These heal rather slowly after injury because joint nourishment is limited; meanwhile the rough surfaces abrade each other more than usual even in gentle movement, which tends to prolong the injury. Your capacity for healing may therefore be overwhelmed, and you will need to break the resulting stalemate.

HELPING YOURSELF

Elbow: * Picking up your child by his forearms may dislocate one of the bones painfully, making him reluctant to use it. If there seems no possibility that he has broken anything, bend his elbow to a right-angle and, holding his elbow in one hand and his wrist in the other, *gently* turn his palm upwards, as if to receive a coin. *Do not proceed if the pain seems severe or the movement is not free.* The joint re-locates with a click you can feel, relieving the pain immediately; otherwise consult a doctor. If he confirms the dislocation, ask to be shown how to reduce it; they tend to recur.

Hip: * Stubborn bruising sometimes troubles sportsmen, and heals with Comfrey tablets plus Vitamin C supplementing a predominantly vegetable diet.

Destructive osteo-ARTHRITIS is the commonest problem. Podiatric treatment or osteopathy may help, but surgical replacement of the joint is often the fastest way back to good function. The operation is now routine, usually gives excellent results, and can be offered to quite elderly people.

Knee: * Most joints are very simple, but your knee is a two-decker sandwich, your cartilage the slice in the middle. Being mobile it is easily pinched and torn, especially in a wrenching injury under pressure. The medical treatment is good, especially if reinforced with good DIET, Comfrey Tablets or tea and extra Vitamin C. But if surgical removal of a damaged cartilage is suggested, put it off for as many years as you can. If you use it carefully, keep slim and supplement your diet for healing, it may improve: keep hoping. Once the cartilage is removed your joint will wear faster, giving early Osteo-ARTHRITIS; and knee replacement is not so successful. If we could graft new cartilage to replace the old, things might be different.

Neck: * Almost anything wrong in your neck is better treated by a *Chiropractor,* * *Osteopath* * or *Chartered Physiotherapist* * than by a doctor, though an X-ray first is sometimes an advantage. Displaced joints must be manipulated back before resting them, or they heal out of place and are much more liable to impaction.

Ribs: * The cartilage joints at the front of your chest bruise easily and take time to heal; Arnica Ointment externally and tablets internally are helpful immediately, and Comfrey tea or tablets with extra Vitamin C accelerates progress afterwards. Exercise the joints deliberately with chest breathing to stop them stiffening.

Shoulder: * Follow treatment for a dislocated shoulder with Comfrey tablets or tea and Vitamin C for three months; this will help you to heal up strongly the surrounding capsule of the joint, which is inevitably torn by this injury, and guards against the recurrences a weakened capsule would risk.

Frozen shoulder is a variety of RHEUMATISM, and requires a cleansing DIET plus massage and manipulative treatment. Accept no more than two injections from your doctor, and stop any tablets within ten days; they suppress the symptoms and let their cause progress.

MEASLES

Measles is a means-tested VIRUS INFECTION. Your experience of it is directly related to your general health. It still kills many under-nourished Third World children but has become a mild disease in countries where most people have enough to eat. Even the subtler malnutrition that comes of depending on industrially processed food does not seem to let measles back in, but perhaps IMMUNIZATION has thinned out susceptible children enough to make cross-INFECTION more difficult, thereby masking the weaker general defences some children now seem to have against COLDS and other infections. The introduction of live measles vaccine in 1964 contributed little otherwise to the decline of the disease in Britain, already well under way by then.

It is highly INFECTIOUS and tends to occur in winter when the scarcity of living food leaves your child's general IMMUNITY at a low ebb. *Antibodies** you gave him before he was born protect a baby until he is around five months old, and BREAST FEEDING adds general resistance for as long as you persevere. However decay of this endowment, coupled with increasing exposure as a toddler's social circle widens, makes it likely that he will meet the disease again at an age when he is no longer protected. Most children have had it by ten. Before IMMUNIZATION there was usually an *epidemic** every second year, each one immunizing naturally most of the children born since the last.

It takes up to 15 days for the virus that infects you to multiply, or *incubate.** You then get a miserable heavy COLD, COUGH and moderate FEVER for a few days during which tiny red spots with paler dots like grains of salt may appear inside your cheek. You pass the virus on in the tiny droplets of atomized CATARRH that explode into the air around you whenever you cough.

The fever seems to relent, then comes back even more strongly as you begin to react against the virus with the antibodies you have been making. A rash of small dull red patches begins around your neck and chest, then spreads and coalesces into larger blotches all over your body. Within a few days the fever has subsided, the cold has stopped and you feel brighter – unless BRONCHITIS or EARACHE sets in as a complication. The illness lasts a week to ten days overall, and gives you IMMUNITY for the rest of your life.

All this can be very severe or very slight, according to your constitution and general vitality at the time of the attack. Doctors have no routine treatment for it but deal with any *bacterial** complications that take advantage of your weakened condition.

IMMUNIZATION prevents it fairly reliably, but may itself cause a brief feverish illness ten days after the injection. This is because it consists of a milder live version of the measles virus which takes those ten days to incubate and imitate the onset of natural infection. Absence of this reaction does not mean that the immunization has not taken. However quite an appreciable minority of immunized children go on to have a mild attack of measles when they are subsequently exposed. For them the injection may seem to have been wasted, but it does make *encephalitis** far less likely.

HELPING YOURSELF

BREAST FEED your babies, then wean them to the healthy DIET you eat yourself. Include some raw fresh vegetable food at the start of at least one meal every day throughout the winter; the seed-sprout RECIPE is a reliable stand-by.

Be sensible about exposing small children to the coughs and catarrh of their playmates. They can cope with any amount of it when they are brilliantly well, but in a measles epidemic be more cautious. How much virus they inhale partly determines how ill they will be.

If an already sick child is threatened with measles your doctor can prevent it with an antibody injection. Ask him about this urgently.

When a robust child starts with CATARRH during a measles outbreak, give him drinks of Barley Water RECIPE acidified with crystalline Vitamin C instead of lemon juice – up to 1500mg ($\frac{1}{2}$ level teaspoon of crystalline powder) per 500ml, which is ample for a day.

Homoeopathic* Bryonia 6 is worth while during incubation of the disease, or until the rash breaks out. Give everyone else in the house who is susceptible alternating doses of Aconite 3 and Pulsatilla 3, one of each twice daily. Morbillinum 12, one tablet twice daily, is more specific if you have it.

There is no need to confine a measles child to bed or in the dark unless his symptoms warrant it.

Tell your doctor at the beginning of the attack so that he can notify the case, but he may not need to come unless the child is very ill, or irritable with a terrible HEADACHE – brain involvement (encephalitis) is rare, but serious.

If a few days later his chest worsens or he gets EARACHE, bacterial infection may have set in; you may need the doctor then, if not before.

All Education Authorities require exclusion from school of every case of measles, however mild, to check its spread. Keep your child out of school for seven days from the start of the rash, however well he may be.

If he takes ages to get properly better give him one tablet of Morbillinum 100 on two nights each week until he recovers his health; an experienced homoeopathic practitioner could help you decide for how long.

Measles IMMUNIZATION is for a healthy child the least essential of those available; but a feeble child gains by being immunized when he is relatively well, if only to prevent encephalitis. Follow on with Morbillinum 100, as in the previous paragraph.

MEDICAL CHECK-UP

If you want to take out a life insurance policy, the company you choose will (with your permission) obtain your medical history from your doctor, and may ask you to attend a doctor they nominate for a medical examination. On the basis of your answers to his questions and his findings from examining you, they have to weigh up your chances of surviving to pay all your premiums.

This procedure is by now about half a century out of date. It gives reasonable information about your present position, but very little about your future prospects – beyond the shrewd guesswork of a seasoned physician. Obviously, he will not back anyone in their forties with an established chronic disease, who SMOKES heavily, is OVERWEIGHT or has a very high BLOOD PRESSURE. But a lot of people without these handicaps prove to be poor risks too, and some with medical black marks do very well. About the most useful assessment your examining doctor can make is how good you look for your age, which forecasts your personal outlook better than most modern technological assessments can.

With the physiological and medical knowledge available today we could do a lot better than that. In many centres throughout the world work has gone on for decades now to explore what keeps people well, so as to overcome disease as elegantly as possible. What is being discovered in this way also gives strong leads towards positive health maintenance and promotion, and reliable predictive medicine. With these we could discover the STRESSES acting on you now that will eventually produce disease, and be able to relieve these in homely non-medical ways long before that consequence is inevitable.

This contrasts radically with the best that a good preventative medicine clinic can achieve. You already know your SMOKING habits, ALCOHOL consumption, DIET and EXERCISE pattern; the clinic relies on you to tell them. Even an assessment of your weight, urine and BLOOD PRESSURE, and physiological measurements of your fitness and BREATHING capacity, mean very little on their own. BREAST examination and *cervical smear** are undoubtedly useful ways to detect serious disease early but do nothing to prevent it. The whole exercise focuses unwelcome attention on selected minority aspects of your disease potential, which should never be made to preoccupy a healthy individual. The carefree confidence of positive WELLBEING is to be promoted, not undermined.

We require a complete *'colour'** change in our outlook on prevention. Instead of continual apprehensive searching for early signs of every imaginable disease, we need to recognize and cultivate the basis of good health. There is every reason to believe that this activity prevents disease comprehensively, as well as promoting happiness. The traditional preferences of a very conservative profession are all that stand in our way.

A few independent organizations such as Templegarth Trust (ADDRESS) are working for this change, but they have yet to interest life insurance companies and the medical profession as a whole. You can contribute a great deal to progress by exploring the possibilities for yourself.

HELPING YOURSELF

Ask to know your *pulse pressure*,* which is the gap between the highest and lowest pressure in each pulse wave. If it is regularly over 50mm of Mercury (7kPa) and you are not significantly OVERWEIGHT or under STRESS, your arteries may be beginning to lose their elasticity. Check yourself for COLDNESS and take the DIET and SUPPLEMENTS recommended for ARTERIOSCLEROSIS.

Pinch the skin of a finger or toe and see how long it takes to pink up after you release your grip. If this is more than two seconds, your CIRCULATION is appreciably impaired. Look up that topic for the health promotive steps you can consider.

Assess the general condition of your skin. If it is dry and rough, blemishes frequently and heals poorly, it reflects poorly on the rest of you. Your HAIR and nails are likely to follow suit, and provide a record of your general health over the past two months. Correct the flaws with the DIET for health, SUPPLEMENTED at first with a wide range of Vitamins, Minerals and Essential Fatty Acids.

Keep your TEETH in good repair. Active decay requires correction of a faulty DIET, *not* misguided short-cuts like fluoride.

Check that you can BREATHE freely through each nostril, and exhale a full breath forcefully and freely without coughing – a sighing noise is not unhealthy. If you do not pass, consider whether you COUGH regularly and produce any CATARRH from your chest. Chronic BRONCHITIS cripples people wholesale and shortens their lives. Put your habits right, and see a doctor for further tests if you are worried about your chest.

Eat half a packet of dried figs and see how long it takes for pips to show in your faeces. If three days or more elapse you are CONSTIPATED, whatever you may think. Confirm that some days you do not go at all; that your faeces look brittle and lumpy, and seldom float; that you sometimes take ages to pass them, or need to strain. Look through the advice on this topic.

Check your *basal temperature** for a few mornings. Shake the mercury well down the scale of your clinical thermometer and leave it easily accessible on your beside table while you sleep (without a heated overblanket). On waking, with the minimum of effort, slip the thermometer under your armpit and keep it there for ten minutes, remaining covered up in bed. Record the reading before securing the thermometer in its case. If it never exceeds 97.8°F (36.6°C), your metabolism is too slow – see COLDNESS.

If you daily use ALCOHOL, coffee, cola or sweets, break that daily routine. If this proves very hard, you were very much in the habit of consuming them, if not actually addicted. Get yourself right out of the habit for three weeks or more before having it again, and avoid getting into a daily habit ever again.

MENOPAUSE, change of life

Your female fertility comes to an end as your *ovaries** cease to function, over a period of months or years some time during your fifth or sixth decade of life. You may scarcely notice it, or suffer miserably for months at a time. Because of the strong *'colour'** content of the symptoms male doctors are inclined to underestimate their true importance; they are often simply put down to NERVES or TENSION.

This explanation gets very near the truth of their *'mono'** mechanism. Hot flushes occur because of disturbance in the way your temperature is controlled within your nervous system. You behave as if you were much too hot, and divert your CIRCULATION into your skin to cool it down. The skin goes red and perspires, drenching your bed or clothing and embarrassing you dreadfully. It is no comfort to be told that they are nothing like as conspicuous to others as they feel to you.

This disturbance evidently arises from wild fluctuations in amount of the various *steroid** chemicals involved with making *oestrogen** (woman-hormone). These can occur very suddenly, and are in consequence quite difficult to study. Even so, biochemical research into the basis of menopausal symptoms seems to have a very low priority. It must have some significance that research policy is decided almost exclusively by men. They cannot even argue that no-one ever dies of it, since a proportion of *suicides** take place against its background. Even discounting this, it is hardly fair to leave preventable conditions unrelieved just because they do not immediately threaten your life.

Once your menopause is over, your outlook for two categories of degenerative disease – ARTERIOSCLEROSIS and OSTEOPOROSIS – increases to an unwelcome degree. It is as if loss of fertility deprives you of some of your instinctive purposiveness, weakening your IMMUNITY. However these changes are not inevitable, and you can take advantage of the best in traditional foods and modern knowledge to postpone these *ageing** processes.

Unfortunately some forms of SURGERY accelerate them, and can have quite important effects on your outlook for health in old age if you accept one of these operations when you are still young. Removal of your ovaries is an obvious example, not lightly undertaken. But many surgeons consider removal of your womb (*hysterectomy**) and *sterilization** to be safe in this respect. My experience is otherwise. Many young women seem to experience an early menopause after hysterectomy, and a few develop more erratic menstrual patterns after sterilization. It is as if your ovaries give up, either because of interference with their blood supply or for lack of a 'colour' purpose.

Cases like this sometimes justify medical treatment with an artificial oestrogen supplement, which would be unwise during or after a natural menopause. It makes you more vulnerable to high BLOOD PRESSURE, CORONARY or *stroke** from inappropriate blood clotting and CANCER of your womb or

210

BREAST. By this time your risk of these catastrophes is much greater than it is for younger women taking the CONTRACEPTIVE pill.

HELPING YOURSELF

If you are offered hysterectomy, find out from your doctor whether this is simply to control BLEEDING or for a more dangerous reason such as CANCER. Some surgeons are far too eager to perform this operation on young women who do not have life-threatening disease without adequate consideration for your full circumstances and prospects. Do not accept it until you have tried controlling your bleeding problem by the more conservative means suggested under that topic, unless you are already very weak because of it and are approaching menopausal age in any case.

If your hot flushes are severe and frequent fast for up to two days, taking only fruit juices and home-made Lemon Barley Water RECIPE. Then start on the DIET for health, avoiding meat and poultry; this may contain residues of steroid growth promoters which would upset your condition further. Coffee, strong tea, SMOKING and ALCOHOL are all likely to aggravate your symptoms.

Take 200–400 IU Vitamin E Complex (Mixed Tocopherols) with 1000mg Vitamin C (Ascorbic Acid BP) and two tablets of Dolomite twice each day for a week. Halve the Vitamin E and Dolomite dosage after the hot flushes have disappeared, which should be within a week. Continue at this level for several weeks at a time, resuming if the flushes return.

Stabilize your circulation by finishing every hot bath with thirty seconds of cold water. At other times, brush your skin all over vigorously instead, using a dry loofa or soft brush. Do one or the other twice each day.

HYPOGLYCAEMIA sometimes plays a part in menopausal symptoms; check that topic if the above measures fail.

Siberian ginseng (Eleutherococcus senticosus) tends to normalize unbalanced or STRESSED metabolism but is a more expensive approach. Panax ginseng is a good second best; buy the red roots and prepare them without heat.

If your symptoms are still hard to control, add Vitamin B_5 (Pantothenic Acid 50mg daily) to your SUPPLEMENTS. Support it with six to nine tablets daily of Brewer's Yeast.

There are several *homoeopathic** preparations that may help you. Try for yourself Ignatia 3 six hourly, Sepia 6 six hourly, and Graphites 30 four hourly. Take each for three consecutive days and pause for the rest of the week before trying the next. Then consult a homoeopathic practitioner (ADDRESS) for further advice, taking with you a note of what you have tried.

A *Medical Herbalist** or *Traditional Chinese Medicine** Practitioner may be able to help you further if all these measures fail (ADDRESSES).

MIGRAINE

Migraine is a very particular and severe kind of headache which occurs repeatedly at irregular intervals according to the same pattern and to which some people are particularly prone. Each attack is foreshadowed by a tense, irritable mood which may build up to characteristic warning symptoms; these give way suddenly to terrific heat and TENSION in your head, often confined to one side. This attack disables you for hours or a day before gradually subsiding. Once you have had one, it is unmistakable.

The naturalistic physicians of fifty years ago had much better ideas about its cause than prevail today. They studied the way your blood deals with *waste acids** from *metabolic** breakdown of meat and other foods, which can only be cleared from your tissues through your blood to your kidneys if there is enough *alkali** (like bicarbonate) to dissolve them in. All is well if your food provides plenty of alkali, and little that will turn to acid when digested; your blood then has plenty of surplus alkali to pick up the waste acids from metabolism and carry them safely to your kidneys.

Problems arise from two sources. If you eat a lot of meat, eggs and meat stock you make a lot of waste acid, and to dissolve it you need all the alkali your blood can hold; but blood bloated with waste acid, even safely dissolved, irritates the vessels it passes through. They open up, but the circulation only slows down, clogging your tissues with waste-laden blood; fresh air cannot get through the traffic jam, however well you breathe.

This condition makes you feel ill and sluggish, and may cause chronic VARICOSE VEINS, PILES, *sinusitis,** GALLSTONES, heavy PERIODS, EPILEPSY, ANGINA or *cramp** if it becomes a habit. You seek relief for your discomfort, and may find it in coffee, tea, chocolate, cola, headache tablets or SMOKING.

That is your second mistake. These stimulants work because they are acids themselves, but with a keener appetite for alkali than the waste acids can muster. So the wastes are dumped from solution, their places taken by the stimulants.

With no waste acids in your blood you feel much better, a new person. But they are still being formed by metabolism, and have to be excreted somehow; otherwise they would build up in your tissues and eventually cause RHEUMA-TISM or ARTHRITIS. So they take every opportunity to get out of there into your bloodstream again, which gets you back to where you were; you take another dose of stimulant to make you feel better again.

If you have migraine, you cannot get away with this. The tension between stimulant acids and waste acids builds up, and your reserves of alkali fall; you pass lots of clear urine, with no waste acid in it. Your blood vessels pick up the tension and cringe, so that your warning symptoms start. Eventually the storm breaks, waste acids pour into your blood in spite of everything and relax the vessels again: a migraine has begun. In your kidneys the sluggish blood flow reduces the urine formed, but now it is loaded with waste acids. For a time they can get out, as in health they must.

HELPING YOURSELF

Migraine is a safety valve you should be glad to have. It gives you early warning of your mistake, before it can build up chronic illness that would wither you away and take you much longer to get rid of. Above all it does what no minor symptom can – impress you enough to do something radical about it.

Immediately begin a special cleansing DIET, avoiding especially coffee, Indian tea, cola drinks, cocoa and chocolate, alcohol and all pain-killing drugs; try Bidor 5% (Weleda) instead and feverfew tablets or tea. Use home-made lemon barley water RECIPE to boost your alkali reserve. It will take you six months to two years to get right, but your health improves all along the way.

If attacks continue despite your diet, look for a particular irritant such as heavy THRUSH infection or some other food you are sensitive or ALLERGIC to and have overlooked; check for it by the exclusion tests described in the special DIET for allergy, and avoid any that prove able to cause you headaches.

Sometimes TENSION in the muscles around your jaw can cause migraine. This may originate from dietary STRESSES as already described, but is sometimes caused by poor alignment of your TEETH so that your lower jaw can never get settled comfortably on the upper. You may find yourself gnashing or fidgeting your teeth a lot in consequence, and the muscles at the back of your mouth on either side may be extremely tender to touch with your finger. If so, you should consult a dental surgeon with experience in dental *Kinesiology*,* who will understand this state of affairs and be able to make helpful adjustments. But you may be liable for private charges to have this done; get the contractual arrangement clear before you start.

Negative electricity helps you to overcome migraine. See ELECTRICITY DISEASE.

Garlic Oil is a powerful cleanser and sometimes boosts excretion of waste acids enough to improve a migrainous tendency dramatically. Take two capsules daily on Saturday and Sunday for six successive weeks, but take care to replace the nutrient minerals this will also flush out accidentally. Two of Nature's Own Multimineral daily from Monday to Friday would be satisfactory.

MISCARRIAGE

See also PREGNANCY, FAMILY PLANNING

WHAT HAPPENS

There always were occasions when a pregnancy did not unfold ideally but nowadays one pregnancy in eight is likely to end in accidental miscarriage. This reflects the wide variety of pitfalls conception is now subject to, especially since non-nutrient chemicals began to intrude more intimately upon our lives, although your body devotes a great deal of attention and resourcefulness to overcoming these obstacles, and usually succeeds. When it cannot, miscarriage is the healthiest way out of an impossible situation.

It is seldom your personal fault, and could not safely have been prevented once the pregnancy had begun to take its course. The seeds of difficulty were probably sown between eight and four weeks before conception, at least a month before any routine test could demonstrate your pregnancy. Exposure at that stage to ALCOHOL, SMOKE, toxic chemicals or nutritional hardship can have a devastating effect on the development of your egg and sperms. Most sex-cells that are badly affected are completely infertile, and no pregnancy ever results. But a few that are damaged only slightly may succeed in starting a pregnancy which is from the beginning unlikely to proceed far.

Your nurture of this pregnancy from then on may be entirely beyond reproach, though still subject to all the same disturbing influences that continually impinge on you despite your best intentions otherwise. Their influence over so new a life runs dangerously deep, and further compounds a faulty start. If there is no major malformation in the formative folds of the developing egg, more subtle imbalances in the 'colour'* blueprint may prompt growth out of proportion to the power of the baby's heart or liver, which at a later stage can still make survival impossible.

So a miscarriage during those first three months when such matters are decided, fully justifies your grief. Were our cultures more civilized we should all feel your pain as our own; no wound in the tissue of life would leave us unmoved, let alone in so tender and innocent a part of it. We should all wonder in humble honesty by what collective folly such things can be, and comfort you with the sincere resolve to set it right.

Meanwhile you face the slow evolution of events. BLEEDING is not a sure sign, since you may menstruate harmlessly at period time from the part of your womb your pregnancy has not yet filled. But it is usually the first, and does not settle properly with rest. Pain usually comes second, and intensifies until the pregnancy is lost. Clotted blood is seldom as hard and distinctly formed as a *concepsus*;* if you doubt what you see, it is probably a clot.

Habitual miscarriage – two or more in succession – may not however be inevitable. If pain precedes bleeding, you may be physically unable to keep the neck of your womb closed firmly enough to keep your baby in. Or you may repeatedly make too little *progesterone** (pregnancy hormone) in those vital early weeks. Both of these can be prevented next time by suitable treatment.

214

HELPING YOURSELF

Negotiate with your doctor where you should be. Home is safe for an early uncomplicated miscarriage, provided you and your medical attendants agree. Rutin and Vitamin C SUPPLEMENTS help to control BLEEDING, reinforcing any medication you are offered.

If your miscarriage is incomplete, or your baby has died but does not miscarry, do not submit to SURGERY if you really cannot face it: collect your thoughts first. In other cultures a disappointed mother usually waits until her body is ready to complete the process naturally. Her womb shrinks, salvaging its contents to replenish her reserves. Her body eventually rejects the much smaller residue in a brief INFLAMMATORY illness that may be FEVERISH. This mechanism is available to you, and worked well in the several cases I have witnessed. Complications that require surgical treatment are rare, but can occur; if your obstetrician has specific fears based on the details of your own case, listen to him. If on the contrary his advice is based only on his standard general policy, and you are for the time being quite well, the dangers of surgery may be more real than those of biding your time. There is no automatic need for a 'D and C', which is in any case rather a crude operation.

Face your grief, and share it with your husband or confidant. Say all that is in you, even the things you know are unreasonable. Ann Oakley's BOOK gives detailed answers to most of the questions that occur to you.

Then search rationally for something to do differently next time. Go over your FAMILY PLANNING carefully for factors deserving more attention. Set about rebuilding the stores you lost with the miscarried pregnancy, giving yourself six months to accomplish this before you try again.

Any wholesome gesture that brightens the 'colour'* of your outlook is worthwhile, however irrational it may be; it need only convince you, no-one else. Anything goes, from a new hat through a change of doctor to open defiance of what usually passes for good sense, provided it gives you the clean sweep you need.

If you have had two or more miscarriages, see your doctor well before you plan your next pregnancy. You may need to see a gynaecologist to investigate the cause, on which your treatment will depend; all this could take several months to arrange.

When you do conceive again, keep it to yourselves until you are clear of the first three months. It is very demoralizing to have to tell people if things go wrong.

MOUTH ULCER, aphthous ulcer

The basic attitude of every living thing, however primitive, is self-preservation. Their outer tissues are organized in flat resistant sheets like the walls of a fortress, renewed as they wear by growth from inside. They have no intention of being plundered easily.

In direct contrast, everything about your intestine is designed for interaction, from the pumping, mixing and kneading action of its muscles to the vertical development and outreach of its skin. This set-up makes no provision at all for self-defence. You therefore cannot afford to let anything enter this specially intimate environment still able to assert itself. Plants organized in life for self-preservation must be disorganized and softened sufficiently to present no physical threat and yield passively to your digestion.

That is what chewing is for, and why it requires time and attention from a rather special organ. It must cope with the harsh textures, angular forms and tough resistant skins of a 'mono'* structure, and yet absorb the flood of 'colour'* that chewing releases from living foods, notifying its spectrum to your APPETITE. Clearly rigid structures like your TEETH cannot combine all these functions. The elastic flexibility of your tongue and cheeks is indispensable to your mouth's purpose, sensitive enough to pick up the quality of each mouthful yet sufficiently tough and muscular to manoeuvre hard lumps of food into place between your teeth.

The skin of your mouth and gums gets burnt, scratched, stabbed and stretched mercilessly in the course of this, and has to protect itself strongly to resist being torn or eroded. It has therefore the same fortress arrangement of tough layers as the plant food you are chewing, and is mounted on an elastic foundation richly supplied with blood.

If you bite it accidentally it ulcerates sorely, making you cautious during the week it takes to heal. This usually happens to your cheek, just where your teeth can catch it as they close. Accidents of this kind are usually one-off, although the INFLAMMATORY swelling they cause makes the wound protrude into your mouth a little more than usual, setting it up to be bitten again.

Artificial colourings in food (most of E100–E155) can erode your mouth in a rather different way. The ulcers are more numerous, selecting especially the sheltered creases of skin between your gums and your cheek, where food residues can linger most easily. Coloured sweets are particularly erosive because of the sugar and acids they usually contain as well.

Sometimes however you may notice breakdowns of the skin all over your mouth for no obvious reason. These usually mean that your general vitality has declined for some reason. You will therefore have some difficulty getting them to heal, since this is harder work than preventing them in the first place. Besides which, whenever you eat they are bathed in digestive saliva and are physically abused as you chew.

Chew a tablet of Comfrey Root into crumbs, and plug the ulcer with the gelatinous mass these become. It will adhere firmly and last for several hours unless you deliberately remove it. Not only does this dress and soothe the wound, but the allantoin in the comfrey accelerates healing too. You can manage two or three ulcers at a time in this way, those deep in the crease between your gums and your cheeks being particularly suitable.

Red sage tea can be drunk or gargled to soothe sore mouth ulcers; it has a mildly antiseptic effect as well. Potassium Chlorate and Phenol Gargle BPC also makes an excellent antiseptic mouth-wash which pickles your skin and numbs any sore patches. Dilute it 50:50 with hot water before use, and do not swallow the washings. Either of these will keep your mouth clean and comfortable while it heals.

Once the ulcers have healed soundly, increase the vegetable content of your DIET and cook it less. If you are accustomed to refined cereals and bread, change to whole-grain versions. The skin of your mouth gets a share of the extra nourishment, and the increased abrasion from chewing challenges it to grow tougher and thicker. The scraping also keeps it clean and makes infection much less likely.

Avoid sweets; they encourage bacterial infection of your mouth, which can cause inflammatory ulcers or colonize any you already have. Sour pickles or highly spiced food will aggravate an existing ulcer and seem to predispose some people to them.

The artificial food colourings which have been shown sometimes to cause mouth ulcers are those derived from coal tar. They are being removed from many manufactured foods under consumer pressure, but sweets will be among the last to change. Avoid buying brightly coloured boiled sweets or gums, especially if they have an acid tang to them. Colouring ingredients are now often identified on packaging by their proper chemical names, since many customers are now too wary of E numbers for the manufacturers' liking. Lawrence's BOOK overcomes this problem for you by listing the full names and numbers together.

There are many medicinal preparations for sores in your mouth, most of them available from the chemist without prescription. Carmellose Sodium is a safe barrier paste, available also in powder form. Be wary of the *steroid** preparations you may be prescribed if you press your doctor too heavily for an effective remedy; they dampen INFLAMMATION but do nothing to heal your fundamental problem, and give THRUSH and other infections more of a chance.

MULTIPLE SCLEROSIS, disseminated sclerosis

The great sophistication of your NERVOUS system depends heavily on the speed with which electrical messages can pass down your main trunk nerves, from head to foot in a fraction of a second. It would take much longer but for the nerve's insulating sheath, which enables messages to take seven-league strides. That sheath consists of a train of specialized *cells,** each one flattened and wrapped round the nerve like a Swiss roll. Lined up close-packed along the nerve they look rather like a string of sausages.

The insulating property of this sheath derives from many layers of the skin or *membrane** of these cells. Any defect of these membranes therefore has disastrous effects on nerve cell insulation, and these may be its only obvious consequence.

Multiple sclerosis is such a disease. INFLAMMATORY patches appear on the insulating sheaths somewhere in your brain or spinal cord, slowing conduction there and causing havoc in your nervous functions downstream. The patch arises under stress of some kind such as TENSION, *fatigue,** exposure to *microwaves,** sun-bathing or acute DIETARY imbalance. Your body usually heals it afterwards with a little scarring, so that you RECOVER almost completely in a matter of weeks. But similar patches may occur again elsewhere in your nervous system, and the slight residual effects add up over the decades. Therefore if disease starts in your teens, it requires more urgent attention than the much milder effects that can begin in middle life. On the other hand, very slight neurological symptoms frequently arise in older people, which never progress to disabling proportions and are often brushed aside when you seek medical advice about them. These may turn out to be a very mild form of multiple sclerosis, surfacing as a feature of *ageing** in people who have successfully held the disease at bay throughout their youth.

Despite the vast efforts being made by charitable research foundations to establish the cause of the disease, this remains controversial. Unfortunately in many laboratories that effort is focused too finely on minute aspects of its biochemistry, hiding the wood behind the trees. Rivalry between some of the personalities involved has further hindered progress. The work of the Naomi Bramson Trust is particularly promising, however. Their findings are strikingly consistent, and suggest a practical approach to preventing the disease – along with many others, notably the most stubborn ALLERGIES.

These diseases can only arise if you have inherited a clumsy way of making cell membranes, and may not break out even then. The clumsiness can be masked and corrected by DIETARY precautions. It can also be reliably detected by an electrical test on your red blood cells researched by Professor E. J. Field and confirmed by workers in four other laboratories up to now. This test will one day enable doctors to identify those who inherit the clumsiness and women who can convey it to their children. With this information we should eventually be able to prevent multiple sclerosis by dietary vigilance or SUPPLEMENTATION throughout childhood, and perhaps throughout life.

HELPING YOURSELF

If you have the disease make contact with Action for Research into Multiple Sclerosis, The Naomi Bramson Trust and the Multiple Sclerosis Society at the ADDRESSES given. Their approaches differ, and they do not at all see eye to eye. You will have to decide for yourself how to fit them to your own temperament and inclinations.

ARMS have sponsored the development of Hyperbaric Oxygen Treatment, now available at various centres throughout Britain. It is based on similarity of the inflammatory patches in multiple sclerosis with those of decompression sickness (diver's bends), which led to the same treatment being tried for both. In some hands it has been very successful; 'colour'* input may very much affect the result. Whether or not its 'mono'* basis is sound, it does no harm; and the 'colour' boost given by sharing in a positive self-help activity more than justifies it.

Eat the DIET for health, keeping especially low on animal fats. Essential SUPPLEMENTS are Blackcurrant Seed Oil (Glanolin – Lane's), 500mg 2–3 times daily with Vitamin E 100 IU and ample water, half an hour before meals. This routine seems to reduce the severity, frequency and duration of attacks. Less essential but prudent additions are Vitamin C 1000 mg twice or thrice daily, one strong B Complex or six Brewers' Yeast tablets daily and a good multimineral. Vitamin B_{12} (Hydroxocobalamin, 100 microgm daily) and Folic Acid (5mg daily) seem to be particularly important and should be adequately represented in the Vitamin B supplement you choose.

Be wary of meetings with other sufferers to hear lectures from experts. Many who congregate there are far worse than you are ever going to be and may present you with a gloomy picture of the future. Active meetings for self-help or fellowship are much more wholesome.

Physiotherapy* or osteopathy* help a lot if you can afford it; learn the most useful exercise to continue at home. Yoga* tailored to your needs by a sufficiently experienced teacher is more economical, develops your 'colour' resources and fosters your self-reliance.

The Naomi Bramson Trust have developed the 'erythrocyte unsaturated fatty acid' test, which can determine whether any of your family could mother a multiple sclerosis child and discover personal potential for the disease in anyone else. This test is still under research but seems to be highly reliable. It is well worth while if the disease affects any of your blood relatives, because the best chance of preventing it occurs in children under 16 years of age who have not yet shown signs of their weakness. A full programme of the diet and essential supplements listed above should be maintained until their early twenties.

Beware of microwaves* and radar, strong sunlight, very hot baths and STRESSFUL situations. All these are suspected or known to trigger attacks of multiple sclerosis in people who are genetically susceptible.

MUMPS

WHAT HAPPENS

The VIRUS of mumps is in a class by itself, with a singular preference for your metabolic glands (*not* your lymph GLANDS) which makes its independent survival precarious. Without the salivary glands in your mouth it could not be an INFECTIOUS disease at all – it would be self-eradicating. It does not make you cough, which is how other more infectious diseases are transferred. It depends instead on the transfer of infected saliva, which requires more intimate contact than most school-children habitually make with each other outside the family circle. Since most cases occur in late winter and spring when people are less robust for lack of fresh live food and sunlight, it is puzzling how the virus survives the summer months. Perhaps it arises spontaneously from transformation of STRESSED glandular cells, as *Béchamp*** believed, and only then becomes infectious.

It takes three weeks to *incubate,** after which it usually declares itself as pain in front of your ear that you may misinterpret as EARACHE. That is followed quite quickly by a pronounced swelling there which may be large enough to completely obliterate the hollow between your jaw and your neck, and protrudes upwards in front of your ear. Unlike lymph GLANDS or other swellings in the hollow of your neck it is wrapped around the back of your jaw, so that you cannot feel its bony corner. Furthermore, if you eat anything sour, or strongly enough flavoured to draw saliva into your mouth normally, a mumps swelling hurts with the effort of trying to respond.

Mumps often appears on one side first but develops over a few days to involve other salivary glands. You mouth becomes dry and unhealthy, and the discomfort may be quite distressing for one or two days, even when you are not trying to eat or drink. After that the INFLAMMATION subsides a little, and the swellings are much easier to put up with during the week each one is likely to last. Occasionally they take turns to appear instead of being present simultaneously.

The only danger arises when other kinds of secretory gland elsewhere in your body become seriously involved, which usually happens just as your salivary glands are recovering. In adolescence or adulthood it occasionally involves an *ovary** or *testis.** When this happens the gland swells to many times its usual size and is very tender. The infection is likely to destroy the gland, which within a few months of RECOVERY will become very small. Fortunately, infection of both sex glands at once is rare. *Mastitis** is unusual unless it coincides with adolescent BREAST development. Rarely it affects your *pancreas,** which may handicap your digestion. *Encephalitis** is rare but serious, and can result in permanent deafness. But most people in good health have a brief uncomplicated illness followed by life-long IMMUNITY.

You are infectious to others during the last week of incubation, and for as long as the salivary swellings last. Kissing, sharing of cutlery and cups, dipping into fruit-bowls, jars and serving dishes and borrowing tooth-brushes or used handkerchiefs are the main routes by which the virus spreads.

Rest from physical activity during mumps, especially if you have it during or after adolescence and your TEENAGE years. It relapses most often in people who try to hasten their RECOVERY. Keep a small child from boredom with drawing, television, board games and the like.

Home-made barley water RECIPE is best in the first few days, with only enough Vitamin C (instead of lemon juice) to neutralize the flavour. Any sour food or drink, or anything else which normally makes your saliva run, makes the swollen salivary glands too uncomfortable.

Make no attempt to prevent spread of the disease among healthy primary age children, since this is the age they cope with it best. It would be sensible to pass it deliberately amongst your neighbours' children, with their agreement, by having them to tea. Kissing, sharing your child's pencils, and foods like nuts and popcorn served in large communal bowls promote the necessary contact.

Once you as an adult have the salivary swellings yourself, take *homoeopathic** Parotidinum 30 every 2–3 hours and give it every 8 hours to any adolescents and sickly children in your household – combining it with an hourly Aconite 3 for anyone who appears to be starting the disease. Keep tooth-brushes separate, and be careful whom you kiss.

If a testis swells take homoeopathic Pulsatilla 3x every two hours; support your scrotum well without squeezing it, using firm underclothing; and rest absolutely in bed.

Mumps vaccine is available, but is not very useful. Being a live altered virus given by injection, it is hazardous for anyone with suppressed IMMUNITY or CANCER, or on *steroid** therapy – just the group you may wish to protect from natural infection. But your doctor may be willing to give a vulnerable person injections of *antibody** which will protect him to some degree during an epidemic. Homoeopathic measures will also help anyone not on steroids.

Anyone who does not seem to RECOVER to their usual vigour within a week or two may benefit from further homoeopathic treatment, perhaps with Parotidinum in a much higher potency. For this you should consult an experienced homoeopathic practitioner, and it would be as well in this case if they were also medically qualified.

NAPPY RASH

In traditional communities, particularly in warm climates, a mother who carries her baby around with her constantly develops great intimacy with him, and senses instinctively when he is about to empty his bladder or bowel; she has time to remove his clothing and let him void somewhere appropriate. In these circumstances his skin is easily cleaned and remains well ventilated, cool and dry; unhealthy rashes are practically unthinkable.

Economic development inevitably complicates all this. Not only do many individual mothers develop a distance from their children, but their whole community distances itself from naked patches of earth. The child cannot tell his mother what he needs, and there are few places she can take him where it is hygienic or polite to let him drop his excreta. The napkin is society's answer. It is in effect a portable latrine, which solves these two problems only by creating new ones to replace them.

In the first place, the skin covered by nappies is kept warmer and damper than is good for it, with hardly any ventilation. This makes it very susceptible to FUNGUS INFECTION. The most readily available is usually *Candida albicans** or THRUSH, which may already be thriving in his intestine and therefore present in the faeces held by the nappy against his skin. If he has been treated for infection with an ANTIBIOTIC, the colony of thrush is likely to be larger and more assertive – especially if he has been artificially fed with dried cow's milk preparations that cannot sustain his IMMUNITY so well.

Secondly, faeces and urine are allowed to mix with each other for several hours, after being voided separately. Urine is free of *microbes** when it is passed, but faeces always teem with them. *Bifidus bacteria** predominate until you finish exclusive BREAST FEEDING, and are highly protective against INFECTION. But artificial or mixed feeding encourages the growth in your baby's COLON of *coliform** bacteria, which overgrow and replace his colonies of *bifidus** bacteria. Coliforms are much more likely to cause trouble generally, and are in particular able to feed by breaking down the urea in his urine-soaked nappy, releasing appreciable amounts of ammonia. This gas stays dissolved in the dampness as a very caustic *alkali,** which burns his skin.

Most nappy rashes arise from one or other of these problems, or a combination of them. If you can detect a strong odour of rotten fish when you change your baby's nappy, then ammonia is playing some part. The rash looks like a BURN, with a uniform sore red surface which wrinkles easily. The edge is flat, indistinct rather than clear-cut, and no more livid than parts further in. Particularly bad patches may *ulcerate** and become INFECTED with bacteria, which may then discharge offensive pusy material which stains the nappy.

THRUSH, on the other hand, is blotchy and has abrupt margins where the fungus is most active that are slightly thickened and raised. The blotches tend to start small as livid spots and broaden over the course of several days into patches with irregular outlines. Bacterial spots and sores often develop if the skin is sufficiently disturbed.

HELPING YOURSELF

Revel in intimacy with your infant, from PREGNANCY on. Bathe with him, have him naked in bed with you, and feed him at your BREAST. Carry him with you everywhere you can in a sling or back-pack. This may not enable you to do without nappies but does undo a fundamental error in developed culture which tarnishes parenthood, deprives your children of you and diminishes the potential of your entire family life.

BREAST FEEDING is strongly protective against infection of any kind, and nappy rashes in particular. You will notice unpleasant changes in your infant's faeces within two weeks of changing to cow's milk, unless by then he can cope with eating fibrous vegetable food as well.

Disposable nappies go against the grain of thrifty people, but they have now surpassed cotton fabric in efficiency and no longer much exceed them in real cost. Composting the bio-degradable part, or burning it as fuel, will appease your conscience honestly if incompletely.

If a rotten fish smell rises from overnight nappies, obtain some Borax (Boracic Acid BP) from the chemist and dissolve a teaspoonful in a pint of warm water. Sprinkle this on a batch of nappies and allow them to dry. Keep these for night-time or any other long stage. The borax neutralizes ammonia as it is formed, and solves the problem. (If you have a redundant scent spray, dissolve as much borax as you can in much less hot water, and dilute it a little before use; a fine mist of this is sufficient and takes less drying.)

Heal ammonia BURNS with Comfrey or Calendula Ointment. Zinc and Castor Oil Cream protects healthy skin from getting soggy. Antiseptics may irritate, and are more likely to be harmful if they are absorbed through your baby's skin and stored in his fat.

THRUSH is cured by Gentian Violet 1% in water, sucked daily by your baby off a piece of sponge; treat your nipples too. But it dyes everything purple; your doctor can prescribe more convenient (and much more expensive) alternatives.

In the first summer after he learns to walk, let your child run around at home with his FEET and bottom naked, indoors and out. Let him wee and poo on your garden soil, and help you to bury poos shallow in its surface with a trowel. This is a completely hygienic fertilizer, and a thoroughly wholesome lesson for everyone: it can no longer disgust you, and your child – who knows his poo is useful – never learns to believe that it is dirty. Potty training then follows on quite naturally and without effort, in an entirely positive and cooperative atmosphere. BED-WETTING is then unlikely to be a problem.

NERVES

Your brain is organized like a pair of semi-detached houses on two floors, with double doors connecting them upstairs. On the ground floor is all the semi-automatic equipment of your *primal adaptive system*,* with junction boxes on the trunk cables from upstairs which pass through *en route* for your spine. Your *'mono'** reasoning happens on the left hand side upstairs, and your *'colour'** feeling goes on next door.

Your 'mono' and 'colour' departments maintain a dialogue through the double doors, but the trunk cables respond most directly to conscious 'mono' control. Your ground floor has many 'colour' connections, however, which tone this conscious traffic and work through an unconscious conditioning network of nerves which are laid alongside the trunk cables. These regulate every part of you that is not under conscious control. Their influence is slow but profound, arousing you to vigorous activity at one extreme or settling you into *recreation** and RECOVERY at the other.

Threats to your health arouse your 'colour' sensibility – to the point of outrage, if need be. Moral indignation 'colours' your 'mono' actions, animating you to challenge and surmount the threat. You can for a while generate extraordinary effort to assert yourself sufficiently, over-riding all your usual self-conservative restraints. So long as the challenge that upset you is itself living and responsive, this vigorous response will overwhelm it and secure your vital interests once more.

Unfortunately, many modern threats take unnaturally stubborn 'mono' forms. They tend to arise at the points where the centralized and 'mono'-lithic structures of contemporary society clash with the living values of individual people. It does not matter whether it is concrete or bureaucracy that thwarts your legitimate intentions. Either way, your 'colour' indignation lacks an appropriate channel and is futile and fruitless. At first this only intensifies your 'colour' fury, spurring you on to prolong and intensify your efforts. Unless you manage to find a healthy outlet for this energy, it too is spent totally in vain. What is worse, resentment and negative feelings reverberate destructively within you, throwing your 'mono' affairs into chaos. *Anxiety*,* SLEEPLESSNESS, TENSION, INDIGESTION or HEADACHES conspire to irritate and exhaust you, with chronic TIREDNESS, apathy and DEPRESSION the eventual results.

'Mono'-cultural development is overwhelmingly responsible for introducing massive unnatural STRESSES into the lives of most ordinary people alive today. It can even explain it scientifically. But such a culture cannot cope with its own 'colour' consequences, and its most prominent and powerful members are the very last to admit this fact. 'Mono' medication is their preferred solution, and considerable industrial effort has gone into developing it in the last thirty years; but these medicines can only ever mask 'colour' symptoms. 'Colour' solutions are always simple and readily available, but may call for major changes in your outlook on life before health can be restored.

HELPING YOURSELF

If your condition corresponds to frustrated arousal it is urgent for you to find out why, and channel your indignation appropriately before you are worn out by it. This may not be easy on your own; a confidant outside your predicament can often see clearly what is obscure to you.

Do not be afraid of doing what seems necessary just because you cannot see where it will lead. Healthy action can change your situation unexpectedly, opening up possibilities you cannot now foresee. Just follow the thread your needs suggest, looking for the wholesome consequences of each step.

Meanwhile you can ease your symptoms. Substitute lemon barley water RECIPE, elderflower or linden (lime blossom) tea for stimulants such as coffee, Indian tea, chocolate, cola, ALCOHOL or tobacco SMOKING. Eat the DIET for health, SUPPLEMENTED for STRESS. Use good BREATHING and lavender-scented baths to ease TENSION, and deal urgently with SLEEPLESSNESS.

If your companion is willing, massage for ten minutes one or more times daily is very soothing, and positively promotes your WELLBEING. It is not necessary to be expert, only to care for the person you are massaging, and to do for him or her what you would like to have done yourself. Deep kneading of all your large masses of muscle is always effective, lingering sensitively over those that are tender and tight. Use a little lavender oil or any sweet smelling essential oil that takes your fancy.

Until you feel easier again, drop inessential activities that distract your attention and dissipate your effort. Television is the worst, because it is not true *recreation**.

Biofeedback*, *hypnotherapy**, *relaxation**, *yoga** and *meditation** are all effective ways to make your resources coherent again. Look up local contacts through the ADDRESSES given.

If you are already TIRED or DEPRESSED by your past exertions, there is no substitute for a prolonged restful RECOVERY lasting several months. Without this you cannot summon up the energy to change your predicament. Medication to arrest your adverse brain biochemistry may be appropriate, or a suitable *Bach Flower remedy** may ease your mental attitude onto more hopeful lines. Then persevere until your vitality rekindles, and apply it to reordering your affairs along the foregoing lines.

The fellowship of others in a similar plight may be good for your morale, but beware of any gathering with self-pitying, negative or dependent undertones. Keep the accent on active and practical self-help. Letters of protest and lobbying demonstrations are rarely anywhere near so productive, and tend to confirm bitterness and resentment rather than foster hope.

NITS, head lice

WHAT HAPPENS

The human head louse is a very resourceful insect that lives 5–6 weeks, exclusively in human hair. It starts life as an egg the colour of your scalp, attached to a hair very near its root. The hairs over your ears, at the nape of your neck and under your fringe are favoured because they keep warmer; the eggs need to incubate at 30–31°C for a full week, by which time your hair has grown 3mm. The pearly white nit (empty egg-shell) is now much easier to see, clinging to your hair as far from your scalp as it has grown since the egg was laid – about a centimetre for every month.

Meanwhile the louse matures within ten days, and mates; four out of five are female. Each then lays six to eight eggs daily for the rest of her life. She moves very quickly through your hair close to your scalp, using her six large claws to hang on firmly whenever you comb it or bathe. You have to be quick to spot one, because they are sensitive to light and avoid exposure to it. They do not fly or jump, but are quick to transfer to another head whenever close enough contact occurs; a few seconds is enough. One louse can visit several heads in a day, if opportunity offers!

It feeds several times a day from the CIRCULATION in your scalp with its long retractable mouth, injecting a little anaesthetic saliva as it probes. This prevents you discovering the insect immediately, but gives it away in the long run; sensitivity to these accumulating injections is what eventually makes you itch, after two months or more of INFECTION.

If you do not then deal with it, or are constantly reinfested, after about a year you become much more profoundly sensitized. Your muscles become uncomfortable, especially in your legs, and you feel generally unwell – 'lousy' in fact. A 'nit-wit' is a child so affected that he cannot concentrate or think straight!

Children in nursery and infant schools are the main reservoir of head-lice, girls more especially; but short hair is not an advantage. The insects prefer a clean scalp, so frequent washing does not protect you. Indirect transfer never occurs; only an insect already half dead would drop from your head onto clothing or a chair-back.

Although lice may at times run wild through whole schools, infesting practically every pupil and many of their families, infestations are nowadays seldom prolonged; school nurses react urgently to any reported outbreaks. But they rely increasingly on shampoos and lotions containing one of two potent insecticides – Cabaryl and Malathion – to kill the lice they find.

Consequently lice are becoming resistant to insecticides, just as *bacteria** have decoded many ANTIBIOTICS. The insecticide is easily destroyed by heat or sunlight so that the dose actually received may be less than intended; this helps give the insect time to develop resistance. Meanwhile we neglect the simple measures we relied on for centuries, which cost practically nothing and are totally harmless. We had better re-explore these methods, rather than be tempted to use other insecticides that are less safe.

HELPING YOURSELF

Grooming your hair daily with a strong undamaged comb is the best simple hygienic protection. That makes life dangerous for any lice you acquire. A damaged limb makes them much less functional; they cease to lay, feed less well and quickly perish.

Search your children's hair for nits every time you wash it, at least once a week. To spot insects part the hair quickly with a comb, and move the parting systematically across the scalp; watch for the louse retreating fast!

Obtain from the chemist a fine-toothed metal comb designed to strip eggs and nits from human hair; every family medicine chest should have one. Whenever you discover lice or nits wash or rinse your hair, and groom it thoroughly with an ordinary comb. Then work systematically over your scalp, using the nit comb several times on each lock of your hair, from the scalp upwards as far as your nits are visible. Some combs have teeth cut square only on one side and are bevelled on the other; the square side does the stripping, so should face away from your scalp. Clear the scrapings from the comb frequently to prevent it clogging. Repeat this procedure every week while the outbreak lasts.

Rue (Ruta graveolens) makes an excellent deterrent to lice which is perfectly safe for people. Apply it as a lotion in the evening and wash it off the following morning. An alternative lotion is Sabadilla tincture, diluted one-in-ten with water. *Homoeopathic** Nat mur 6 can be taken four hourly through an outbreak, alongside either lotion.

The insecticides Carbaryl and Malathion are used medicinally in lotions and shampoos at 0.5% concentration, to kill lice and eggs outright. If you decide you have to use them make it once only, and follow the instructions meticulously; note particularly that heat, sunlight and chlorine destroy them. Afterwards, depend on harmless lotions and weekly vigilance.

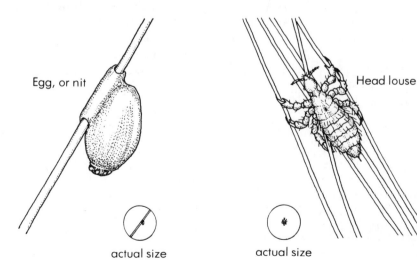

Egg, or nit

Head louse

actual size   actual size

NOISES IN YOUR HEAD, tinnitus; vertigo; Menière's Syndrome

Unless EAR WAX is pressing on your ear-drum and distorting it, or INFLAMMA-TION in your throat has swollen to audible proportions the torrent of blood CIRCULATING past your ear, persistent head noises (*tinnitus**) indicate some interference in the workings of your inner ear. This is a tiny but complicated cave deep in your skull on each side, lined with delicate sensors to detect vibration and rotary movement in the *lymph** that fills the cave. It converts these mechanical movements into NERVOUS impulses to your brain by which you are able to appreciate sound and control your balance.

In the past, damage to your inner ear could often be traced to severe BOILS or chronic destructive INFECTION of your middle ear. These problems are now much less common, partly thanks to ANTIBIOTIC treatment. DIETARY imbalance and chemical pollution of foodstuffs are much more likely nowadays to congest and irritate delicate sensory organs, silting up your CIRCULATION and lymph drainage channels just as they do in RHEUMATISM and ARTHRITIS. Because your inner ear tissues are micro-engineered, they cannot tolerate pollution nearly as long as your JOINTS can before their function breaks down. Tinnitus, or disturbance of your balance with a false sense of rotation (*vertigo**) or any combination of EARACHE and deafness with these (*Menière's Syndrome**) are the misleading sensations you start to suffer as a result.

Your inner ear has one major advantage over your joints, a direct and relatively rich CIRCULATION. Its blood and lymph vessels correspond with your ear in their small size, which has further functional advantages – by the time blood reaches your ear its pulsations and turbulence are abolished and cannot cause movement or vibration to mislead your sense organs. Though fine blood vessels silt up more easily, being directly present makes restoration of their health and correction of your symptoms a much more hopeful prospect.

Medical treatment of this condition is confined to controlling the false sensations and is rather limited in scope. Destructive SURGERY is only contemplated rarely and as a last resort. So most people who are affected must put up with waiting for their ears to deteriorate, palliated more or less successfully with suppressive drugs. They are only likely to be free of trouble when the diseased ear apparatus has destroyed itself completely, by which time they may be very deaf.

Yet naturopaths have for a century recognized and taught the connection between inner ear problems and CATARRH or degenerative disorders elsewhere in your body. None of the natural treatment methods they have recommended since then in any way contradict established medical teaching – on the contrary, they complement it perfectly. Their only drawback is the time they may take to produce results; but in a condition as chronic as this, you have plenty of that.

In areas like this where medicinal treatment is thin on the ground, doctors are exceedingly remiss not to explore and promote every safe measure that offers hope of genuine improvement.

HELPING YOURSELF

Getting rid of middle ear degeneration requires sustained and energetic measures, but corrects all manner of other maladies along the way – some of which you may not yet know you have.

Get rid of any hardened EAR WAX that may be blocking your ears; you may need your doctor's help for this.

Adopt the DIET and SUPPLEMENTS for cleansing, for six weeks at a time. Alternate these with a healthy DIET reinforced only with mineral RECIPES – Egg Nog, home-made Lemon Barley Water and Honey-Cider-Vinegar. Cut out all sugars, white bread and other refined flour products, animal fats and chemically processed foods; use *'organic'** produce whenever you can.

Check the advice on ARTERIOSCLEROSIS. A twice daily SUPPLEMENT of Nicotinamide BP 50mg gently opens your peripheral circulation and may improve blood flow to your ear.

ALCOHOL will not improve CIRCULATION through damaged blood vessels and impairs your balance anyway: avoid it.

SMOKING directly hinders blood flow in small vessels. You need to stop if you smoke yourself and should avoid regular exposure to other people's smoke. If you must share a workplace with smokers, try asking for an *ionizer** to be installed there to remove the smoke and keep everyone alert and productive.

After bathing sluice your head with cold water at mains temperature, more and more boldly as you become accustomed to it. A shower nozzle is the ideal tool. You will feel the passages in your head clearing as you do it; the tonic effect on your blood vessels is less obvious but just as pronounced. Reinforce this internally by gargling every morning with hot and cold water alternately, half a minute each for up to three cycles, always finishing with cold.

Each evening for ten minutes apply hot and cold packs alternately to each side of your neck just below the ears. Hot packs last one minute, cold only thirty seconds; finish with cold. Then (four or five nights a week) apply to your neck a strip of linen 8cm wide, slightly damp with cold water, and fastened fairly tightly with a pin; cover it with a dry woollen scarf. Apply an exactly similar compress around your waist, like a cummerbund 20cm wide. After the initial chill, these heat up within a few minutes. If this is not obvious to your touch within ten minutes, take them off; otherwise wear them all night. Their effect is to scavenge to your *abdomen** blood and lymph from your neck, helping everything that drains through there – including your inner ear.

Take the trouble to BREATHE deeply and efficiently through your nose, at least five times on several separate occasions daily.

EXERCISE in the open air, vigorously enough to prevent conversation, for ten minutes each day – or at least three times each week.

OSTEOPOROSIS, Soft Bones

WHAT HAPPENS

The essential feature of *ageing** is reduced *'mono'** IMMUNITY – a decline in the vigour with which your body holds its own against all the pressures that tend to disorganize it. The process begins imperceptibly in middle life, but depends very much on circumstance. By forty you may have some inkling how fast you are ageing, and by fifty it is usually obvious.

A major feature of physical ageing is gradual loss of protein from your body, which brings with it a loss of calcium. This is far the most abundant mineral you have, around 1.1 kilogram in all. Nearly all of it is deposited in your bones as crystals of a complex phosphate of calcium called *hydroxyapatite.** These are rod-shaped and hard, very suitable for reinforcing the protein skeleton of your bones without making them too heavy, brittle or permanent. These features allow your bones to grow and to heal, and leave plenty of space in their structure for blood vessels and the *cells** that construct and remould the mineral architecture.

That remoulding is continuous, though it proceeds very slowly. You absorb and excrete about 100mg of calcium each day, which means that one thousandth of your calcium stores are remoulded daily. About 400mg of bone calcium is easily accessible at any time, a quarter of which is exchanged with your environment daily.

From middle life you begin to shed more of this than you absorb, losing a tiny fraction of your calcium annually. After your MENOPAUSE the rate can rise dramatically, ranging up towards three per cent each year. Many factors have some bearing on the pace of this process. If you use your body little it maintains itself less vigorously; dwindling *hormones,** reduced sexual interest and an early MENOPAUSE are among the possible results. SMOKING aggravates matters, apparently by accelerating your sexual decline.

But your DIET is important too, and the demands your life has made on it. BREAST FEEDING several babies represents quite a challenge for your calcium reserves, which need time and opportunity to recover. Eating much meat, and drinking more than two cups of coffee every day, both make this difficult. Insufficient fresh food and general digestive inefficiency aggravate your tendency to scavenge for calcium less avidly as you get older.

The consequence is thinning of the mineral lacework which gives your bones their strength. Men have much stronger bones to start with, which protects them initially from the worst effects. Even so, by seventy your spine may hunch forward, bending from the middle of your back and shortening you by several centimetres. This pushes your chest contents downwards, making your *abdomen** stick out. *Steroid** medicines for ARTHRITIS or ASTHMA make matters worse. At least a quarter of women by 60, and both sexes ten years later, are significantly affected. Trivial injuries then easily lead to major fractures that heal poorly, and may prove to be the occasion for you to become an invalid more or less permanently.

Yet prevention is elementary, if you start young and keep it up.

HELPING YOURSELF

Adopt the DIET for health, which contains all the protein you need even before you garnish it with occasional meat meals. Fortify this with the RECIPE for Egg Nog three or four times weekly, especially if you prefer not to consume dairy produce or are ALLERGIC to the cow. Limit your coffee intake to one or two cups on only a few days each week.

Lemon Barley Water and Honey-Cider-Vinegar RECIPES cut down the acidity of your blood, which helps you retain all the calcium you need and keeps it dissolved, preventing GALLSTONE and kidney stone formation.

Give up SMOKING.

EXERCISE regularly in any case, but daily after age 50, for an hour if you can. Work challenges your bones to stay strong.

For six months after BREAST FEEDING, and after your MENOPAUSE or age 50, SUPPLEMENT your diet with two tablets daily of Calcium with Vitamin D BP and three of Dolomite 500mg. This provides you with more than a quarter of your total Calcium requirement and all the Vitamin D you need to make use of it, plus a useful amount of Magnesium to top up your Egg Nog and other food. Vitamin C 1000mg with each dose of mineral supplement, at two main mealtimes, helps you absorb enough Zinc and Manganese from your food as well as the Magnesium and Calcium – all four contribute to mineralizing your bones. The cost of all this works out at 16p daily or £60 per year – a very cost-effective insurance policy. Your doctor can prescribe them under the National Health Service, if you are exempt from the charge; otherwise it is cheaper to buy.

If you notice you are beginning to stoop or get shorter, or if your TEETH start loosening, you are probably developing osteoporosis. You should consult your doctor, but institute all the measures advised here too.

OVERWEIGHT, dieting

See also UNDERWEIGHT

WHAT HAPPENS

It is easy to understand why you get fat. A rich DIET of counterfeit food has deranged your APPETITE; you crave exactly the wrong things because they have you hooked. You EXERCISE little because you have no time to walk or cycle everywhere, and live too far from work and the best shops. Yet constant STRESS makes you long for relief sometimes, and nice food is an inexpensive and portable substitute for anything more appropriate and fundamental. And it is far safer and more socially acceptable than ALCOHOL.

You join a large minority of Westerners of all ages who are five to fifteen kilograms overweight with lumps of fat under your shoulder-blades, on your buttocks and thighs and around your waist. Your complexion is waxier than you would like, marred further by cheesy *black-heads** or septic spots. This is a far cry from the fashionable lean limbed image most people sigh for – though remembering the massive daily effort it takes to keep a model looking good might make you feel a little better.

So you start on a reducing diet – regularly. The initial weight loss is impressive but unreal; you have simply used up your *liver's** stores of easily available starch, intended for ready use. Burning off old fat is not so easy. Some of it may have been laid down years ago to support BREAST FEEDING, which you either gave up early or chose not to do; that is very difficult to shift in any other way.

But your *carbohydrate** balance is only the beginning of your difficulties. You meet head on your reason for eating too much and must find a better way of dealing with it. Hard work may help, unless you are already over-TIRED. More SLEEP is not easy to get. Other *recreations** take extra effort to organize.

If you clear that hurdle, you may start feeling dreadful as the fat burns off. Poisons dissolved in it out of harm's way are turned out as the fat dwindles and re-enter your CIRCULATION where they can upset your *metabolism.** Excreting them properly is difficult and time-consuming, which is why they got into your fat in the first place.

Then comes another shock. When you get to the weight you want to be, you cannot go back on the diet you would like without gaining weight again. Dieting is permanent, and a new personality goes with it which you or your family may dislike.

Or dieting may make you slow and stupid, with COLDNESS of your limbs, rather than reduce your weight. Your body has taken your small food intake to mean that there is a famine, or a long hard winter in prospect. Some people of Northern European descent inherit from their ancestors the ability to adapt to such conditions by hibernating. Your *thyroid** activity slows, you cool down slightly and use up your stores of energy only very slowly. In these circumstances, however, movement is less vital than insulation; so you burn off muscle rather than fat. The result is undesirable and counter-productive.

HELPING YOURSELF

Your weight is not a disease but a high reading on the 'barometer' which reflects your general unease in life. Do not try to reduce it directly, or for its own sake, unless your life is threatened by its medical consequences; let it rise and fall with your fortunes.

Go by whether you are fat rather than your standing in weight charts, which cannot cater for individual build. Skin-fold thickness calipers are a better investment than scales, and cost about the same.

Do not try to diet during PREGNANCY. You will do better well covered and lose it after about four months' lactation; so keep on BREAST FEEDING for at least six months instead.

Avoid all refined fatty, starchy and sugary foods but substitute something legitimate – raw carrot, freshly baked potato, wholemeal toast, Brazil nuts, fresh fruit, dried apricots.

Start every meal with a generous raw salad or coleslaw, using olive oil with cider vinegar or lemon juice as a dressing. Chew it well and slowly, and pause for a few minutes before eating your next course.

Eat most of your energy food – cereals, fats and nut butters – at breakfast, and little or none at night. Meat and fish are more appropriate then if you desire them, eaten without bread or potato to improve their digestion.

EXERCISE gently for ten minutes three times a week at first, to get reasonably fit; then work it up to thirty minutes. This will keep you burning fat and stop you hibernating. Exercise reduces your APPETITE, so try it instead of lunch. Choose something you enjoy, vary it if you get bored, and try to make it useful. Perhaps you could cycle to work, after all.

Shower off your perspiration afterwards; finish with cold water to retone your skin. This powerfully reinforces excretion of any problem toxins that begin to show as you dissolve away the fat.

Avoid coffee, tea, cocoa and cola which spoil toxin excretion, though they make you urinate more. Substitute parsley piert, broom or juniper berry tea. Home made Lemon Barley Water and Honey Cider Vinegar RECIPES are more substantial and tasty ways of doing the same thing.

If you feel COLD and slow, check your body temperature before getting up. Your thyroid gland may be under-active; you can SUPPLEMENT that temporarily if necessary.

BOOKS by Cannon and Melville give the best advice on dieting, if you want to read more.

PAIN

When your flesh is heated, stretched, pierced, crushed or threatened in any other way you automatically withdraw it, thanks to the reflex behaviour built into your NERVOUS system. This is one of the purest 'mono'* mechanisms you possess, quite devoid of any feeling. If it coincides with intense preoccupation you may not even notice, far less experience pain of any kind.

Pain is the 'colour'* of the event, which you experience at quite a different level. It usually starts a split second after the action is all over, which is the time it takes your mind to notice. Its tone is much more variable than the INJURY it relates to. In anger a wound hurts much less, especially if acquired in venting it. If the blow touches your pride as well as your body, it hurts much more. Pain is amplified enormously by anticipation, which good doctors strive to mitigate and torturers deliberately exploit.

It arises alongside the ability to override your defences wilfully, if the stakes are high enough. Pain 'colours' a complicated threat, mounting in proportion to its importance, defying you to ignore it. Sometimes you will, even so. But in health a serious danger usually generates pain impressive enough to make you deal with it.

At first the pain is coded straightforwardly to make you withdraw from further injury. INFLAMMATION, congestion and pressure all demand protection, rest and cooling for your affected part; TENSION calls for relaxation and heat. But if you ignore and override this simple corrective it soon breaks down. Unrelieved pressure crushing a nerve in your BACK tightens painfully the muscles surrounding it, compounding the injury and your agony. A blocked bowel or congested nasal passage soon becomes inflamed and infected, superimposing on colic* the profoundly debilitating ache of peritonitis* or sinusitis.* In long-running CANCER, ARTHRITIS and RHEUMATISM the pain eventually has no straightforward purpose at all, and may be quite out of proportion to the 'mono' pathology. Terrible destruction, clearly visible on X-rays, may not hurt at all; or disabling pain may arise in joints that appear almost normal. Worry, TIREDNESS, isolation and hopelessness are then often more significant factors in your pain than the disease itself.

The pain of childbirth* is more or less directly related to your fear of it. Often the presence of a trusted and loving companion relieves it as well as an injection, and far more safely. POSTURE and activity make an enormous difference too; if you are free to move about and try different attitudes during your contractions, you will find that the most comfortable varies according to your stage. Standing upright, or squatting on all fours, may take more effort but is usually much less painful. And when the baby finally comes, the sharp pain of a tear is avoided if you take your time to stretch properly and refuse to be hastened.

When you or your doctor responds to pain merely by suppressing it with drugs, you vastly under-estimate its meaning and waste a valuable opportunity.

HELPING YOURSELF

New pains in your HEAD, chest or *abdomen,** prolonged or severe enough to worry you, deserve attention from your doctor within 24 hours of onset.

The pressure of *sinusitis** or EARACHE is eased by an ice-pack across your brow or cheeks, or the back of your head where your neck muscles are attached. A handful of broken ice-cubes wrapped in a damp face-cloth will do nicely. If you need decongestant medicines from your doctor or chemist to sustain this relief, confine yourself to using them continuously for three or four days only. Follow that with *Homoeopathic* Aconite 6, Nat mur 6, or Merc sol 6 if necessary; one of these may work just as well for you and cannot let you down in the long run.

A *Priessnitz pack** – a hot bath before wrapping a cold damp cloth tightly around your body and covering it with a woollen pullover – will help to relieve pain in your *abdomen** which the doctor has assured you will pass. HEADACHE is often eased this way, or by a foot-bath – hot if your FEET feel cold, and *vice versa.*

Activity helps PERIOD pain and most JOINTS. Massage from a caring friend helps pain almost anywhere; every parent has eased her children this way many times.

Beware of depending continuously on pain-killing drugs; their relief eventually weakens, but their side-effects tend to accumulate. Soothe away TENSIONS which complicate the pain, and learn to *relax** in spite of it. If you can cultivate detachment, by *hypnotherapy,** *yoga** or *visualization** if necessary, your agony will cease. Look up ADDRESSES for local contacts.

Metabolic congestion causes MIGRAINE and contributes to pain in other *tissues.** Adopt a cleansing DIET during your worst attacks; it will probably help relieve their cause as well.

Osteopaths,* *Chartered Physiotherapists** and practitioners of *Traditional Chinese Medicine** and *Homoeopathy** each have much to offer in the management of pain, particularly if your doctor seems totally baffled by it. You may approach any of them directly, but get your doctor's blessing if you can.

In a few special circumstances either very powerful pain relieving medicines or anaesthetic injections have a useful place. Your doctor can refer you to a local NHS Pain Clinic if this applies to you.

Confide your fears and griefs to a relative, friend, counsellor or priest. Sharing eases them, and they may prove to be groundless. Chronic pain can often be reduced from agony to hard work, simply by dealing with your fears.

PERIOD PROBLEMS

Whenever your body prepares for a PREGNANCY that does not follow, menstruation occurs in order to undo those preparations. As its *hormonal** support is withdrawn, the engorged and vascular lining to your womb breaks down and is shed along with some blood. This usually involves muscular contractions of your womb, which are painless if they are well coordinated. If your CIRCULATION is clean and your genital organs healthy, your loss is usually slight and trouble free.

It is surprising that so many women have regular and easy menstrual function for most of their lives. At best it is a poor compromise between FAMILY PLANNING and CONTRACEPTION; many other animal species manage things much better. Some individual women do as well, either as an active independent and mobile young adult or else later, once your experience has matured you as a whole person. In either case your periods may occur seldom or cease altogether, yet you remain able to conceive a pregnancy whenever you really want to. Your chief problem then is lack of confidence in the situation, which undermines it; you may well prefer the reassurance of a regular monthly flow.

This begins with *ovulation*,* an event which depends on hormonal regulation by your *pituitary gland** and is therefore subject to control by your *primal adaptive system*:* that is how you are able to suppress useless reproductive effort during extremes of starvation or athletic physical exertion, or through sheer personal wholeness. Otherwise, ovulation sets off a programme of events that leads automatically to PREGNANCY if your egg is fertilized, or to menstruation if not. Your body knows which way things are going almost immediately, so the interval from ovulation to your period is regular – between 10–14 days according to your nature. Erratic behaviour of your ovaries is the variable feature which underlies *irregular periods*.

Heavy or painful periods arise either because your womb is inadequately supplied or your CIRCULATION is loaded with irritants; both unbalance and fatigue your NERVOUS system and womb muscle. The little toxin you manage to shed with your menstrual flow is poor compensation; 'cleansing' is an idea that misrepresents the truth.

Endometriosis* is inappropriate growth of the lining skin of your womb, and may arise either inside or outside your womb as non-CANCEROUS lumps which gradually enlarge with each period but dwindle at your MENOPAUSE. This condition is closely associated with Western-style civilization, and mainly affects people who are better off. It is likely to begin in your thirties, and by blocking your fallopian tubes may seriously impair your chances of further pregnancy. It usually causes PAIN and tenderness during your menstrual flow if the problem lies inside your womb, or beforehand if it has spread outside. The flow itself is usually much increased, more erratic and more frequent. You may in addition feel permanently bloated or heavier in your *abdomen** than previously, throughout your menstrual cycle.

HELPING YOURSELF

All menstrual problems will respond to healthy corrections in your DIET, especially reduction of your meat intake. *Steroid** growth-promoters used in animal husbandry can affect your genital function, and are not well enough regulated to ensure that they are absent from all meat sold for consumption. Try to confine yourself to *'organic'** livestock, or avoid it altogether.

SUPPLEMENTS as for BLEEDING (Rutin and Vitamin C) help control the amount of your flow but are best taken throughout the month. Vitamins B_3 (Niacin), B_6 (Pyridoxine), C and E are all essential to the health of your womb and ovaries, along with Essential Fatty Acids; SUPPLEMENTS of all these are worth trying for a few months, according to your means; but remember to support the B Vitamins with at least three tablets of Brewer's Yeast daily. They will more quickly restore your reserves to levels that a healthy DIET based on fruit, vegetables and whole-grain cereals can maintain.

A daily cold *Sitz Bath** is a simple way to improve the nervous coordination of your womb contractions and the circulation to your ovaries and womb muscle, all of which helps gradually restore prolonged, heavy or erratic periods to a regular and manageable pattern. Increase the frequency of the bath to three or four times daily, from two days into your period to two days after it has stopped. Firm massage to your lower spine for ten minutes daily reinforces the effect, if your partner will do this.

If your periods are usually PAINFUL, fast on the day before they begin, taking only home-made Lemon Barley Water RECIPE and hot Peppermint Tea. Finish the day with a hot bath, and take hot Sitz Baths at intervals during the period to relieve your pain. Raspberry leaf tea or tablets are usually helpful during painful periods, taken several times daily.

If a gynaecologist says that endometriosis is part of the reason for your distressingly painful periods, lie down for fifteen minutes every three hours to relieve congestion of the pelvic organs that are INFLAMED by the menstrual back-flow. Otherwise work on your diet consistently, and establish a regular programme of daily Sitz baths. You need to distance yourself in these ways from the features of Western life that are most likely to engender the disease.

Many other herbs and homoeopathic medicines may be helpful according to your temperament and constitutional needs: consult a *Medical Herbalist** or *Homoeopathic Practitioner** for further assistance in choosing them. *Osteopathic** problems in your spine should be corrected. 'Women's Health Concern' may be able to put you in touch with sympathetic practitioners. (ADDRESSES.)

None of these methods is likely to produce dramatic results within the first month. Expect gradual improvement over about six months to a year.

PERTUSSIS, whooping cough

WHAT HAPPENS

Whooping cough is unusual among the infections of childhood. Breast feeding conveys no specific protection against it, although your milk strongly upholds your baby's general IMMUNITY and maximizes his chances of an uncomplicated RECOVERY from the disease. It is usually caused by a *bacterium** which is very insensitive to ANTIBIOTICS, so that conventional treatment is very unsatisfactory. Its worst effects arise not from the *microbe** directly, but from a chemical toxin produced by it which makes the NERVES in your windpipe extremely sensitive, causing the spasmodic cough which gives the disease its nickname. COUGHING spreads the germ about a good deal, especially within your family.

You are INFECTIOUS from a few days after you catch the germ, which grows in your wind-pipe producing CATARRH, slight FEVER and COUGHING within another week. After two weeks of this the infection settles, but the cough really gets into its stride. You simply cannot stop once you have started, until you are so empty of air that your face goes blue and you are about to faint; then a long whistling breath in sets you up for the next coughing spasm. Once you have seen it, the pattern is quite unmistakable.

The cough is so intense that your eye or nose may BLEED, and its weakening effect open you up to all sorts of complications – EARACHE, BRONCHITIS and *pneumonia,** EPILEPTIC fits and *ulceration** of traumatized parts of your throat. If the catarrh gets too thick to be expelled the force of the cough recoils on your lungs, rupturing some of the gas exchange bubbles and over-inflating the small tubes leading to them. This is *bronchiectasis,** a life-long sump where pus collects unless you up-end your chest regularly to empty it.

You are out of circulation for at least five weeks, and may take another three months to recover anywhere near your best. But the toxin can persist in your wind-pipe for several months more, long after the infection has died out, giving an *encore* whenever a cold rekindles it.

Whooping cough ranks with *meningitis** and antibiotic-resistant bacterial FOOD POISONING, the last infections left which commonly cause severe problems in Western countries. Ten thousand cases are reported annually: only five die, but many more have some permanent damage, and all lose three months of their lives to the disease. Prevention offers the only effective control, and a vaccine for this purpose became available in Britain during 1957.

Whilst in principle this seemed like the answer at first, it has drawbacks in practice. The vaccine is not perfectly effective; one recipient in five gets little or no protection. And there are more positive drawbacks. About one baby in 100,000 who receives the full course of three injections may suffer permanent brain damage – less rare than with any other commonly injected vaccine. Publicity about this risk has drastically reduced uptake of pertussis vaccine, and there is no doubt that babies who have ever had brain damage, neurological symptoms or irritability should not be given it.

HELPING YOURSELF

Do not wait until vaccination age to begin protecting your children against pertussis. There are many things you can do right from birth.

Take all the precautions you would use to prepare for and buttress other IMMUNIZATIONS.

Homeopathic* potencies have been prepared from the CATARRH of pertussis patients and used to prevent the disease. It is given as drops or a tablet at long intervals, contains no *'mono'** substance or microbes, and appears to be utterly harmless. Insufficient research has been done in this country to establish its effectiveness, but 70% protection is claimed from experience abroad, which is close to the best the injection achieves. It cannot be obtained except on prescription, however, and public policy is firmly against it. This is a pity, because it should be explored. Maybe your doctor would consider it, if you or your health visitor were to discuss it with him. It could be used to protect your baby until he is old enough to take injections reasonably well.

Wait until your baby begins to WEAN himself (about six months) before starting injections; but in any case get at least two completed before playgroup or school entry unless there are overwhelming reasons not to. This helps to protect younger members of your family who are not yet old enough to be immunized actively.

Public policy at present favours commencing immunization at three months, to start protection as young as possible. But your baby's immune system is not yet ready at this age, and many other measures are available to cover this period. To inject tiny babies with anything is inhumane, and many are obviously very upset by it. After getting over that a minority again become generally unsettled, uncomfortable and sometimes FEVERISH for a day or two. A few have a more localized type of physical reaction, a tender hot swelling at the site of the injection which may last a week. This often turns out to be a reaction to the aluminium compound used to intensify the effect of most injected vaccines; it can be excluded from later doses to prevent repetition.

None of these upsets are permanent or confined to pertussis vaccine, but very occasional severe reactions can be. You should be cautious if your baby may have inherited a tendency to EPILEPSY from a close member of his family, was premature or showed any sign of NERVOUS irritability, feebleness, or brain damage. If in doubt, immunize later rather than sooner.

Pertussis infection in a healthy child need be no worse than a COLD, but for the COUGHING bouts. Early ANTIBIOTIC treatment may help prevent them, but ordinary cough medicines are no use at all. Try Drosera 3 2-hourly and give it or Pertussin 30 to everyone else night and morning as a preventative. Otherwise try *anthroposophic** Pertudoron (Weleda UK Ltd ADDRESS). At the catarrhal stage try Aconite 3 every two hours; once spasmodic coughing has begun try Ipecac 3 instead. Use the Honey Cider Vinegar RECIPE as refreshment after coughing bouts. Pertussin 30 is useful during RECOVERY.

PILES: Haemorrhoids

WHAT HAPPENS

CONSTIPATION produces faeces that are too dry and too small to slip easily along the last thirty centimetres of your bowel, especially once chronic COLITIS has stiffened its kinks. Overdistension weakens the grip of your bowel muscles, despite stimulation from medicines. If you hope to move your bowel at all, you are going to have to push.

In health, all the propulsion your faeces need comes from your bowel itself. A wave of contraction presses from behind, and the bowel in front relaxes out of the way. But that is not all. The propulsive wave needs to get a grip on something, like a roller-skater trying to move a heavy bin. The only anchor available is the relaxed bowel in front of the faeces you are trying to move, and pulling on that draws it back over your faeces as if peeling the bowel skin off them. That not only gets the tunnel your faeces must pass through wide open and out of their way, but leaves stale blood free to flow away from your bowel, back into CIRCULATION towards your heart and lungs. Nothing in this process can possibly cause congestion.

Straining alters these forces radically. Propulsion now comes from your *diaphragm** and the sheets of muscle round your *abdomen,** which press inwards on everything they contain. If your bottom is relaxed it cannot resist this pressure from within, and anything nearby pouts out. That includes all the flesh surrounding your anus and the last part of your bowel, as well as any faeces inside them. Sustained high pressure also traps blood in your legs and lower bowel by blocking the main vein that drains them; blood even tends to flow in the wrong direction. So engorgement and congestion of the flesh round your anus is added to the stretching and scraping they get. Irritation from accumulating faeces perpetuates the congestion between bowel actions, so your bottom gets no rest. ITCHING and ECZEMA are the immediate consequences, and piles the long-term structural results. They may take only twenty years to form, especially if PREGNANCY is allowed to aggravate matters.

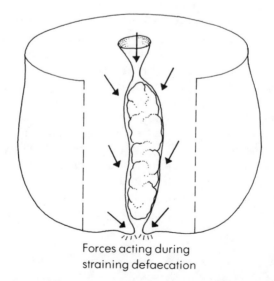

Forces acting during
straining defaecation

HELPING YOURSELF

The English pedestal toilet is appallingly designed because of the POSTURE needed to use it. To act your bowel well you need to squat, your knees apart and thighs firmly against your belly, your back well arched. That lines up your bowel, giving faeces a straight run out.

Always act when pangs tell you your bowel is willing and never postpone it. Adopt a good posture, relax your bottom thoroughly, and BREATHE deeply with your diaphragm, holding your breath in briefly but *not straining*. This massages and energizes your bowel, reinforcing and harmonizing its action. It is quickly unloaded, easing and satisfying the whole of you.

Piles get painful when blood clots in them; otherwise they are sore and irritable. Grease them with vaseline or anaesthetizing ointment before your bowel opens, and soothe them afterwards with a generous flow of cold water. A bidet is ideal, but a short hose adapted to your cold bath tap works just as well. Really acute discomfort responds to ice; sit gently on a cube for several minutes, letting it melt into the shape of your anal cleavage. Afterwards pat yourself dry, and apply Calendula or Hamamelis Ointment to soothe soreness and irritation. Arnica Ointment is better for aching pain, but avoid using it on any scratches or fissuring.

If you are obviously CONSTIPATED, act accordingly. Curing this is vital to reducing your piles and getting defaecation comfortable again.

Never get out of a hot bath without chilling your bottom thoroughly, as if it had just acted. Give those tissues no excuse to stay bloated and relaxed; it undermines all your other efforts.

Several ointments and suppositories available from your doctor are fine, but try to keep off any containing cortisone or other *steroids,** or antispetics.

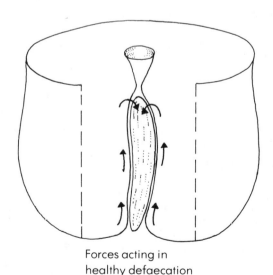

Forces acting in
healthy defaecation

WHAT HAPPENS

Everything on our earth has to cope with its gravitational pull in some way or another or it would collapse. Plants grow their semi-permanent architecture with gravity in mind so that its pull helps to determine their form. You move about too much to do that, but can brace your muscles of movement against gravity and balance yourself in any series of positions you choose.

Think of yourself performing a dance or walking across a room. Your *'colour'** intention directs the succession of postures and movements from one to the next as a graceful and economical progression. Your *'mono'** NERVOUS system then coordinates the tone and movement of every muscle to play its part in the manoeuvre. So in ordinary life, your 'mono' movements answer a 'colour' intention.

Not all disciplines of movement are used like that. 'Keep Fit', Aerobics and Remedial Gymnastics are taught for their own sake, a 'mono' means to a 'mono' end; exactly how they make you feel better is usually not pursued. Even sport gymnastics may be taught as disciplined 'mono' movement for its own sake, though like any sport it could be set to serve a 'colour' purpose.

Dance, drama, yoga and eurhythmy are quite different. They deliberately use 'mono' movement as a means to pursue a 'colour' purpose that is clearly defined in advance. As pure 'mono' EXERCISE they do not make much sense, and amuse otherwise intelligent people who misunderstand this. These kinds of movement exercise your 'colour' faculties; if that feels strange at first, it just shows how little exercise they get!

The grace of healthy posture and movement is beautiful to see, and easier to appreciate once you realize these principles. On the other hand, clumsy movement and poor posture take on far greater significance. They do not only mean that your body is being inefficient, with strain in JOINTS and painful TENSION in postural muscles. Defects like these hinder your 'colour' development or may themselves arise from your faulty 'colour' signature. Explore them therefore. If you cannot swing a golf-club exactly as you intend, or your riding instructor complains constantly about your seat, find out why. If spinal PAINS and stiffness tend to relapse after appropriate treatment, look deeper.

The problem may be as simple as CONCUSSION or an old INJURY which has jammed some part of your spine or skull, so that the slow rhythmic pulsations which should flow freely from your brain through your limbs are unable to pass. Since this pulsation seems to be involved in your mechanism for posture coordination, hindrance of this kind has long-term consequences and is well worth dealing with.

Or the 'mono' and 'colour' departments of your brain may be in conflict, so that your 'colour' intention is hindered by hesitancy or non-spontaneity in the way you carry it out. This cramps your style in everything; dealing with it will release you to discover at last how free living is meant to be.

HELPING YOURSELF

Explore with a Podiatrist problems concerning your FEET or walking.

Take any stiffness or PAIN in your spine and limbs to an *Osteopath** or *Chiropractor,** after checking with your doctor that there is no cause he can help you with. (ADDRESSES.)

If treatment drags on or your problem keeps recurring, ask yourself and your therapist why. If you tend to thrust your chin forward and get a stiff neck, the set of your TEETH may be wrong; seek out a dentist who understands dental kinesiology and jaw JOINT problems. There is an ADDRESS to help you.

A teacher of Alexander Technique (ADDRESS) understands posture and movement in this way, and will help you discover and correct your underlying problem.

Some sports coaches are now teaching the 'inner game', deliberately exposing conflict between your 'colour' intention and your 'mono' execution of the skills in your game. If you seem incomprehensibly erratic or unable to progress, enrol on a suitable course.

Once your ease of movement is restored, practise it. Ballroom *dance** may appeal to you if *yoga** seems exotic; *ballet** comes hard unless you learnt it when young, and *eurhythmy** may not be available nearby (ADDRESSES). Drama is comfortably conventional for grown-ups, but must be handled imaginatively; take soundings about the group or teacher before committing yourself. Several provincial theatres now run community workshops to popularize drama; enquire at your nearest theatre company.

Choose your sport for its 'colour' content as well as for 'mono' EXERCISE. *Riding** is specially suitable because it teaches attunement to an individual animal. Small boat *sailing** and *windsurfing,** especially on the sea, attune you similarly to wind and water. All are available extensively, see ADDRESSES.

PREGNANCY

WHAT SHOULD HAPPEN

To have a baby is the most creative opportunity available to most people, and the finishing-school for your adult life – not just for parenthood. Every child is a unique living expression of the wholeness of his parents' union, which he helps you to fulfil. You are not doomed necessarily to repeat any mistakes your parents made. Each new child's growing unfolds the unspoilt truth before your senses, exposing any half-truths and illusions you were brought up to. If only you will look, and dare to act on what you see, new growth can heal your own shortcomings.

Pregnancy is not a disease but an accomplishment of health. It unfolds naturally as part of your family life. Good Midwives and Family Doctors sincerely respect your preferences and inclinations, and cater for them as fully as they can. They make no attempt to fit you into a statistical category, but study your individual potential, cultivate it and watch it unfold. If and when you come under STRESS which threatens the security of your pregnancy they advise you how to ease it, separating you from your home only in the last resort. They seek the assistance of an Obstetrician – a specialist in the medicine and surgery of diseased pregnancies – only when they judge that your own capacities are exhausted, or soon will be.

If you approach your delivery in good health, there is no need to provoke it; your baby will initiate his birth when he is ready. Throughout its early stages you can remain actively occupied at home under your midwife's surveillance, eating and drinking normally and regularly while you can. Feel free to move, POSTURE, shout or rest as the impulse takes you; a close female companion, or your husband, can indulge your whims. Only when your labour is well established need you transfer to hospital, accompanied by your midwife, if that is your plan.

A good maternity ward runs more like a hotel than a hospital, allowing you privacy under discreet surveillance. Your midwife avoids at all costs disrupting your confident frame of mind, allowing you to progress in your own way, at your natural pace. You are never unattended. Medicines are avoided so that you and your baby remain alert. Delivery takes place in whatever posture is most comfortable, quietly in subdued indirect light. The cord is only cut if its tightness impedes delivery, and any womb-shrinking injection is postponed until after your placenta has ceased to function. You are given your baby as soon as he is born, to hold skin-to-skin while you are attended to. Natural delivery of your placenta is awaited, aided only by your baby's suckling; but your cord is cut for convenience when it shrivels and ceases to function. You are permitted to get up and bathe your baby if you wish, with your placenta still unborn if necessary, so long as you are not BLEEDING.

You let your baby get used to BREAST FEEDING before you go home, within a few hours if all else is well. Your baby stays in bed with you, overnight if you wish. Facilities are provided for your husband and your other children to stay as well, if you wish.

244

HELPING YOURSELVES

Before contemplating pregnancy explore yourselves thoroughly, create your home and settle down in it. Do not panic about your age!

Start positive FAMILY PLANNING at least six months before you hope to conceive. Meanwhile muse together over how you would like your pregnancy to be, what you want from your attendants and what you expect of family life.

Know that the law permits you to have your baby in any way you choose, provided you summon a midwife or doctor in good time before the birth takes place. You can register under the NHS with the Maternity Medical Practitioner of your choice, who need not be your own doctor. See him together to register, and explain your aspirations from the beginning. If you would like to have your baby at home, say so. He will not give promises, but his reaction to your suggestions will indicate the attitude you can expect.

Make friends with your midwife, and cooperate in your antenatal care. If you visit the obstetrician, take with you a note of your wishes to be incorporated into your hospital records. Keep a copy for yourselves.

Register with a good parenthood class. The National Childbirth Trust and The Birth Centre (ADDRESSES) offer well-conceived courses which take full account of your point of view; your Health Visitor or midwife will have arrangements too, which may expound things from a more medical point of view. But these courses will vary as much as the people organizing them. Shop around a bit and go to one of each kind if you can, especially first time.

Explore *homoeopathic** remedies for the simple ailments of pregnancy, rather than drugs. The BOOKLET published by the HOMOEOPATHIC Development Trust will help you choose.

Vitamin B_6 (Pyridoxine, 50–100mg twice daily) often helps in pregnancy SICKNESS, and Brewer's Yeast often helps you over a TIRED patch. A good general daily multimineral and multivitamin SUPPLEMENT (eg Nature's Own, or Lambert's Health Insurance Plus) is well worth while, from your pre-conceptional interval onwards.

You can ignore generalized warnings or forecasts of trouble that are based only on statistical attributes like your height, age or weight. People do not behave that predictably, and you are entitled to be treated as a unique individual for so long as you are actually well. However you should take seriously all professional advice that is based on factors in your own present condition or past history. Simply ask why you are being advised to adopt any particular course of action you distrust. A specific reason will be promptly and confidently given, and you can easily distinguish the vague, uncertain or evasive excuses that will be offered if no good reason exists.

PREMENSTRUAL TENSION

This is a topic doctors no longer ignore, but cannot agree about. Its sheer frequency has forced them to accept that it exists, though many remain reluctant to admit it. None of the wide variety of drug treatments offered is reliable. Even if they were, their cost, side-effects and potential long-term complications would restrict their usefulness to the women most severely affected.

Yet very few doctors so far have given the problem a fraction of the attention it deserves. Fewer still have paused to wonder why so many women nowadays – estimates range from three to nine out of ten – should be mentally and physically disturbed in some degree while awaiting their menstrual PERIODS. When eventually they are persuaded to exercise their collective common sense on the problem, they will quickly realize that long-term medication could never in any case be an appropriate response to so common a condition.

Your biological history illuminates this phenomenon better than twentieth-century biochemistry. Menstrual PERIODS are customary, but not altogether natural; they are the debris of PREGNANCIES that your body planned and you frustrated. There must be better means of FAMILY PLANNING and CONTRACEPTION available to us, because many less sophisticated species employ them routinely. But few, even of those women who do experience more selective menstrual function, are comfortable with it.

Most settle for a complex monthly conflict between your 'mono'* and 'colour'* natures, on several levels within you. Instinctive 'colour' wistfulness for motherhood conflicts in your thoughts and feelings with equally reasonable cultural aspirations, and 'mono' economic ambitions. Ambivalence at this level leaves your primal adaptive system* without a clear-cut purpose, so that your primitive reproductive urge never adapts to modern circumstances. This leaves your 'mono' genital apparatus without firm 'colour' guidance; it carries on functioning at its most primitive level, of attempting pregnancy as soon and often as possible.

Premenstrual tension occurs during the monthly physical struggle to hold a pregnancy you do not want or have failed to conceive. Your body already knows your egg is not fertile, long before menstruation reassures your mind. Exactly how the TENSION shows depends on your particular weaknesses. Four main symptom groups with distinct origins are distinguished by Dr Guy Abraham, an American gynaecologist who has taken a special interest in the condition. Your main symptoms may indicate disturbed mental functioning – either over-arousal with anxiety, restlessness and irritability; or depression, with forgetfulness, tears, and confusion. Some people show disturbances of fluid balance most prominently – WEIGHT gain, BREAST tenderness and pelvic swelling. The final group have APPETITE disturbance with cravings and the symptoms of HYPOGLYCAEMIA. Correct whichever of these apply, and the physical component of your tension will ease or resolve completely.

HELPING YOURSELF

A DIET for health is essential, avoiding sugar, refined flour and dairy products in particular. Coffee, tea, chocolate and cola are likely to aggravate your symptoms. Stop SMOKING or reduce your intake drastically. Avoid ALCOHOL during your symptoms.

Daily SUPPLEMENTS of Vitamin B6 (Pyridoxine) 150mg, Brewer's Yeast six to nine tablets, and Magnesium (as three tablets of Dolomite) are always worthwhile and harmless. If these are disappointing Essential Fatty Acid SUPPLEMENTS are the next to try; they are appreciably more expensive. These aim to restore quickly your hormone metabolism, of which great demands are made each month. After four to six months you should be able to cope on a healthy DIET alone.

If NERVOUS TENSION, irritability and mood swings are your main symptoms, the above should cover your needs.

If weight gain, fluid swelling or bloating with GAS or BREAST PROBLEMS predominate, add Vitamin E to all this – up to 200 IU daily. Coffee, tea, cocoa and cola are particularly liable to aggravate symptoms of this kind.

If hunger, sugar cravings, FAINTNESS, HEADACHES or TIREDNESS figure largely in your premenstrual symptoms, HYPOGLYCAEMIA may be their cause. Add Chromium Orotate 1mg three times daily to your SUPPLEMENTS.

If DEPRESSION, SLEEPLESSNESS, tearfulness, confusion or forgetfulness are important features, include Vitamin C (1000mg three times daily) among your SUPPLEMENTS.

Beyond this you will need the help of a *Naturopath,** *Holistic Doctor,** *Homoeopath** or *Traditional Chinese Medicine** practitioner. The Premenstrual Tension Advisory Service and Women's Health Concern offer experienced guidance (ADDRESSES).

Keep your own doctor informed, ask his advice in advance, and see if he will cooperate by prescribing the more expensive supplements – certain brands (eg Nature's Own, Lambert's) can be made available under National Health Service arrangements.

Deep-seated personal conflicts may underlie your physical symptoms. List your ambitions, and rank them honestly: are they unrealistic or mutually incompatible? Your partner, a friend, a *Counsellor** or *Clinical Psychologist** can help you do this. If your state of mind is clear, try the corresponding *Bach Flower Remedy** (ADDRESS).

The only medical treatment with a long track record of success is human progesterone ('Cyclogest'), which was pioneered by Dr Katharina Dalton. Its effect is sometimes dramatic, and it appears to produce very few side-effects. There is no harm in asking your doctor for a trial of this, though the odds are he will prefer a synthetic alternative that has been sold harder by its manufacturers and is therefore more familiar to him.

PROSTATE PROBLEMS

Your prostate gland is wrapped round the urinary pipe as it leaves your bladder, about the size of a small tomato. It lies right next to the last part of your bowel, which is one reason why doctors sometimes feel this area with a gloved finger inserted through your anus.

It matures at puberty as part of your male sexual apparatus. Whenever you ejaculate, sperms out of storage behind your bladder are mixed with a mucoid fluid which pumps from your prostate, flushing them down your urethra. It is particularly rich in zinc, and contains an *enzyme** to activate the sperms and citric acid to prime it, plus protein-splitting enzymes that liquefy the fluid and enable the sperms to swim through it. This prostatic fluid makes up most of your semen, which is why *vasectomy** (to prevent sperm getting out to join your semen) does not alter its volume or appearance much.

Half your prostate consists of the glands for making the fluid, which accumulates continuously in its *cells** and ducts between ejaculations; another quarter is muscle for pumping it out during each one. The glands are arranged in three layers, the innermost of which are very prone to swell gradually as you *age.** The material which engorges them is rich with protein, and can with patience be massaged out during a prolonged rectal examination – though this is not practical as a form of treatment.

The swelling can accumulate to many times the size of your original gland, or the size of an average orange. If this swelling is mostly outward it may not interfere with your urination until it is quite large. Often, however, a small hump can develop inwards from the start, before your prostate has enlarged appreciably otherwise. This restricts your urinary flow to a dribble without any force behind it and makes it difficult to get the flow started. The frequent need to urinate at night can often be traced to this cause.

CANCER and INFECTION (including THRUSH) can both complicate this condition, but protein accumulation by itself is the commonest form of prostate disorder. It affects a large minority of men in developed countries from the age of forty, and seems to be a consequence of eating meat in any quantity. Zinc deficiency plays some part, since diseased prostates and their semen contain strikingly less of it and SUPPLEMENTS can be corrective.

Doctors know little about prostate health, confining their interest to distinguishing the CANCERS and SURGICAL treatment of the non-cancerous glandular swellings. The medical situation is therefore very much the same as with CATARACT, VARICOSE VEINS, PILES and NOISES IN YOUR HEAD. If you seek preventive medical advice or early diagnosis it is quite likely you will merely be told to return when your condition is bad enough to warrant surgery. And yet there are several simple and harmless things you can do while you are waiting which would do no violence to any essential medical principle and may save you an operation. That doctors do not take the trouble to explore and adopt this wisdom is grossly negligent of the medical profession as a whole.

HELPING YOURSELF

Prevention hangs on eating the DIET for health, with meat meals restricted to no more than one or two occasions each week. Wholemeal cereals, legumes (pea family) and root vegetables not only contain ample protein but are rich in Zinc, too.

When some degree of non-CANCEROUS prostate swelling is discovered, embark on a special cleansing DIET of raw vegetables and fruits for three weeks, and repeat it for one week each month. Avoid all meat, fish, poultry and hard cheese for six months. This will prevent any further protein accumulation in your prostate.

SUPPLEMENT this with Zinc 15mg and Vitamin C 1000mg, twice daily at mealtimes. This rapidly corrects any prostatic zinc deficiency, enabling it to function better and contribute to its own recovery.

Obtain from a *herbalist** Tincture of Echinacea and take three drops in a teaspoonful of cold water every night; this helps get rid of the swelling.

Sponge just behind your scrotum alternately with hot water (one minute) and cold (thirty seconds) for three cycles finishing with cold. Repeat this night and morning to stimulate contraction of the muscle in your prostate, which will extrude some of the fluid congestion each time.

Have ten minutes of firm massage to your lower spine (as far as your buttocks) whenever your companion can manage it – daily if possible. Each massaging stroke should approach your mid-line upwards and inwards from both sides, successively starting a little lower down. Taken together, the strokes are like the branches of a herring-bone laid along your spine, tail downwards. They stimulate the NERVES that control your prostate muscle, to reinforce the effect of sponging.

Cooperate with your doctor to identify the nature of your swelling, but only agree to SURGERY if six months of the above gives no improvement.

If your prostate dwelling is cancerous you are more likely to be offered female *hormone** treatment than surgery. Consult a doctor registered with New Approaches to Cancer (ADDRESS), who will recommend additional SUPPLEMENTS you cannot buy without a prescription. In general, however, the same principles apply.

PSORIASIS

WHAT HAPPENS

Your skin is not just a container but a remarkably sophisticated organ which regulates losses of heat and moisture from your body, can store and excrete surpluses from metabolism and receives sensory impressions. Despite its permeability it is a very effective barrier against *microbes** and moisture, and can regulate the penetration of sunlight to the tissues inside. It wears tirelessly, and will grow into a form appropriate to the physical work expected of it. Its elasticity enables it to cope with changes over the years in your shape and size.

It has idiosyncrasies too. Enormous individual variations occur in thickness, texture, hardness and colour, most of which are inherent in you. A few rare skin diseases seem to be inherited directly in this way, and are inevitable; but none of the common ones are in this category, although they are particularly common in some families. What you inherit is not the disease but a weakness for it. This means that when your skin is under stress it will probably break down more readily than other people's, and in your particular way.

Psoriasis is like this. The weakness is in you all the time, but the actual disease can come and go. The healthy cadence of changes in your skin structure, from its foundations to its surface, is disrupted as in ECZEMA but in the opposite direction; cells grow too fast in both diseases, but in psoriasis they heap up in silvery crusts and usually stay dry. This mainly affects skin that grows fast normally and forms crusts to resist wear, such as your scalp and the rough hardened skin on the outside of your JOINTS; but it can go anywhere except your face. These patches may sometimes ITCH, but chiefly offend by their prominent and unhealthy INFLAMED appearance. When your scalp is severely involved it can cause temporary HAIR LOSS. It is one of the commonest skin diseases in Europe, and affects one or two per cent of people in Western countries.

The disease is your peculiar way of responding to the excessive *waste acids** produced when you habitually over-eat protein or suffer from mineral imbalance; but it can result from food ALLERGY, chemical *intolerance** or heavy metal poisoning. Food from the cow is a particularly common irritant. It is made very much worse by STRESS or TIREDNESS, if either is severe enough to preoccupy your coping capacity and leave your skin less well defended. That it affects your whole body is clear when it accompanies rheumatoid ARTHRITIS or when the destructive kind of arthritis peculiar to psoriasis develops instead.

You would not therefore expect external treatments to heal it radically, and they do not. If you want a sustained effect you will need to apply them intermittently for an indefinite period, and they will not always work. To overcome your susceptibility to psoriasis you will have to work from the inside, using the same cleansing therapies that will cure the arthritis it sometimes accompanies.

HELPING YOURSELF

Keep your skin healthy by ventilating it well, taking every opportunity to bathe in the air and the sun. If you use an ultra-violet lamp in winter be very sparing, only one or two minutes daily at the prescribed distance. Cool your skin afterwards with cold water.

Have a daily dry friction rub, using a loofa or soft grooming brush, either just before a hot shower (finished with cold) or whenever you can stay naked or lightly clothed for ten minutes afterwards.

A cleansing DIET of raw food is very successful, but may need to be sustained for many months; be patient. Check at the outset whether you are ALLERGIC to food from the cow, which is commonly associated; it will be more difficult to confirm after months of abstinence.

Arsenicum album up to 30th potency is a *Homoeopathic** remedy you can try yourself; if it fails you will need professional assistance to select something more appropriate for you.

Your doctor has at his disposal creams for removing the silvery scales, and coal tar lotions and shampoo to deal with your scalp. These are quite good supportive measures while you are curing yourself. Tell him your intentions; he will be interested in your progress, though he may not admit it.

Specialists sometimes use immunosuppressive therapy for severe psoriasis. I cannot recommend this because of its drastically weakening effect on your IMMUNE system. Start an intensive raw diet instead, supported by the other measures already given.

SUPPLEMENTS of Zinc (15–30mg daily), Vitamin E (200IU twice daily), Selenium (400mcg twice daily), Vitamin C (500mg three times daily) and Essential Fatty Acids may be helpful for two or three months; thereafter your diet should maintain you.

ARTHRITIS responds to the same cleansing methods, but particular JOINTS may need passive movement, and hot wax or alternating hot and cold water baths to promote the traffic of healing. Treat them energetically to prevent erosion and destruction of the joint surfaces.

RADIATION

WHAT HAPPENS

Ionizing radiations from nuclear reactions are, unlike ELECTRICITY DISEASE, part of the background against which life continues to evolve on earth. Lovelock points out in his BOOK that primitive life forms had to cope with about ten times the background radiation we now endure, some of it arising from hot spots – natural nuclear reactors – in the earth's crust. Evidently we should be able to tolerate appreciable degrees of radiation STRESS without being adversely affected.

Nevertheless we know that dense pulses of radiation are lethal, and that sub-lethal doses *age** you prematurely and may cause CANCER and birth defects many years later. Radiation is the only known cause of LEUKAEMIA,* a blood cancer whose frequency varies a lot from place to place and is unusually high near the Sellafield Nuclear Reprocessing Plant in Cumbria and a number of atomic energy research establishments. The radioactivity of the main isotopes concerned persists for periods ranging from 25,000 years upwards, so that the opportunities and implications of leakage and accident cannot be discounted. And our security against the possibility of nuclear war is far less still.

These issues must be resolved by public debate and democratic process, but there are two practical matters you can act on for yourself.

Most atmospheric and geological radiation is inescapable and amounts to a third of your total background exposure. But another third derives from Radon and Thoron, radioactive gases that leak from the earth into the atmosphere. They can pass through conventional building materials and accumulate in buildings that are inadequately ventilated or air conditioned. This enormously increases the concentration of these gases in modern offices and homes, so that their contribution to your annual radiation exposure becomes very significant. The background radiation dosage to people in exceptionally affected houses may be as much as 100 times higher than the average, which in Britain is around 2 milliSieverts annually.

This radiation harms you mainly by producing *free radicals,** which are viciously reactive chemical fragments like splinters of broken glass smashed forcefully off any protein *molecules** or *genes** that happen to intercept a particle of radiation. These free radicals are highly mischievous, able to set off chain reactions that reverberate through your tissues doing widespread damage. Extensive random damage is bound eventually to include important sites, destruction of which interferes disproportionately with your *metabolism** or *cell** reproduction. When cells are damaged only slightly in this way they may remain viable but be incapable of responding normally to your *'colour'** control. This is how radiation can cause CANCER, MISCARRIAGES and birth defects to increase.

This damage depends on the concentration in your tissues of free radical scavengers, which prevent chain reactions. Supplements of these greatly increase your resistance to radiation damage. Whatever scientists may say about the safety of nuclear accidents, this precaution is well worthwhile.

HELPING YOURSELF

Read the British Medical Association's two BOOKS on the medical effects of nuclear war, and the National Radiological Protection Board's BOOKLET. Our radiological protection standards are highly dependent on statistical averages and theoretical projections from limited experimental evidence. They make no allowance for the wide variations from average values that are likely to occur in practice, even within small localities. Reassurances of this kind must consequently be treated with caution.

Ventilate your home thoroughly in all seasons, whenever the weather permits. This applies whether or not you live on the ground floor.

Avoid using aerosol sprays for any purpose; even most spray-can medications are available in alternative forms. This helps slow down the build-up of halocarbon propellants in the upper atmosphere, where they destroy ozone – our shield against cosmic rays.

Eat the DIET for health, keeping flesh foods to a minimum. Meat animals scavenge radioactive chemical pollutants over a large area in the course of their growth, whereas root vegetables are somewhat protected from atmospheric fallout and even leaves collect only from a limited area.

SUPPLEMENT this with 1000–5000mg Vitamin C daily, according to your means and the risk you are exposed to. This is the cheapest harmless free radical scavenger available. If necessary, a *Naturopathic Practitioner** or *Clinical Ecologist** can test your urine to discover how much Vitamin C you can make use of in this way. Vitamins B_5 (Pantothenic Acid, 50mg twice daily) and B_6 (Pyridoxine, 50mg twice daily) both help to protect skin and other tissues from radiation damage.

In emergency make up a *Bach Flower Remedy** as follows: half a teaspoon of sea salt and two drops each of the Tinctures Cherry Plum, Gentian, Rock Rose, Star of Bethlehem, Vine, Walnut and Wild Oat, all dissolved in 100ml of natural spring water. Four times daily take four drops in a teaspoon of water, savoured well for a few seconds before you swallow it.

It does no good to worry about things you cannot personally change. Hopefulness and optimism maintain your own purposiveness and IMMUNITY, and they favourably influence other people. Enough of us, all thinking positively as ardently as we can, exert considerable 'colour' influence on world events.

RECIPES

Brose

Mix one cup of coarse oatmeal with two cups of broad bran and a handful of raisins. Sprinkle this mixture into four cups of boiling water and allow it to stand for ten to fifteen minutes. This is a completely safe and very effective way to take bran as a remedy for INDIGESTION or CONSTIPATION.

Coleslaw

Shortly before your meal take equal parts of fresh raw onion, carrot and cabbage, and shred them finely. Mix them in a bowl with just enough Salad Dressing RECIPE to coat all the shreds evenly. This dish is intended to be eaten very fresh: make only enough for the forthcoming meal and discard any remains that will have to be kept overnight.

Egg Nog

Take the waste shell from a clean free-range hen's egg and crumple it into a tablespoonful of 'organic'* Cider Vinegar. Overnight this will dissolve the greater part of the shell, at the same time losing its sourness. Strain the fluid from the solid residue. Rinse this repeatedly with hot water, adding the washings to the strained fluid.

Make this palatable with a tablespoon of honey or black strap molasses, and dilute the whole to a mugful. It slightly resembles coffee, and cannot altogether be described as pleasant. But it is an excellent and comprehensive mineral supplement which is practically free, and takes good advantage of a wasted food resource.

Emergency Maintenance Fluid

> Ingredients:
> Water (preferably spring water) one pint
> Salt (preferably sea-salt) ½ level teaspoon
> Molasses (best), Malt, Honey, Brown or
> (worst) White Sugar – 2 level tsp.

Stir to dissolve, and warm to body heat. It should taste of nothing in particular; otherwise check your quantities. If in doubt, dilute further to taste.

Garlic Lozenge

From a plump firm bulb of garlic detach one clove, complete with its crisp outer skin. Tidy any debris away from its 'root'. Insert the whole clove in your cheek and leave it there for two hours. Do not suck, chew or bruise it. With care one clove will serve for eight hours of intermittent use.

Honey Cider Vinegar

Mix equal quantities of a good organically grown Cider Vinegar and locally produced or organic honey. Dilute with hot water to taste. Try a tablespoon measure of each for a mugful. Will keep in a sealed vacuum flask but is better made up freshly when you want it.

Lemon Barley Water

Cover 60gm (2oz) pearl or pot barley with cold water and bring to the boil. Strain off and discard surplus fluid. Pour 500ml (17fl oz) of freshly boiling water on the swollen grain, stir and allow to steep for $\frac{1}{2}$–1 minute, when a misty grey-blue appearance develops. Strain and retain both grain and fluid. A second longer steeping gives a useful fluid, but of lesser quality. Oversteeping gives a fluid that sets on cooling.

Sour the fluid to taste with lemon juice or Ascorbic Acid. A little honey, molasses, malt or fruit juice may be added if necessary.

Live Yoghurt

Heat 500ml (17fl oz) fresh milk to 82°C (simmering), then cool to 37°C (blood heat). (Yoghurt is native to goat's milk, which gives the best results.) Mix in a tbsp of live natural yoghurt, or a starter, and keep in a scalded vacuum flask for 4–6 hours. Chill the yoghurt to conserve it.

Mayonnaise

Ingredients:
2 free-range egg yolks
a few twists of milled sea salt
$\frac{3}{4}$ teaspoon dry mustard
$\frac{1}{8}$ teaspoon freshly milled pepper
230ml (8fl oz) cold pressed olive oil
15ml (1 tbsp) white wine vinegar or lemon juice

Put the yolks, mustard and seasonings in a mixing bowl and whisk them into a uniform consistency. Add the oil a drop at a time while you continue to beat the mixture steadily, until it begins to thicken and stabilize; you can then trickle the oil in faster. Add a dash of vinegar occasionally to stop the emulsion from solidifying. When all the oil is combined, add the rest of the vinegar. Adjust the seasonings to taste, and store in a screw-topped jar.

This sauce can be made thick enough to act as a substitute for butter and margarine, and will surpass the nutritional quality of both if you choose your ingredients well.

Müesli

Bircher-Benner's original recipe is:
>2–3 small apples or one big one
>1 tablespoon walnuts, hazel nuts or almonds
>1 level tablespoon organically grown rolled oats, soaked beforehand for 12 hours in 3 tablespoons of water
>1 tablespoon sweetened condensed milk
>Juice of ½ lemon

Prepare freshly, just before serving. Rub the apples clean with a dry cloth; do not core or peel them. Mix condensed milk and juice with the oats, grate the apples quickly and stir into the mixture. Serve, offering the nuts freshly ground as a separate garnish.

Possible Modifications: Brazil nuts are good value at present; peanuts **do not really count** as properly speaking they are pea-family, not nuts at all. Make up a mixture of rolled grains from whatever you can get organically grown: oats, wheat, rye and barley are usually available. Omit the sweetened condensed milk unless you are UNDERWEIGHT (as many of Bircher-Benner's patients were); substitute a tablespoon of chopped dried fruit, soaked overnight and mashed if necessary. You need not grate the apples if you are prepared to eat them along with the grains, which you can moisten by other means. *Otherwise the details matter – especially the fresh raw fruit.*

Preserves

Make jam and marmalade by all means, but rely more on the fruit. Use any traditional recipe, but halve the quantity of sugar and boil the mixture down to jamming temperature. You get a much more fruity result and the marmalade has more bitterness; but it fills fewer jars. However it's good, and will not tempt you to excess. Refrigerate each jar after you have opened it or the surface will go mouldy.

For marmalade go to the expense of obtaining 'organic'* fruits, or at least ensure that they have not been sprayed. The chemicals used to protect the peel from rotting are only permitted under EEC regulations on the assumption that they will not be consumed. I for one got stomach pain after home-made marmalade using sprayed oranges – but not since unsprayed fruit came our way. We would never again use anything else.

Salad Dressing

> Ingredients:
> 50ml (3 tbsp) cold pressed olive oil
> 15ml (1 tbsp) 'organic' cider or wine vinegar
> a few twists each of freshly milled sea-salt and black pepper

Mix all the ingredients in a small bowl and beat them until they are well emulsified. Alternatively, put them in a sealed jar and shake it vigorously for about twenty seconds. Only make what you can use today.

Sprouting Seeds

One-fifth fill a jar with wheat, whole lentils, peas, cress or any other viable seed *not chemically dressed for planting*. Soak overnight with plenty of warm water. Drain the swollen seeds, through a sieve or gauze to keep them in the jar; then rinse with warm water and drain again before standing them in a warm place. Rinse and drain twice a day: large seeds need rinsing more often, small seeds need prolonged draining. Start eating the sprouts when their shoots are as long as the seed. After a few days more they fill the whole jar.

For small children, liquidize sprouts into soup just before serving.

Vegetable Water

Rinse the vegetables thoroughly, cleaning off soil and insects. Cook diced roots in the minimum of unsalted water in a closed pan of stainless steel, glass or ceramic – not aluminium; steam chopped greens simultaneously on a stainless steel basket. Strain off the water and save it. It makes a wholesome and pleasant drink, which can be cooled and given to babies from a few months old instead of 'juice'. It will mask the sourness of a Vitamin C dose dissolved in it.

WHAT HAPPENS

Illness is rather like a train strike – the official dispute is only the public part of a much longer process. Bad feeling accumulates inconspicuously for months or years before the strike erupts. When a deal is done to end it, all the trains and staff are in the wrong places, dirty and short of supplies. It can take weeks to restore normal operations, and months to assimilate the new state of affairs in the industry.

If we handle industrial disputes badly, we cope with illness worse. Not only do we ignore the trends which lead up to it, but we seldom allow ourselves the time and resources for proper recovery, or *convalescence.**

Common VIRUS INFECTIONS are probably the worst example. The obvious symptoms of 'FLU last only a few days, during which time virus particles are multiplying inside your *cells,** bursting out and destroying them, and moving on to attack further cells in the same way. Once your *antibody** response is mobilized their advance is checked and you start to feel a bit better, but there is a trail of destruction still to be cleared up. Healing that devastation takes you at least twice as long again, and requires as much effort as to heal a large SURGICAL scar. It is no less real for being spread about your body in microscopic portions. During that time your stamina, tolerance and concentration are poor, but to anyone else you just look a bit pale. You feel a fraud, and everyone is so eager to have you back in harness that you are tempted to return before you really have the energy to last the day. Giving in prolongs your convalescence and keeps you vulnerable to further illness.

The need for convalescence arises primarily from the depletion of your reserves, spent on the extra effort of fighting off the illness. You may actually lose weight, indicating that 'mono' energy has been pouring out faster than you could replace it. But the effects may be much more subtle, and more difficult to make good. Vitamins, fatty acids and minerals may all be used faster in illness and take many days or several weeks to replace at the fastest rate your body can cope with absorbing them. Digestive processes may be upset. A backlog of fluid, minerals, and *waste acids** from the decomposition of damaged tissues may accumulate for excretion. The electrical and *'colour'* vitality of tissues that survive the disease will require recharging.

The orderliness and energy of your healing depend in the first place on a vivid 'colour' blueprint for the parts concerned, maintained by your *primal adaptive system** as architect of your recovery. Energy and materials for the work must be supplied from your food or existing reserves and reduce your energy for living while your convalescence lasts.

TEENAGERS take longer to convalesce, because growth takes precedence over routine defence during your growth spurt if your DIET cannot supply both. Only in severe and protracted illness will growth yield precedence to recovery; most of the headway you lose in consequence is regained afterwards.

Make lemon barley water from the RECIPE if you cannot at first eat much; this drink will nourish you lightly, fortify your *alkaline reserve,** rekindle your metabolism and thus your appetite.

Fresh fruit such as grapes, ripe apples and over-ripe bananas are suitable foods to start with. Add live yoghurt RECIPE if your digestion has been upset.

Then eat a simple DIET for health, SUPPLEMENTED for convalescence. Vitamin B_{15} (Pangamic Acid, 50mg three times daily) is especially useful in promoting recovery. Take each dose with a tablet of Brewer's Yeast.

Comfrey Tea, or 400mg tablets of the Root (two three times daily) is a useful stimulant to your healing blood-cells if there is still flesh to repair, bruising to clear away or pus actively forming. Limit your use of the root to a maximum of one or two months; it is safe to eat fresh leaves and brew tea indefinitely.

Be active for short periods when you feel you can, but stop when your stamina runs out. These rests will gradually get briefer and less frequent, but are essential meanwhile to divert energy from your budget for living into your healing effort.

Do not fret about things you feel you should be doing – this wastes your mental energy and disintegrates your healing effort. Settle your mind lightly on thoughts of getting better, visualizing how the work is proceeding in your affected parts. Ask by all means for the healing process to be explained to you, so that you can visualize it more realistically; but it does not matter if the image in your mind's eye is a little fanciful!

Keep the air around you fresh, freely ventilated to the outside. BREATHE deeply, consciously using your *diaphragm** to the full, for at least ten breaths several times each day. This is something you can always do, even if you can manage little else.

Bathe your naked body in fresh air for five or ten minutes twice daily, shaded from the sun until you are acclimatized. Sunbathe a little too when you can, but not through windows. Start with five minutes of direct sunlight to each side, gradually increasing your daily dose to twenty minutes. Keep your head shaded. Red silk filters the harsher rays out of strong sunlight, safer if you are fair skinned or red-headed. Finish with a brief cool shower.

Shower with hot water until you are warm and relaxed, then play cold water on your limbs for thirty seconds. Repeat this daily, including your face and body in the cold phase when you are ready. Rub yourself dry vigorously.

Think out what your illness has taught you, and what changes in your life will strengthen the weakness it revealed. Then act on your conclusions.

WHAT HAPPENS

Most people in developed countries reach thirty in the prime of life – all TEENAGE qualms over, your youth still blooming and embellished with experience enough to tackle your main life choices maturely. By forty some of your options have fallen away, exchanged for the experience to base sound judgements on. Your body and mind remain alert, supple and strong, with plenty of stamina and reasonable speed; there is still very little to distinguish people who will last another forty years from others who are fading.

By fifty however your ways have parted, and differences in ageing are conspicuous. Many people are worn out long before retirement; yet a pension starts others on a whole new life that remains vigorous for another twenty years. What makes the difference?

The first requirement is food of adequate quality. For several generations we have valued foodstuffs almost entirely by their weight and appearance, mistaking perfect form for quality. And we have assumed as of right, for several generations, that food should be cheap. This tenet originates from days when enough food was beyond the means of the poor, and the argument had force. But it has resulted in overproduction of the second rate, on which you cannot expect to survive into old age in good form.

Yet we know very well that in everything else, from soft furnishings to shoe leather, long life must be paid for. Such quality is alien to modern foods but distinguishes the naturally grown produce of healthy soil. Genuine 'organic'* quality conveys long life not only to the produce but also to the people who consume it. It is becoming more readily available in supermarkets, and in retirement you have all the time you need to grow it for yourself.

Good food sets you up for strong personal IMMUNITY, which is your greatest asset. It underpins your enthusiasm, confidence and common sense, on which you can base a healthy *action pattern** for tackling everything you do. You flow along with life, at odds with nothing else living; resourceful enough to deal equally with awkward people and the potentially negative feelings they arouse. This entirely positive outlook on everything is powerful, versatile, self-respecting and self-reinforcing. It is the essential hallmark of health and WELLBEING.

Even so, good food and a wholesome approach to life are your means, not ends in themselves; you need them to set about '*colour*'* aspirations that are worthy of you. No purely '*mono*'* ambition withstands unemployment or retirement; even with a comfortable home and adequate income you need a personal purpose to engage your talents fully. It is for you to explore and to choose, free of any constraint by others. What is more, you can by now really let your hair down, if you want to. There are no sanctions that will be brought to bear against you – provided you stay within the law, and just this side of madness. Society may not take much notice of you, but will indulge and tolerate your whims.

HELPING YOURSELF

Eat the DIET for health, throughout your life. Choose 'organic' quality foods whenever you can, and pay willingly the premium prices they command. Buy less if necessary, since their quality makes up for it.

Get Hills' BOOK and grow food this way for yourself, in window-boxes, flower pots, garden and allotment. However humble your first crops may appear, you know their quality is honest: build up the health of your garden soil and watch that quality improve.

Eat low on the food chain – mainly things that grow directly in or on the soil. These keep your blood clean and only produce *waste acids** at the rate you can comfortably cope with. Flesh foods upset this, and the diseases of waste acid accumulation easily follow – MIGRAINE, ARTERIOSCLEROSIS, RHEU-MATISM and ARTHRITIS among them. Meat-eating people age faster, other things being equal; life-long vegetarians outlive their neighbours by up to ten years.

SUPPLEMENT this with up to 3000mg Vitamin C daily, the least expensive efficient *free radical** scavenger available. This offsets the ageing effects of prolonged physical STRESSES such as chemical pollutants and RADIATION.

Treat ALCOHOL with respect, and keep off SMOKING altogether. Spirit drinking ages you rapidly, and anything regularly or in quantity makes you OVERWEIGHT.

EXERCISE for an hour every day, vigorously enough to make conversation difficult. Regular full use is the best way to keep your CIRCULATION and BREATHING efficient and your limbs supple; full living depends on all these. Purposeful activity is best – sawing logs, carpentry, gardening, and walking or cycling about your business. Only pursue sports you enjoy in themselves; there is no need any longer to do anything you actively dislike just for the sake of appearances. Try *yoga** if nothing else appeals to you (ADDRESS and Volin's BOOK).

Attend to the quality of your SLEEP, so that you awaken naturally and refreshed. It is worth spending your first six months of retirement getting this right, since nothing new comes easily to a chronically TIRED mind.

Make your retirement a process of unfettered exploration. Pursue those skills and fascinations that were never suitable as *recreation,** not profitable in themselves; a pension is licence to indulge in them, without regard to the time they take. The University of the Third Age (ADDRESS) may appeal to you.

Reflect positively on the meaning and purpose of your life, and on the prospect of DYING. If you come to practical conclusions, act on them.

RHEUMATISM

The story of this single word tells a great deal of the history of medicine's decline into inappropriate technology, all by itself.

It began with the idea of a watery flowing humour, which by contaminating or clogging up your muscles and ligaments would cause them to INFLAME and hurt. PAINFUL conditions of this kind would be treated by all means fashionable, in every age; but there was never very much to show for them before the seventeenth century. No archaeological study, by the way, has ever revealed evidence in the ancients of two major modern diseases – *rheumatoid ARTHRITIS** and *ankylosing spondylitis** – even though a sizeable minority survived long enough to acquire them.

Pasteur's well-publicized misinterpretations of Béchamp's nineteenth-century studies of INFECTION led the medical world to deal with everything in terms of germs and vaccines; that influence remains predominant today. Watery humours were out and the spas declined – at the very moment when the biological science of Howard and McCarrison was justifying the natural-istic medical teachings handed down to twentieth-century physicians like Bircher-Benner, Haig, Lindlahr, Picton and Waerland (BOOKS). By the time germ theories of rheumatism were discredited, chemists were developing drug treatments for its most obvious consequences – the conspicuous inflam-matory changes it causes in joints – which have been big business ever since.

These drugs give fast results easily compared with the best spa cures – months of harsh DIETS and bathing routines. But generations of users have now discovered the underlying truth, that drugs only go symptom-deep. They make no difference to the progress of the disease itself, and may even accelerate it.

Your fundamental problem is slow accumulation in your *tissues** of *waste acids** and other chemicals. This comes about because you cannot excrete them as fast as they arrive, in chemically processed food and meat, which you have become accustomed to eating too often and in too large a quantity. In excess these waste acids can form a sticky colloidal gel in your CIRCULATION, which cannot then flow freely through your tissues. This severely restricts *metabolic** work, forcing you to replace damaged active *cells** with inactive fibrous tissues. That is the beginning of the destruction rheumatism can cause, slowly over several decades, in comfortable people lulled temporarily by their drugs.

Vague and fleeting though the symptoms of this process are, doctors were never justified in ignoring it. They have simply refused to take any active part in the one debate that matters, the quality and balance of your DIET. Nutrition takes practically no place in the medical curriculum, and even there consists of entirely dead *'mono'** technical information.

Reversal of the accumulation process is your best chance of preventing far worse diseases doctors understand little and treat poorly – ARTHRITIS, BLOOD PRESSURE, CATARACT and MIGRAINE are only a few.

HELPING YOURSELF

If you have bouts of troublesome pain, *tenderness** and stiffness that arise repeatedly in widely different parts of your body, but with no changes in your blood or visible on X-rays that impress your doctor, you have rheumatism. Do *not* form the habit of taking anti-inflammatory medicines – Aspirin, Codeine, Ibuprofen, Paracetamol and their combinations – whether medically prescribed or not. These only hinder even further your excretion of the waste acids that are causing the trouble. At best, they turn off PAIN (your alarm signal) and INFLAMMATION (your healing effort) for a time. At worst they accelerate the degenerative process of the disease. Other *stimulants** have the same effect – ALCOHOL, coffee, SMOKING in particular, tea and chocolate somewhat less.

Instead adopt the special cleansing DIET for three weeks, and repeat it for one week in every month thereafter. Stick carefully to the DIET for health otherwise. Eat little or no meat of any kind, including poultry and game; a little fresh fish occasionally is about the limit. Rely mostly on fresh vegetables and ripe fruits, half of them eaten raw, with whole-grain cereals in the second line. There is no need to go hungry or feel restrained – explore the enormous variety of exotic and interesting foods available now.

Expect to lose weight quite quickly, as mucilaginous fluid is dispersed and excreted. Occasionally you will have a COLD or 'FLU, MIGRAINE or a bad HEADACHE, when acids are flowing in torrents through your bloodstream and kidneys; you are rid of them for good. Eat nothing substantial on these days; home-made Lemon Barley Water RECIPE will keep you going and help the acids out. Excuse yourself as unfit for work if the symptoms are severe.

Promote excretion by bathing regularly, always finishing with cold water for half a minute. At other times brush your skin well to tone it and remove loose scales. BREATHE well in a deliberate fashion for a few minutes several times daily, and EXERCISE for ten minutes or more several times a week, briskly enough for conversation to be difficult. After you have stopped perspiring, a brief cold shower and change of clothing is very beneficial.

A *Naturopath** will understand what you are doing and is the one to consult if you have difficulty. Otherwise, massage by an *Aromatherapist,** *Osteopath** or *Chartered Physiotherapist** (ADDRESSES) will help to ease the tissues worst affected. Within six months you will have fuller movement, greater stamina and less or no reliance on drugs – true rejuvenation.

SCHIZOPHRENIA, Psychosis

In a *neurotic** mental illness you retain contact with the same sense of reality as everybody else, and are aware that your emotional reactions to STRESS are exaggerated and out of control. Psychosis is very different. Your mental contact with other people is no longer on these terms, so that you are more likely to think that everybody else is disturbed and you the only sane one among them. Schizophrenia is the commonest psychosis affecting young people, in which part of your mind keeps its bearings and part is out of touch. You may hear voices or see visions from outside *'mono'** reality and not realize the distinction.

Your mental behaviour is not in itself extraordinary, however, despite what your doctors and society in general may think. Many 'sane' people have similar *'colour'**-only experiences throughout their lives. Everyone does in childhood, unless and until their parents or teachers talk them out of it. Very old people seem to as well, but may by then have lost some of their communicative faculties and it is difficult to tell. One clear-minded old lady once described this as like living in a tent whose walls are getting thinner, so that you can see vague shapes moving outside it; when rain soaks the canvas you can see through it more clearly for a time. She was quite looking forward to DYING, so that she could step outside her 'mono' tent and enjoy the 'colour' landscape! People like this are accustomed to their knowledge, know the difference between 'mono' and 'colour', and keep it to themselves. Inability to regulate your thoughts and maintain a consistent and orderly view of the world is the real nature of the disturbance.

At one time many victims of this disorder spent all their adult life in hospital but the invention of effective drugs revolutionized its outlook – even though they may leave your mind dull and confused. But drugs brought doctors no nearer to understanding its cause, except to recognize how strongly it runs in families. This does not mean that schizophrenia is inherited, however: medical sociologists have independently shown how closely it associates with the mental and social background against which you grew up.

The most promising development this century took place at the Brain Bio Centre in Princeton, New Jersey in 1971. A patient called Sara made a dramatic and complete recovery from schizophrenia after intensive nutritional treatment. Dr Carl Pfeiffer (BOOKS) went on to characterize three main chemical types of the disease. Half of all its victims lack *histamine,** a chemical messenger in your brain; these people have too much copper and too little folic acid, and are the most likely to have extraordinary 'colour' perceptions such as *paranoia** and *hallucinations.** A fifth have the opposite problem – too much histamine, with low stocks of copper – and are inclined to suicidal DEPRESSIONS. The remainder (30%) have an inherited metabolic defect called *pyroluria** which makes them short of zinc and Vitamin B_6. Correction of these imbalances can set matters right within 5–10 days, in Pfeiffer's experience covering hundreds of cases. Medical recognition of his work is long overdue, though some penal reformers are beginning to realize its value.

HELPING YOURSELF

Whether or not your doctor is prepared to cooperate in all this, do keep him informed of your efforts, and set out by asking his advice about them. He can prescribe a lot of the supplements under the National Health Service, and may be able to refer you to an appropriate NHS specialist.

Make contact with the Schizophrenia Association of Great Britain (ADDRESS) and read Hoffer's BOOK, which they distribute.

Adopt the DIET for health, avoiding meat and peanuts which reduce your stocks of an essential fatty acid. Follow the principles set out for HYPOGLYCAEMIA.

Take SUPPLEMENTS of Zinc 60mg and Vitamin B_6 (Pyridoxine) 1000mg daily for one month. This will cure pyroluria and does no harm if that is not your problem.

If this fails, check your symptoms against Pfeiffer's classification and act accordingly:

Paranoia, over-excitement, hallucinations and delusions suggest insufficient brain histamine. Take Zinc 30mg and Manganese 10mg daily; the copper-shedding SUPPLEMENT is suitable. Vitamins B_3 (Niacin) 250mg, B_{12} (Hydroxocobalamin) 100 microg and Folic Acid 2mg daily complete the programme. You may improve well initially, then become depressed; stop the Zinc and Manganese.

Depressions and suicidal thoughts suggest you have too much brain histamine. You need the help of a *Clinical Ecologist* or specialist in Orthomolecular Medicine, if you can find one and afford him (environmental medicine ADDRESS). Otherwise, if you really want to persevere, attempt the measures which follow.

Try the special gluten-free and milk-free DIET simultaneously for a month. Only go beyond that with the aid of a nutritionist or dietician.

Add to your SUPPLEMENTS Essential Fatty Acids (eg Glanolin 500mg) and Vitamin C 1000mg, three times daily. Two each of Efavite and Efamol three times daily were formulated to satisfy all these requirements. The amino-acid L-Cysteine Hydrochloride (1.5gm daily) may overcome a block in your use of Vitamin B_6, which will unleash your mechanism for shedding excess copper.

Some people labelled 'schizophrenic' are irrepressibly psychic or clairvoyant but have never had this explained to them or learnt to handle their gift. You should contact an experienced *healer** or school of natural healing. Westbank Natural Health Centre, The Pegasus Trust and The Wrekin Trust (ADDRESSES) are three bodies who will understand your situation.

With reasonable luck some combination of these measures will help you. Be methodical and determined, and keep on believing in yourself.

SHINGLES, Herpes Zoster

If at the time you had CHICKENPOX – perhaps many years ago – your IMMUNITY was not at its best, you may have failed to suppress that VIRUS INFECTION completely. In that case small remnants of it can lie dormant in your spinal NERVE roots until aroused by further exposure to chickenpox at a time when your immunity is low once more.

How this occurs is imperfectly understood. The virus may remain dormant for decades in very specific junction boxes on your sensory nerves. It usually sticks to one side only, but may affect these junctions on two or three adjacent nerve trunks arising at consecutive levels in your spine, which in turn serve serial slices of your body and the skin overlying each. Most of your sensory nerves arise in the skin, of course, anything up to half a metre away from the junction boxes where the virus lies hidden.

Current medical theory has to propose that this virus, once re-activated by renewed external exposure to it, can multiply in the junction boxes and travel down the nerve fibres fast enough to appear in your skin after only a few days. This is far faster than cell substance can travel the same route when the nerve is RECOVERING from INJURY and is scarcely credible. It may be that chicken-pox is (like MUMPS) one of the diseases which challenge our usual theories of INFECTION beyond their useful scope.

The illness that follows reactivation of chickenpox is quite different. It begins with severe pain in the part of your body served by the infected NERVES – often a stripe round your body or a part of your face, usually limited to one side. When it affects your chest it can easily be mistaken for a CORONARY, until a red rash covers the painful area and draws your attention to the truth. By that time virus particles have (according to theory) tracked down the nerves to your skin, where they multiply. The result is a series of daily crops of small blisters on the flat red base, similar to CHICKENPOX.

These blisters can affect your CONJUNCTIVAE, and rarely the nerve inside your ear that controls the muscle of your cheek. Occasionally they can produce a very dangerous brain infection. Any part of your body that is under particular immune pressure – a limb containing CANCER or severe infection, for example – may be especially singled out for shingles involvement.

However troublesome and painful the rash may be, the debilitating effect shingles can have on you for months after the rash has cleared is far beyond what most people expect. Your brain is fagged and DEPRESSED, just as if you were severely CONCUSSED. *Neuralgic** PAIN often accompanies this – a stubborn and severe malfunction in the sensory nerves of the rash-affected area which may never really heal.

Doctors tend to regard shingles as untreatable, and accept rather fatalisti-cally the protracted misery it causes. It is hard to understand why simple remedies offered within other traditions are not at least tried, since they can do no harm. Fortunately, it is fairly easy to do the work yourself.

HELPING YOURSELF

Maintain your IMMUNITY at all times with a healthy DIET, SUPPLEMENTED if necessary when you are run down or repeatedly unwell. Be especially wary of visiting grandchildren with chickenpox when you are not vigorously well yourself.

At the very first sign or hint that your pain may be shingles, take homoeopathic Variolinum 6, one dose four hourly. I have seen the disease stop short at the red rash stage with this. Arsenicum album 3 can be given 4 hourly if the disease develops; Rhus tox may be preferable if you are well under retirement age. You are unlikely to have the other possible remedies readily to hand, but could consult a homoeopathic practitioner for further help.

Take lots of Vitamin C (3000mg daily) and a Vitamin B Complex Strong (eg Nature's Own), to support your nervous system under such pressure. Home-made Lemon Barley Water and Honey-Cider-Vinegar RECIPES accompanying a DIET based on fresh fruit and juices is best throughout the acute disease, until your APPETITE returns.

Calamine Lotion BP with 1% Liquefied Phenol BP is an excellent pain-relieving lotion. It is mildly caustic, so avoid getting it near your lips, eyes and genital skin, and do not apply it too often.

Cider Vinegar may be preferred or used alternately with this, applied undiluted to the rash every three hours. Not only is this very soothing, but it may help heal the rash faster and is quite harmless.

Comfrey oil keeps your skin moist and helps heal the scabs more quickly.

*Bach Mustard Flower Remedy** often helps shingles sufferers through the pain and depression that drags on after the rash has gone.

A practitioner of *Traditional Chinese Medicine** (ADDRESS) may be able to relieve neuralgia, if that should follow.

SICKNESS & DIARRHOEA in children

WHAT HAPPENS

A healthy child eating a wholesome DIET is rarely aware of his bowel except to empty it. The climate of your intestines is remarkably stable, considering the various foods and moods with which it has to cope. But it can be upset by a binge, and routine dietary lapses undermine it permanently. This leaves you much more susceptible to changes in WATER, emotional TENSION or excitement, unwisely mixed foods or small doses of dirt that would not otherwise upset you. Small children are more readily affected anyway, because they have only just got their intestines fully operational and easily make mistakes. COLDS, FEVER and CATARRH may consequently upset them but not affect adults.

When the climate goes wrong digestion is automatically upset, making foul messes and GAS by accident. A child reacts just as an adult would in FOOD POISONING, with sickness and diarrhoea. This is a healthy part of the cure, and to suppress it immediately will undermine his recovery. But you cannot afford to let it run on for long, as you could in yourself; THRUSH may get established and be difficult to dislodge.

If blood or slime appears in your child's faeces, and the diarrhoea seems to be running on for weeks, he may have been INFECTED with *campylobacter** which is a common gastro-enteritis *bacterium** among children nowadays. You should consult your doctor, who will be able to treat it and may want to ensure that others of your family do not have it.

HELPING YOURSELF

Let his intestines rest. Accept his lack of appetite, but offer Emergency Maintenance Fluid RECIPE, in small sips at body temperature, well washed round his mouth before he swallows it. Be content if he manages half a glass in an hour; do not rush him. Rest in bed with a hot water bottle on his stomach is soothing; anxiety, chill or activity aggravates the condition.

Once he can keep this down without nausea, progress to *home-made** Lemon Barley Water RECIPE which replaces lost minerals, and gives easily digestible energy. This may be necessary for a day or two, while any unhelpful colonies of germs or yeasts are starved down to manageable size.

His appetite will return before the diarrhoea stops. Stewed apple is a good first meal, sweetened only with raisins. Live Yoghurt RECIPE eaten with it provides a vigorous colony of bacteria that combats THRUSH and helps re-establish healthy digestion, especially of milk.

Now you can add other fresh washed fruit and vegetables, according to appetite. Cereals and wholemeal bread follow next; after that eggs, fish, milk and soft cheese should come easily in small portions, according to preference. Poultry, hard cheese and meat should come last, as they tax digestion the most.

If at any stage this routine is not working, or your child is FEVERISH, lifeless or ill-looking, or blood appears in his diarrhoea, consult your doctor as a matter of urgency.

NAUSEA, sickness of PREGNANCY

WHAT HAPPENS

During the first four months of your pregnancy the *hormones** that maintain it come from the *ovary** that made the egg which is becoming your baby. If you have had time to do your FAMILY PLANNING well, you can cope with the boisterous reorganization of your hormones, and supply every need; otherwise slightly over-exuberant or unbalanced hormone growth may unsettle the part of your *primal adaptive system** which regulates your intestines and appetite. You may vomit or feel sick regularly until the imbalance settles. That coincides with decay of the hormone factory in your ovary, and take-over of its function by your baby's *placenta**.

HELPING YOURSELF

Avoid getting weary, angry or flustered. Rest often to let these moods pass, with fresh air on your face. Read Pickard's BOOK.

Practise good BREATHING, and EXERCISE gently.

Eat lightly and often; fresh fruit, plain buttered wholemeal toast, a small coleslaw, a baked potato. Coffee, tea, rich confectionery and ALCOHOL are all best avoided.

Homoeopathic* Ipecacuanha 6 or 30 may help ease nausea. Vitamin B_6 (Pyridoxine, 100mg twice daily) may help. Try medication if these fail.

TRAVEL SICKNESS, motion sickness

WHAT HAPPENS

This can happen to anyone whose sense of balance is sufficiently over-stimulated, though some are much more easily affected than others. It is much worse when you are tired, unwell, NERVOUS or apprehensive, or have over-indulged in rich food or ALCOHOL. You acclimatize eventually, but only after several days – which is really only any good to you during long voyages at sea. Journeys by air or road can be a perfect nuisance to you, unless you find an easily portable and harmless remedy which works for you.

HELPING YOURSELF

Eat as the preceding paragraph before and during your journey. Avoid SMOKE, fatty smells, the odour of vomit and the company of seasick travellers.

Keep still and warm, in gently moving fresh air and in sight of the horizon.

On car journeys take an interest in sights outside, and stop regularly. Consider fitting an *ionizer** inside the car or a less expensive earthing strap outside.

Try homoeopathic Cocculus Indicus 3 or Petroleum 3, 8 hourly beforehand and 2 hourly during the journey. Crystallized ginger is an effective option.

SLEEPLESSNESS

WHAT HAPPENS

Your body may need rest when it is TIRED, but has no use for sleep. That is exclusively a *'colour'** requirement of your whole being, to give time for your daily experience to settle into perspective. Your need for sleep therefore varies considerably throughout your life and according to your circumstances. For babies everything is new; they sleep not to avoid it, but to digest what they are learning. Fit RETIRED people tend to need much less, because little of their daily experience is new any longer; everything falls neatly into place according to a well established outlook on life.

At any other age your sleep requirement depends on how rapidly you are growing. If you settle into an accustomed routine, with stable activities along familiar lines within settled relationships, you will find yourself able to manage with less sleep. But as soon as you become bored or understimulated by your present circumstances and begin to explore new interests, your requirement increases. If you move house or change your job the same thing happens temporarily, and calls for a general increase in your *recreational** budget to cope with the rather STRESSFUL pace of change.

Inability to sleep when you are TIRED is a serious matter, as your mental efficiency will rapidly deteriorate. The cause may be something very simple, like drinking stimulants – lightly roasted coffee, strong Indian tea or strong cocoa – too late at night. Otherwise, spend a portion of your wakeful hours working out what is wrong and do something definite about it.

If you are ending each day with your spectrum of 'colour' needs inadequately met, you will not settle to rest at ease. Working late at night makes you unnaturally alert and overstimulated while recreational activity balances the 'colour' spectrum of your efforts for the day instead of aggravating it further. DEPRESSION may wake you early in the morning, feeling gloomy and downhearted. Worst of all is working for too long close to the limits of your STRESS tolerance. You lie awake TENSE with worry, your mind working overtime so as not to lose your grip.

*'Mono'** hypnotic drugs do not meet needs like these. They are marvellous for a few nights, and you think you have solved your problem. But after a week or two you feel much less benefit, because your body treats them as poisons to be detoxified, and has begun to neutralize their effect. So you start to take more to compensate. Eventually you find yourself taking pills in order to sleep only as well as before you started them, but suffering nevertheless their full range of side-effects. This is *habituation,** a benign form of addiction which you should watch for and avoid.

Many people use ALCOHOL instead of drugs as a hypnotic. Apart from being more expensive, it is no more effective and much more dangerous. An habitually overstimulated brain is ripe ground for alcoholism, which is much more destructive than hypnotic drug dependence.

Sooner or later you must face and solve your underlying problems, because you cannot afford to depend habitually on props of any kind.

HELPING YOURSELF

If you awake naturally at a reasonable hour feeling your best and ready for anything, you are getting plenty of sleep. Adults usually fail this test, already heavily in overdraft. Children and TEENAGERS should pass it easily, even if their idea of a respectable hour differs from yours. Act urgently if your child always needs wakening, is surly or slow first thing, complains regularly of HEADACHE or is dull and incurious at school.

Identify what keeps you awake, makes your sleep fitful or arouses you too soon. Deal with DEPRESSION in its own right. Switch off the television two hours earlier. Avoid coffee, tea, cola, chocolate or cocoa late at night. Camomile, basil, lemon verbena or lemon balm tea would be much better.

If your temperament contributes significantly to the problem, a well chosen *Bach Flower Remedy** (ADDRESS) may help you, and can do no harm at all.

If you are under pressure from homework of any kind, work to a reasonable hour and get up earlier to finish it. You are far more efficient in the morning than at night, and will sleep better if you are not over-tired. Problems you cannot solve late often drop out easily in the morning, after sleep has given you a chance to get them into perspective.

A light supper of cereals and milk, a banana or two or a hot milk drink may help if your evening meal is early. All these foods are rich in the *amino-acid** tryptophan, which has useful sedative properties. SUPPLEMENTS of L-Tryptophan are expensive, but anything from 1–15gm could be used in capsule form instead if you prefer. Perhaps the cost will compare favourably with the food items, plus any OVERWEIGHT they may cause!

Always allow at least an hour of recreation before you go to bed. Music, conversation, a good book or some light-hearted television or radio may suit you. A relaxing walk, or even a brisk jog, is sometimes what you need. Sometimes a hot bath with lavender essence, finished with splashes all over of cold water, is the best end to the day. Seek by any of these means to please yourself, in a contrast to your earlier exertions.

If your problem persists try taking Lecithin or sufficient SUPPLEMENTS of Inositol and Choline to make it in your body; Vitamin B_5; and enough Vitamin B_6 (Pyridoxine) to ensure that you recall dreaming pleasantly – but Strong B Complex will keep you awake and alert! Dolomite provides Magnesium, which aids sleep. Siberian Ginseng is worth a month's trial. Change these methodically at weekly intervals or longer, to see which help.

When you cannot get to sleep, try splashing your feet in shallow cold water for a few minutes, then dry them and go back to bed. Better, put on cold damp cotton socks and cover them with dry woollen ones; these should glow comfortably in bed, and come off dry. Or try a *Priessnitz pack.**

Try fresh heather or hops in your pillow, and *homoeopathic** Coffea Cruda 6 or 30, before using hypnotic medicines. Then limit the drug to one week in two, or four doses weekly, for a defined period; then try again without them.

SMOKING

I do not smoke, but cannot claim much credit for that. When I was at the age when most people start I could not afford it. By the time I could, I realized there were better things to spend my limited money on. So I have never faced the ordeal of giving it up. But I know what TIREDNESS feels like, and have often found myself over-eating to stave it off. So I can begin to appreciate the anguished feelings of someone dependent on tobacco and beleaguered for it.

It is inconceivable that you do not know smoking is bad for you. If you still do it, there is a powerful reason. You probably started when you were too young to appreciate the dangers, and now find yourself in a steep-sided trap you cannot easily escape. The hectoring manner and self-righteous attitude of some anti-smoking campaigners is certainly unhelpful, and under-estimates the difficulty of your position. Society offers few respectable outlets for anguish, and does nothing to help you replace this one with something as effective for soothing your NERVES.

The facts are less clear cut than many care to admit. Tobacco smoke is no doubt very STRESSFUL to the skin of your mouth and lungs, and certainly increases your susceptibility to BRONCHITIS and CANCER, other things being equal. But they are not directly and inevitably linked, as cause and effect. Your smoking acquaintances no doubt bear this out, varying greatly in their physical tolerance of it.

Heavy smoking is in some countries associated with much less lung disease than we have in northern Europe and America, if DIET is good enough to compensate. This is not a matter of wealth. Spain is comparatively poor, but protective food – vegetables and fruit – grows abundantly there and is cheap enough for everyone to buy. They are not therefore tempted by the more luxurious items that fail to support the IMMUNITY of wealthier Northern Europeans. This is evidently more than enough to compensate for their heavy tobacco consumption *per capita* and lesser medical resources.

The main problem is that you cannot help sharing your smoke with others, and the children among them are much more vulnerable than you are. This is a pity, since you do not really need the smoke any more than they do. It is nicotine you are after, which you could get at the same price and just as easily, in much more socially acceptable ways. You could be free of the effects of the smoke itself – BODY ODOUR, BRONCHITIS, lung CANCER, COUGHING, and grossly impaired taste and smell. Nicotine will of course continue to restrict your CIRCULATION and increase your risk of raised BLOOD PRESSURE, a STROKE or a CORONARY, but only as much as it does already.

Many people seem to find it easier to get off nicotine chewing-gum than cigarettes, presumably because you can simply make a piece of it last longer and longer each time. Even if you cannot, the benefits of the change seem very well worth exploring.

HELPING YOURSELF

Replace all your cigarettes with nicotine chewing gum. The 2mg size will be sufficient unless you are used to thirty or more cigarettes daily. Start with 10–15 pieces daily, the fewest that satisfy your cravings. Then gradually lengthen the life of each piece – something you cannot really do with cigarettes. This gradually reduces your daily dose of nicotine, and creates the possibility that you can give it up altogether.

Use the gum properly. Chew only until you taste the nicotine, and let this linger in your mouth to be absorbed from there: any you swallow is destroyed in your stomach and wasted. Swallow your saliva when the nicotine taste has gone, then chew out a little more.

Meanwhile you will realize with horror how disgusting all your clothes and soft furnishings smell, and get them cleaned.

A healthy DIET will taste better when smoke stops ruining your APPETITE, and goes some way to helping you cope with nicotine. SUPPLEMENT this with 2000–3000mg Vitamin C daily and lots of Brewer's Yeast; the other STRESS SUPPLEMENTS may also help. Avoid simply increasing your use of alcohol and coffee, which would not be any real advance.

If you become OVERWEIGHT because of your improved appetite, that is for the time being a much lesser evil.

Now the real work begins. You have to discover what you are using nicotine for. If it were just a habit, you could easily have given it up long ago. If you are very attached to the cigarette itself, you need the image it creates: what is the matter with the real you? If you use it to soothe away frustration and emotional pain, are there no other ways you can do this?

You can start by BREATHING better and using lavender essence in your bath to help you relax. *Anthroposophic** Fragador (Weleda UK Ltd) is a wholesome remedy you can try, or a well-chosen *Bach Flower Remedy** may help. Look up the ADDRESS of a local *yoga** or *relaxation** teacher, or ask your doctor for referral to your nearest *clinical psychologist** or *community counsellor** for assistance. Otherwise the chewing gum is the end of your line, for the present.

Nicotine may at the moment help your concentration or mental stamina, which is fine so long as it lasts. You are for the present adapted to it, in the STRESS sense. Unfortunately this adaptation will not last for ever, but will gradually become less and less satisfactory. When it is finally exhausted you will be forced to do something about it, with weaker resources than you possess now. If you can summon up the will, now is the time to act.

SORE THROAT: TONSILS & ADENOIDS

Most of the INFECTIONS that can occur in your MOUTH behave quite unlike COLDS, presumably because your gums, your tongue and the skin inside your cheeks is tougher and less sensitive than the skin that lines your nose. But your throat is susceptible to VIRUS INFECTION and reacts in much the same way as your nose.

The special thing about your throat is the tonsils. These are lymph GLANDS spread out just beneath the skin on each side of your throat. They are closely allied with your adenoids, which are similar glands on either side of your nose near its back entrance where it joins your throat. They are only separated from your tonsils by the thickness of your soft palate, the arch of skin over the top of your throat; it frames the hole you can see in the mirror, over the root of your tongue.

Virus attack in your nose or throat can easily arouse the protective function of both your tonsils and adenoids, making them sore and swollen. This may be your most troublesome cold symptom, or nasal blockage and CATARRH may preponderate; people's patterns differ. But a virus sore throat is commonly accompanied by the other symptoms in some degree, which helps to distinguish it from *bacterial** infections.

These are less common, but are important to recognize. One particular type of bacterium – called *Haemolytic Streptococci** because they are round, multiply in threads or strips and can break up blood *cells** – is able to hang on for long periods in the tonsils and only cause symptoms at intervals. If not overcome properly these bacteria can cause chronic RHEUMATIC problems many years later. Although that is now rare, safety cannot be taken for granted.

Fear of these bacteria puts doctors under pressure to treat with ANTIBIOTICS all sore throats that may conceivably be caused by them. It is possible to take a throat swab for a simple test that will demonstrate whether the bacterium is there or not, but it takes a few days and is regarded as a little over-conscientious. Besides which, most people do not want to wait even a few days to be relieved of their symptoms.

It is well worth becoming an exception, and giving your doctor a break. Frequent courses of antibiotic treatment may open the way to THRUSH, which not infrequently turns up in the throat swab as the cause of your sore throat! While you are waiting for the result, there are several safe and useful remedies on the next page that may solve your problem anyway.

Swollen red INFLAMED tonsils are not usually infected themselves, but actively defending skin under attack somewhere nearby. You deal with most of these attacks locally in the skin itself, and are never made aware of the challenge. But small children come under particularly heavy pressure. Frequent tonsillar swelling is not necessarily unhealthy in your early school years, if you keep well and vigorous despite it. It usually lasts only as long as it takes you to encounter all the *microbes** that are common in your locality and become IMMUNE to them.

HELPING YOURSELF

See COLDS and VIRUS INFECTIONS for many ideas which apply here too.

A DIET including plenty of crisp fibrous food needs a lot of chewing and is mildly abrasive. The muscular massage and scraping this gives your throat at mealtimes keeps the hollows in the tonsil surface clean, and stops your lymph circulation from getting sluggish and congested – far the best direct protection against sore throats. They are usually more nourishing too, adding to your indirect defences.

Avoid sugary and white floury foods like biscuits, which become pasty in the mouth and can stick in the hollows of your tonsils, making them ideal places for germs to grow. They also nourish you less well, indirectly weakening your defences against microbe attack.

Try using red sage tea as a soothing antiseptic gargle; or keep a clove of fresh garlic (RECIPE) in your cheek as a lozenge. The reek is not too obtrusive provided you keep the outer skins on and do not chew or bruise it.

There is no single *homoeopathic** remedy, you will have to experiment or take professional advice.

A good conventional mouthwash is Thymol Glycerine Compound, which can be used neat or diluted with three parts of hot water. Better for pain is Potassium Chlorate and Phenol Gargle, diluted with an equal part of very hot water; but do not swallow this one as it is mildly corrosive. Three Dispersible Aspirin in half a glass of water make another good analgesic gargle, but have no antiseptic properties.

After three days see the doctor; sooner if severe sore throat is your only symptom or fever begins. A throat swab, and antibiotic treatment, may be wise.

Think three times before having your adenoids SURGICALLY removed. It is a messy operation, with an appreciable risk. Work hard at improving their efficiency, by SUPPLEMENTING your diet for IMMUNITY; meanwhile bide your time. Deal with deafness separately (EARACHE).

Tonsillectomy is a neater operation, but rarely necessary unless the glands have become festering wrecks. This is more likely nowadays in adult life. If you get three or four bouts of genuine *tonsillitis** each year, ask your doctor if the advice of an ENT Surgeon is worthwhile.

*Quinsy** is an *abscess** around and beneath your tonsil, which closes your throat, alters your voice and makes swallowing very painful indeed. You will need medical treatment as soon as possible for this one, and may be offered SURGERY to remove your tonsils after only one or two attacks. Surgery is in this case elegant, of low risk and fully curative; you should probably accept it. Otherwise the condition tends to recur.

SPRAINS

The bony parts of your JOINTS only do the mechanical work of hinge and load-bearer. They are firmly held together by tough fibrous *ligaments** shaped as sheets or ropes, that will not stretch along their length but can twist and bend freely otherwise. Additional stability is provided by the *sinews** through which your muscles pull on the bones nearby to move the joint, and by the dense fibrous sheets of *fascia** that separate the muscles from each other and generally box everything up. Some of this fascia surrounds the joint as a lining *capsule,** to seal into it the lubricant that oozes from the blood vessels on the surface of the capsule.

A sprain is an INJURY affecting the capsule or ligaments of your joint, leaving the bones and *cartilages** intact though perhaps *bruised.** In principle any joint can be affected but those in your arms seldom are. They are not stiffly braced with ligaments since they do not constantly bear your weight; this makes them much more supple and mobile than joints in your leg, and much more liable to *dislocation.**

Nevertheless thumb and finger joints are sprained quite frequently, usually by being forcibly bent backwards beyond their normal limit, but sometimes by a bruising blow. Your wrist is liable to a similar injury if during a fall your whole weight is thrown into bending it. Otherwise it is supple enough to cope with most contortions; your fingers are liable to be injured first.

BACKACHE often arises from spraining of the ligaments in your spine or pelvis, but your *hips** are so massively surrounded by muscle that injuries likely to sprain them are usually strong enough to break them too. Your *knees** are also strongly braced, and more liable to cartilage injury. Spraining is serious when it occurs, and must be expertly treated for months to restore full stability.

Your *ankles** suffer the worst of both worlds. On the one hand they must be supple and springy like your wrists, to enable your FEET to cope with uneven ground and absorb shock; on the other they constantly bear your whole weight. So they are quite hard to break, and very liable to spraining.

Usually your feet roll outwards, typically over the edge of a pavement or off the platform of a high-heeled shoe or ice-skating boot. The ligament on the outside of your ankle is stretched, and the capsule is often torn. It is BLEEDING from the blood vessels in this capsule that causes all the bruising and most of the swelling; this may not show until the next day, spread out over your foot and on your lower leg where the greaseproof layers of fascia will allow it to surface.

By the second and third days after a sprain, INFLAMMATION has set in to begin the work of healing. This may stiffen considerably and hurt more than the injury. The worst is over by the fourth day, but it will take another week to heal completely: ligaments are specialized for strength and are rather slow to repair.

HELPING YOURSELF

As soon as you realize you have sprained your ankle, press firmly with all your fingers along the front outside quarter of the crease between your leg bones and your foot, as illustrated. Sit there patiently for ten minutes at least, however foolish you may feel, and do not allow yourself to be diverted. This will stop any bleeding from torn blood vessels, and give them time to clot. These ten minutes greatly reduce the discomfort and inconvenience you will have to put up with over the next ten days.

As soon as you can, immerse your sprained ankle or wrist in cold water until it feels numb. Dry it, apply Arnica or Hamamelis (Witch Hazel) Ointment, and bind it firmly with an elastic or crêpe bandage.

If you feel shocked or unsteady, take a dose of *homoeopathic** Arnica 30 or *Bach Rescue Remedy** (two or three drops of tincture in half a glass of water, sipped occasionally).

You will need to re-apply this bandage twice each day. Repeat the bath while your ankle is painful or swollen, but start with three minutes in hot water before thirty seconds under the cold tap. You can repeat this cycle up to three times, but finish with cold. Then dry, apply Arnica or Hamamelis (Witch Hazel) Ointment, and re-apply the bandage. Use two bandages alternately if possible – the elastic recovers much better if it is rested between applications.

Comfrey appreciably accelerates the healing of bones and ligaments; the allantoin in it stimulates your white blood *cells** to work up to four times as fast without loss of efficiency; it is a pity they are only involved in a part of the effort required for healing! The herb is easy to grow, and produces fleshy leaves and stems you can eat or brew for tea. The root is used to make tablets, but contains a trace of a toxic alkaloid chemical that accumulates in your body; therefore avoid using these for longer than a month or so at a time. A suitable dose is two tablets of Comfrey Root 400mg three times daily, with meals. Take Vitamin C 100mg with every dose of Comfrey tea or tablets, since your white blood cells will use even more of it than usual.

If after two days you still cannot put your foot to the floor, or the bruising is very severe, consult your doctor or hospital accident department to explore the remote possibility of bone fracture. Unless fracture is obvious from the beginning you will do yourself no harm by waiting, and save yourself unnecessary X-ray exposure. If you are in any doubt, at any stage, consult a doctor in any case.

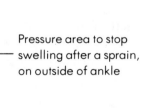

Pressure area to stop swelling after a sprain, on outside of ankle

STRESS

Stress is engineers' jargon for the load on a structure; *strain** is the bending it causes, which may or may not damage the structure permanently. This idea was borrowed by Hans *Selye** when he began to study how animals respond to challenge. But being new to English he confused stress with strain, and set people thinking that stress includes strain automatically. Selye showed, on the contrary, that the level at which a stress produces harmful strain varies according to circumstance – and circumstances can be changed.

So stress is really just another word for challenge, and strain means effort. Any worthwhile objective challenges you to make the effort of reaching for it, in defiance of the odds against success. That goes for the APPETITES that prompt you to maintain yourself from day to day, just as for the more distant hopes that keep you striving from year to year. Any goal or need you hunger for is stressful, in the proper sense.

Only when your goal eludes you does the strain begin to show. You can for a short time stand up to enormous stresses with great vigour. Beyond that you can learn to pace your resistance against moderate prolonged stresses, patiently rolling with the punches for months or years. Selye would have incorporated both of these in his *Phase of Resistance.*

What you can bear indefinitely, however, is limited by the recuperative power you can muster day by day. You may actually need the stress to help you mobilize that recuperative power, and feel lifeless without it. This is Selye's *Phase of Adaptation.* If that is exceeded and you allow the situation to continue on these terms, your vitality will gradually ebb away leaving you apathetic and disillusioned – the *Phase of Exhaustion.*

In health you are free to match your strategy to circumstances, measuring your effort in pursuit of an objective to ensure that you can gain it without exhaustion. When your best personal resources prove totally unequal to the task you need not be daunted: you can choose either to change the objective or to join forces with others who share it.

But society imposes some unnatural stresses you cannot modify like this. They are asserted from outside you, as the duties and obligations of membership. Society owes you in return the opportunity not only to meet these obligations but also to provide for your personal needs and explore your own aspirations. In practice however the resources available are inappropriate and unevenly distributed. You may be helpless both to avoid an obligation and to meet it, stressed beyond your means by a goal you cannot change. Your *primal adaptive system** is then in overdrive, with nowhere to go. Unless you are rescued, or drop out of society altogether, your health will in due course break down catastrophically.

This *stress disease** epitomizes our failure to understand healthy human needs, and underlies all forms of personal and collective violence. It calls for fundamental changes in our social system or it too will break down.

HELPING YOURSELF

If you have stress disease, you need to know. Look for frequent unaccountable TENSION or NERVOUSNESS, *palpitations*,* SLEEPLESSNESS, liability to angry or violent outbursts you do not really intend, or dependence on SMOKING, ALCOHOL or stimulants for energy or relaxation. Total apathy and DEPRESSION mean you are already exhausted and constitute the least destructive form of *breakdown*.*

Identify the challenge that is breaking you down. If your ambitions are inaccessible, confer with your family and change them. Find a healthier outlet for your pent-up energies, which meets your real needs more appropriately. There are less expensive places to live, and happier ways to provide for yourselves. They may be less prestigious and physically harder work, but will correspond much better to your natural tolerance and capabilities.

Next attend to your DIET. Healthy food costs no more, because you need less of it. It greatly increases your ability to cope, and is essential to recovery from stress disease.

SUPPLEMENTS of Brewer's Yeast (9 tablets daily) plus Vitamins B_5 (Pantothenic Acid, 50mg twice daily) and B_{15} (Pangamic Acid, 50mg twice daily) optimize your stress tolerance. Siberian Ginseng (Eleutherococcus Senticosis, 250–500mg up to three times daily) is a more expensive but valuable addition, and preferable to the more readily available oriental or panax ginseng. This is a good second best, but should be bought as whole red or brown roots and prepared for consumption without heat.

If you possibly can, take a holiday break for *recreation**. The stress will still be there afterwards, but you will have recovered some of your stamina for dealing with it. Provided you now tackle your stress more appropriately, you will not simply run down again to the same state as before.

If tension, nervousness, sleeplessness, smoking or dependence on alcohol and stimulants do not ease automatically, deal with each of them in turn. They undermine your capacity for tackling the main problem, however much you feel reliant on them.

If failure brings you face to face with basic problems in your personality, ask for help. The *clinical psychology** department of your local hospital is the place to start; you may first need a letter from your doctor. Otherwise approach a *community counsellor** through your local Social Services Department; trained private counsellors are available in some areas (ADDRESS).

Do not give up hope. That reduces your life to mere *survival*,* which will leave you fundamentally dissatisfied as long as there is any life left in you. Wriggle about as much as you need, and abandon any position you have to, however cherished, in order to stay alive.

SUPPLEMENTS, vitamins, minerals See also DIET

WHAT HAPPENS

Chemical pollution of the air, water and soil on which everything alive depends is already a critical survival issue and will take several generations to correct. Meanwhile we have to defend ourselves against it, and cope personally with the deficiencies and imbalances it causes in our food.

However carefully you buy, you are unlikely to find sufficient perfectly constituted 'organic'* food to subsist on it all year round. Even if you did, it would take up to five years for it to correct every imbalance and deficiency you have acquired from your conception up. If you are aware of severe problems now, you will not want to wait that long. If these problems have weakened you, solving them unaided may be beyond you in any case; getting well takes much more effort than staying there.

The difficulty is keeping the problem in perspective. Some people will not trust their food for anything, and supplement for every nutrient they know about. That is expensive and dangerous; anything left out becomes deficient by comparison with your huge artificial stockpiles, which lack any 'colour'* that would help you balance them up. Make the most of your DIET. It can provide almost everything you need, and is an essential basis for making good use of any supplementary nourishment you need.

The only consistent deficiency arises directly from mineral* imbalances in modern soils. Healthy plants can find most of the major organic elements they need, but are becoming seriously short of minerals we require not as structural materials but to facilitate the construction process. Since every other kind of food depends on plant fodder for its mineral supplies, these basic soil deficiencies affect us whatever we eat. Only fish and sea vegetables can help to redress the imbalance.

If you eat much butter and meat, which are loaded with energy-storage fats,* you are probably deficient in the special essential fatty acids* you need for structural purposes, particularly in the skin of every cell in your body. Not only are these scarce in the diets of food animals, but their benefit is largely offset by the storage kind. You need to cut these down, as well as supplement the essential vegetable fatty acids.

A well-balanced fresh diet will cope much better with vitamins* than these other items, but certain parts are especially rich. Only Vitamin C requires special attention. It is the cheapest and least harmful way to combat free radical* damage caused by RADIATION or chemical pollution. For this you can use several grammes daily, over and above the 200mg or so that you need for nutritive purposes.

If you have no other specific problem or purpose in mind these items are sufficient, and are summarized on the next page under 'Health Maintenance'. For additional items that become especially important in particular conditions, look elsewhere under Special Needs and Purposes. Once you have identified which items you need, read on down the page for Sources and Doses.

SUPPLEMENTS

HELPING YOURSELF — SPECIAL NEEDS AND PURPOSES

Anaemia*:
Iron, Molybdenum, Zinc;
Vitamins C and E.

ARTERIOSCLEROSIS:
Dolomite, Manganese,
Selenium, Zinc; Vitamins
B₆, C and E; Lecithin.

BLEEDING
Vitamin C, Rutin.

BLOOD PRESSURE
Chromium; Vitamins B₃
(Niacin), B₆ (Pyridoxine),
C, E; Essential Fatty
Acids; Garlic; Siberian
Ginseng and Rutin.

CANCER:
Dolomite, Potassium,
Selenium, Zinc; Vitamins
A and D (Halibut Liver
Oil), B₁ (Thiamine), B₅
(Pantothenic Acid) and B₁₅
(Pangamic Acid), Brewer's
Yeast, and C; Essential
Fatty Acids, with Vitamin
E *unless* the cancer
involves your BREAST,
ovary* or womb; Siberian
Ginseng.

Candida* Infection:
Biotin 50–250 microgm
three times daily with
meals.

Cleansing
Garlic Oil and
Multimineral
Combination (see
overleaf); Vitamin C.

CONTRACEPTIVE *Pill*:
Zinc, Vitamin B₆
(Pyridoxine) and Vitamin
C.

Copper-shedding
Manganese, Zinc,
Multimineral; Vitamin B₆
(Pyridoxine), Vitamin C,
Multivitamin.

Health Maintenance:
Vitamin C, Honey Cider
Vinegar RECIPE, Whole Egg
Nog RECIPE.

Healing:
Vitamin C, Comfrey;
Rutin if blood vessels are
involved.

IMMUNITY-*Building*:
Selenium, Zinc,
Multimineral; Vitamin B₆
(Pyridoxine), and Brewer's
Yeast BPC, Vitamins C
and E; Multivitamin;
Essential Fatty Acids.

PREGNANCY
Multimineral,
Multivitamin, Essential
Fatty Acids and Vitamin
E.

RECOVERY
Brewer's Yeast, Vitamins
B₁₂ (Hydroxocobalamin),
B₁₅ (Pangamic Acid),
Vitamin C.

SLEEPLESSNESS
Vitamin E, L-Tryptophan,
Magnesium.

STRESS
Selenium; Vitamins B₅
(Pantothenic Acid), B₁₅
(Pangamic Acid) and B
Complex Strong; Vitamins
C and E; Essential Fatty
Acids; Siberian Ginseng.

HELPING YOURSELF — SOURCES AND DOSES

The next two pages list all the supplements mentioned anywhere in this book, with their best and most economical sources, instructions for taking them and typical amounts you are likely to benefit from. Under professional guidance you may well be given larger amounts of any of these; my recommendations are intended to be utterly safe for self-administration. It is however wise to relate this information to the particular use or topic that interests you, since some may require adaptation to suit the purpose you have in mind.

CANCER in particular is best handled with the help of a sympathetic doctor, although the supplements mentioned on this page can be used safely without that help if necessary.

More on SUPPLEMENTS

Vitamins*

Name	Daily Dose	Remarks
A	Up to 10,000 IU	Present in carrots, apricots, and fish oils. Larger doses only under professional guidance (*Naturopath** or Doctor)
B_1 Thiamine	100mg	Do not take any single Vitamin B supplement without at least three tablets of Brewer's Yeast BPC or a non-yeast B Complex. This or fresh wheatgerm (1–2 tablespoons daily) will often prove to be sufficient supplements in themselves.
B_2 Riboflavin	100mg	
B_3 Niacin	200mg	
B_5 Pantothenic Acid	200mg	
B_6 Pyridoxine	100mg	
B_{12} Hydroxocobalamin	100microgm	Often given as 1000microgm monthly.
B_{15} Pangamic Acid	50mg	
Folic Acid	5mg	
Para-amino Benzoic Acid (PABA)	300mg	
Biotin	750microgm	
Choline	1500mg	Lecithin (made in your body from Choline & Inositol) is cheaper.
Inositol	1500mg	
C Ascorbic Acid	200–10,000mg	Can cause diarrhoea in high dosage.
D Calciferol	200–400 IU	Do not exceed this dose.
E Tocopherol	200–600 IU	Better absorbed if emulsified.

Essential Fatty Acids*

These aim to provide *Gamma*-Linolenic Acid and vary greatly in their content. All are expensive, so look for value for money.

Oil	Name (Manufacturer)	GLA Content %	Dose (mg/day)
Borage Seed	'Galanol' (Lifeplan)	25–27	1000
Blackcurrant Seed	'Glanolin' (G.R. Lane)	17[1]	1500
Evening Primrose Seed	'Efamol'[2] & various	9	3000

[1] plus 16% of its derivatives, which may be advantageous
[2] includes enough Vitamin E (see below)

Take all these on an empty stomach half an hour before meals, with enough water to wash them straight through your stomach, and Vitamin E 100IU to prevent it from being destroyed before you can absorb it; only Efamol has this Vitamin E built in.

Minerals*

The cheapest reasonably comprehensive supplements are the RECIPES for Honey Cider Vinegar and Egg Nog. Kelp is not as good as is sometimes made out, and contains hugely disproportionate amounts of Iodine; but it serves very well as an Iodine supplement at one tablet daily.

Mineral	Daily Dosage	Remarks
Calcium Orotate	500–3000mg	100mg Ca/gm, well absorbed; pricey.
Calcium with Vit D	One tablet	80mg Ca, 500 IU Vit D.
Dolomite	1500mg	200mg Ca & 120mg Mg/gm; best buy.

NB – take all Calcium supplements with 2000+mg of Vitamin C daily, and some Magnesium.

Chromium Orotate	1–3mg	1mg provides 80microg of Chromium.
Iron	10mg	Take with 1000mg Vitamin C.
Magnesium Orotate	500–3000mg	66mg Mg/gm, well absorbed; pricey.
Manganese Orotate	100mg	Provides 14mg Manganese.
Molybdenum	250microg	Combined with Iron (Nature's Own).
Selenium	200–400microg	Take with Vitamin E 200–400 IU.
Zinc	15–30mg	5–10ml of Zinc Sulphate solution (6.6gm hydrous salt/500ml water) or 100–200mg of Zinc Orotate.

Miscellaneous

Garlic Oil: 1000–2000mg daily, no more than two days weekly. Supplement generously with Multimineral to replace those it flushes out.

Lecithin: 2–5gm/day. As granules, or capsules including safflower oil.

L-Tryptophan: 1–15gm/night. Bananas, milk and whole grains are good sources.

Multimineral/vitamin: Choose Nature's Own or Lambert's Health Insurance Plus.

Rutin: Up to 120mg after three meals daily, with ten times as much Vitamin C.

Siberian Ginseng (Eleutherococcus Senticosis): 1000–3000mg/day. Oriental Ginseng is less effective, especially processed forms and immature white roots.

SURGERY

When a surgeon offers to operate on your body, he is giving you an opportunity to restore disordered tissues to a condition from which they are better able to heal back to the function and structure your 'colour' signature intended all along. He cannot cure you, but he can sometimes remove obstacles which prevent you from curing yourself. No good surgeon claims any more than that. But there are two topics that nowadays even good surgeons seldom raise with their patients and which are neglected in the health services generally.

Firstly, your body became disordered because of a long-standing error in its action pattern.* Some of these – congenital* abnormalities, INJURY – have burnt themselves out by the time the surgeon offers his help. More commonly – ARTHRITIS, ARTERIOSCLEROSIS, BREAST lumps, CANCER, EARACHE, GALLSTONES, hernia,* PILES, PROSTATE swelling, VARICOSE VEINS – the error continues. Unless you do something to keep yourself right once corrected, the disorder (or one like it) will gradually reform. It is by no means uncommon for the same operation to be necessary at regular intervals because this elementary point has been overlooked.

A nautical analogy provides another way of looking at this. If you were navigating a ship through hazardous waters, the wrong compass heading would have gradually taken you off course into danger in just the same way. Drastic over-correction of your compass heading (by natural self-healing measures) may still restore you safely to your course – unless you are already among the rocks. The surgeon offers, in effect, to lift you out of your predicament and place you where you should have been. But he does not correct your compass heading – that is still up to you.

Secondly, surgery is a considerable STRESS for which you should carefully prepare, and from which you need to manage your RECOVERY quite deliberately. It is a special form of controlled INJURY. In an emergency it is just as unexpected as any other kind of injury, and gives you no opportunity to prepare yourself for the ordeal. But an operation planned in advance, for which you may have to wait several months, gives you ample time to make ready.

You can at least make your surgeon's job easier by slimming the OVERWEIGHT body he will need to cut. This also makes the anaesthetist's task safer, and there will be that much less fat for the anaesthetic to dissolve into. You will wake up sooner and have not nearly so much anaesthetic gas to exhale over the next few days. This could make a difference to your chances of getting BRONCHITIS or pneumonia* during your RECOVERY; feeble, dopey COUGHING defends your lungs inadequately against INFECTION. Fatness also makes blood clotting more likely afterwards; this is perhaps the most dangerous post-operative threat of all.

You may even manage accidentally to heal your problem partly or completely while you are waiting, by a sufficiently radical change of DIET and appropriate SUPPLEMENTS. You could for example wall off your diseased part with scar tissue,* making it much easier and safer to cut out.

HELPING YOURSELF

As soon as you know you are to be called for an operation, commence the DIET for cleansing for three weeks, then graduate to the DIET for health.

Study the other topics in this book that relate to your reason for surgery, and merge the recommendations there with these general preparations.

SUPPLEMENT this for IMMUNITY until you know the date of your admission, then intensify this to the full supplements for STRESS.

Take *homoeopathic** Arnica 6 (one three times daily) for the second and third weeks before your operation, and the same dosage of Arnica 30 during the last week. Hold one tablet of Arnica M in your mouth for a minute after receiving your pre-operative injection, but spit out the residue of the tablet before you become drowsy.

After the operation maintain the DIET as best you can – hospital food is often sadly inappropriate for convalescence, but relatives can bring you in home-made Lemon Barley Water and Sprouted Seedlings sandwiches (RECIPES), and you can lobby to get home as soon as you can cope. At the least, continue Arnica 30 (one three times daily) or *Bach Rescue Remedy** (a few drops on your tongue every hour; two drops sipped in half a glass of water once you are allowed to drink), a multimineral and multivitamin and the other SUPPLEMENTS for STRESS.

If PAIN is unexpectedly severe, look up the ideas given under that topic.

Get mobile as soon as you can, and massage frequently the INFLAMED skin around the wound. Remember that the inner wounds take longer to heal than your skin, which is specialized for quick healing after INJURY. Programme ample time for RECOVERY so that you do not feel under any pressure to get well fast. Three months is a reasonable allowance after major surgery.

Above all, maintain a positive and confident attitude throughout. Do not let yourself be dismayed by the odds against success. You are not a statistic, and the great property of healthy living is to defy those odds creatively. Whatever disease got you into your present need, you can abolish that process and start to live in health as soon as you make up your mind and actions to it. Once you have, all your resources for living are at work to get you better. Lead them well, with your enthusiastically purposive outlook.

TEENAGE MEDICAL PROBLEMS

There are at least two occasions in your life when everything you are capable of is called upon at once. Your life before birth is the first, and *adolescence** is the second.

Your teenage years seem at first to be dominated by 'mono'* growth – 'hasn't he shot up!' is the kind of comment you keep on hearing. Your body is obviously getting larger and stronger, and if that were all there was to it these years would be straightforward. But you are changing your form as well, and powerful new emotions are stirring in you. That makes you painfully self-conscious, spending many private hours perfecting or agonizing over tiny details of your appearance. What you wear, and where you are seen wearing it, become terribly important to you. Your mind fills with a huge range of imaginative possibilities you cannot yet evaluate, and has untried powers you scarcely dare explore. All the values of your childhood melt in this white heat, to be purified and fashioned in a new idiom you have yet to find.

Up to now you have confidently anchored your whole outlook on the way of life customary in your family, automatically accepting the frame of reference created for you by your parents. They have 'coloured'* every new experience for you, which was an essential means of simplifying things for you at the time. But all along your own personal nature was in bud, waiting to blossom when the time was right. The real you chooses to emerge during all this turmoil. You realize with a shock that parents and teachers are not infallible, and may have misled you sometimes. Life is suddenly revealed as very insecure, with no-one as reliable as they seemed before. You have to piece together a personal basis for your life, and are open to any ideas that friends may come up with, even though none of you has any notion what they are worth.

It is scarcely surprising that things go astray. Your SLEEP is shortened by late wakeful nights; your FEET and HAIR endure the fashions of the hour. However well you are fed at home, cult foods threaten to undermine your nourishment just when you most need it.

Your DIET must satisfy all your needs in three separate departments – growth, IMMUNE defence and repair, and general vitality. A fully 'organic'* diet always can, however fast you grow or move about, because your 'colour' blueprint evolved alongside this kind of food. Were it now at your disposal, you could be sure of satisfying all your various needs completely.

Most modern foodstuffs fall well below this standard; they are primarily grown for chemical quantity, not nutrient quality. However much you eat of them, some nutritional deficit remains. Growth must take the lion's share of what you can get, but all your needs are struggling. COLDS, ACNE, DANDRUFF and INFECTION penetrate more easily. Some bones (especially your *knees** and *hips**) encounter forces they are scarcely strong enough to bear, and may give way to long, PAINFUL and disabling osteochondritis. You are too easily TIRED, moody and DEPRESSED.

It is tragic to allow such things to undermine your most exuberant years.

HELPING YOURSELF

Get enough SLEEP to rise early feeling at your best, wide awake to every opportunity. Nothing you do after midnight can compensate you for losing out on the following morning.

Then you can breakfast heartily on fruit and whole-grain cereals to power you through the day. Go for baked potatoes instead of chips or pies; fresh vegetables rather than beans or mushy peas; fruit or yoghurt in place of chocolate. That cuts down ACNE, BODY ODOUR, BOILS, COLDS and CATARRH, as well as keeping up your energy. And you keep off the kind of chemicals that provoke ASTHMA, ECZEMA, ALLERGIES and HYPERACTIVITY.

Look out for coffee and cola, and don't drink milk pint after pint – too much of any of these can get you down badly.

If you really want to move add Brewer's Yeast (six tablets daily) or Wheat Germ (a dessertspoonful daily), lots of Vitamin C (up to 1000mg daily) and the Honey-Cider-Vinegar RECIPE to firm up on minerals. Leave SMOKING, drugs and ALCOHOL alone – they can ruin your life faster than anything else.

EXERCISE vigorously for *recreation*; don't be tempted just to watch other people doing it. The real fun is in doing lots of different things that interest you, and working out challenges for yourself. Action of this kind always leads to discovery, to personal impressions you can feel sure of.

Eat with your family at least once a day. You may not like everything they do, but you need to keep in touch. You still have a lot you can share, even when you don't think you need it.

Never let school work DEPRESS you. If it does, tell your parents about it, then maybe your teachers. Never work on so late you cannot relax and enjoy part of your evening. Try finishing difficult work early the next day.

If school work seems pointless to you, be honest and tell your teachers and parents so. There are lots of people around now who realize the imperfections of education and will understand your problem; someone may be able to do something worthwhile about it. Otherwise, make a serious hobby of anything else that interests you, and explore it for yourself. If you don't, you will just get fed up and lose any sense of purpose – which you need more than anything else.

Cope with exams by keeping up on your course work all through the year, and setting yourself a deadline a week before the exam to finish all your revision. After that rest and enjoy yourself, just ticking over on the work. Anything you swot up after that will cloud your mind and unbalance everything else you know – which is much more than it feels. What you need now is not knowledge, but a clear mind to recall it all, apply it to the exam questions, and keep it in perspective.

TEETH

Your skeleton grows towards a potential you inherit, but responds at least in part to the use you make of it in childhood. You can as a result influence dramatically how your child's face will develop.

Almost all of the growth of his head is really enlargement of his face. At birth his brain-box makes up nearly all of his skull, and by six months has attained nine-tenths of its adult size. His face, on the other hand, starts out as little more than a moulding with an insignificant chin that scarcely distorts the egg-shaped outline of his skull. But his face hinges forward and goes on growing downwards throughout his childhood, to become a complete façade only late in his TEENS.

During this growth his face spreads sideways too, but only so far as his use of it demands. If his DIET requires a lot of vigorous chewing his jaws will grow stronger to cope with this. Its muscles will be bulkier and take up more space on the side of his skull, making the upper part of his face much wider. The general effect of this is to broaden his jaw strikingly also, which alters the 'colour'* pattern for the whole of his face. The upper part – his nose, *sinuses** and upper jaw – broadens as well.

This creates much more space for his teeth, whose programme of growth is much more closely determined by inheritance. Not only does chewing fibrous food keep them clean and their gums and cement strong, but it ensures space for them to erupt properly. The huge numbers of orthodontic extractions and operations for EARACHE performed on children reared since 1950 reflects the very soft diet they grew up on.

The same generation suffered appalling *caries** – tooth decay – the result of acid erosion of your tooth enamel. These acids are digested from sugar by *bacteria,** which need a sticky *plaque** of sugar and flour, plastered on your teeth, in which to grow. This condition only occurs significantly on residues of refined food; chewing fibrous food scrubs off wholefood residues before plaque has a chance to form.

*Fluoride** hardens enamel that has already been softened by caries, but makes no other contribution to health. There is no justification for regarding it as an essential nutrient. On the contrary, it is known to be poisonous at doses little above what you now consume, and would not meet the criteria normally laid down to determine the safety of a drug. Already a large proportion of school-children have white mottling of their teeth which is probably caused by accidental over-consumption of fluorides, from food as well as from water. Despite its toxicity, there is no Government laboratory prepare ¹ to check fluoride levels in people who may have too much. Detailed justification of all these assertions is set out fully in Waldbott's BOOK.

Promotion of fluoride as a health benefit can only be rationally explained as a means to justify an official policy of dumping it through the water supply. This rids the aluminium and steel industries of a highly toxic and trouble-some effluent which cannot safely be disposed of otherwise.

HELPING YOURSELF

Eat the DIET for health, and rear your children on it right from weaning. This not only ensures full development of their jaws and faces, but keeps all your gums strong and is self-cleaning. Most teeth fall out because of weak gums, not caries.

If you wish to use sweeteners keep to one type of sugar all day, and change it daily. Ordinary sugar (sucrose) can be rotated like this with malt (maltose), honey or dates (fructose) and grape-sugar or raisins (glucose) through a four-day cycle. This inhibits plaque development because no bacterium can digest more than one kind of sugar; your habit starves out the bacterium that grows on each type almost as soon as it has begun to grow. This tactic only works in combination with thorough cleansing to remove all the day's residues, every day.

Brush your teeth regularly, at least once per day. Plaque must be undisturbed for longer if the tooth decay process is to get established. Discard your brush once the bristles are splayed out – do not damage it by attempting to reach places it was not designed for. If you have troublesome cracks or narrow gaps use more appropriate material – dental gloss, toothpicks, or the 'water-pic' (an intermittent high pressure water jet).

Find a dentist sincerely interested in prevention, and get checked by him regularly. Be suspicious if he needs X-rays to see anything wrong with your teeth – caries starts on the surface, and an experienced dentist can spot it without.

Avoid giving fluoridated toothpaste to children too young to spit out all the washings. It is not intended for consumption, and contains far too much fluoride for safety. If your child is ALLERGIC, HYPERACTIVE or whimpers at the least exertion, stop fluoride in any form. Never give tablets in any case, whatever your dentist says.

MIGRAINE or other severe HEADACHES can arise from cramped jaw development. You need the help of a dentist experienced in Dental Kinesiology (ADDRESS) if the muscles just inside your upper back teeth are tender or your jaw joint grates and clicks.

Good dental hygiene is based first and foremost on a healthy DIET, which positively promotes the health not only of your teeth and gums but of the rest of your body as well. Diet alone can prevent 100% of dental caries and *gingivitis** (INFLAMMATORY gum disease). Second comes regular and efficient cleaning, which can prevent most caries and gingivitis but may also damage your gums; it contributes nothing else to your health, however. Fluoride is at best a poor third, has never been shown to prevent more than 30–50% of caries in any trial, does your gums no good and may harm the rest of you.

TENSION

Animals that drift in water have no need to move or brace themselves against gravity, so POSTURE has no meaning for them. You are so accustomed to the task yourself that you do not notice the effort it entails, except after a prolonged period of illness in bed. Nevertheless a large proportion of your muscular work is devoted to opposing gravity, and requires you to maintain a constant moderate tension in all the muscles of your lower limbs and BACK. Even if your arms can hang limply relaxed at rest, they too must brace against gravity as soon as they move into any other position.

This bracing *tone** is controlled by an elaborate network of nervous reflexes, under your overall *'colour'** direction. They operate automatically, and comfortably within your maximum capacity as a rule, but can adapt to all sorts of influences from higher in your *primal adaptive system.** So when you are angry, alarmed, anxious, NERVOUS or under STRESS of any other kind, your tone reflexes get involved. If they get any less active you FAINT and sink to the ground, which does little to solve your problem. Disturbance which increases the tension of your muscles makes much more sense, since it prepares you for swift action to overcome the stress; so in health this is generally the way things go.

Enhanced tension works well for short-term stresses, but very badly if they persist. Muscles tire, which reinforces the tone reflex and makes them even tenser. Eventually their functional limits are exceeded and they start to hurt. Your posture in that region changes and stiffens, which inevitably affects the grace and efficiency of your whole body. You end up working harder to accomplish less, with apparent reductions in your strength and stamina and your tolerance reduced for any kind of stress.

The muscles most accustomed to postural work are the ones most commonly affected. Most BACKACHE is due to muscle tension in the first place, or is intensified by the addition of muscle tension to prior INJURY of the NERVE, bone or ligaments in the area. *Neck** PAIN and many HEADACHES arise mainly in this way, particularly if your POSTURE is out of balance; people who habitually crane their necks forward are especially prone. Severe pain similar to MIGRAINE can originate from tension in the muscles which brace your lower jaw, unsettled by TEETH in poor alignment.

Prolonged tension symptoms are unlikely to remain confined to muscles, but eventually arouse other functions of your automatic nervous system. The CIRCULATION to your stomach lining empties, leaving it unable to make enough protective mucus. But you are liable to make more acid rather than less, which attacks your blanched stomach lining to cause INDIGESTION and its consequences. Meanwhile your COLON tries to empty itself more vigorously when aroused, producing *irritable bowel** symptoms. Your pulse will race and palpitate violently, and may become irregular. In a crisis the arteries around your heart may actually go into spasm, precipitating a CORONARY.

Tension is a hiding to nothing. You need to know how to release it.

HELPING YOURSELF

If you are usually tense, tender or stiff in any muscular part of your body, consult an *Osteopath** in the first place to discover why. He may be able to correct it within a few treatments. If not, look up the other relevant topics listed here for deeper reasons why his treatment fails, and attend to those that apply to you.

General reduction in all avoidable STRESSES, whether or not they are directly implicated, will improve your tolerance of the one which causes your tension. In particular adopt the DIET for health, which on its own can often ease tension back within bounds.

SUPPLEMENTS of Brewer's Yeast (six daily) and Dolomite (usually one tablet two or three times daily) are safe and inexpensive ways of helping your muscles to give of their best.

Good BREATHING always helps, both during bouts of tension and to prevent them. Singing releases tension particularly well; passionate delivery matters more than skill or competence.

*Alexander Technique** deals with tension by attending fundamentally to your POSTURE and movement. It is highly practical and offers in addition many unexpected insights into your nature and motives. This is the most comprehensive approach available, and highly recommended if there is a teacher near you.

If BREATHING provides inadequate self-help, learn how to relax from an expert. *Yoga,** 'Relaxation* for Living', *hypnotherapy,** psychological *counselling** and *biofeedback** are all appropriate ways of doing this. Explore the ADDRESSES and your Yellow Pages to discover which are available locally, enquire what each has to offer and make your choice. 'Relaxation for Living' is the most down-to-earth, if it is available. If not, get Jane Madders' BOOK.

THREADWORMS, pinworms

WHAT HAPPENS

These are far the most common worm infestation of humans, which we do not share with any other animal. Eggs have been found in faeces 10,000 years old, so they have probably been around as long as we have.

About 60% of school children and up to one in five adults are currently affected in developed countries, without much regard for poverty or social class; so most families have them at some time or other. Fortunately they are harmless, but discovering for the first time that you or your children have them is a nasty shock, and symptoms can be quite a nuisance. Getting rid of them is easy, but keeping free requires constant vigilance if you have school age children or if your work puts you regularly in close contact with people.

Adult female worms are white and about 10mm long, so they are quite easy to see; their resemblance to pins or threads accounts for their various names. They live in your COLON and a few get excreted by accident, but they are easily overlooked in your faeces unless you are heavily infested. You will rarely see a male worm; they are smaller and survive only long enough to fertilize a female. Her 11,000 eggs are then laid in relays, during expeditions outside your anus onto the skin of your buttocks, usually in the evening or at night. The worms' wriggling movements set you ITCHING; if you scratch yourself in your sleep the eggs get under your fingernails and all over your hands. From there you quickly spread them to your face, nose, eyes and mouth; others on your bedding and clothes can survive for anything up to two weeks before dying. A child who sucks his thumb can consume a great many eggs in a very few days, and may consequently get so many adult worms in his bowel that they obstruct it and cause *colic** or are mistaken for *appendicitis*.*

The female worms go on laying for four to six weeks before dying, by which time their eggs have had a chance to be consumed and develop in your intestine to adults in their turn; each generation takes about two weeks. So it only takes a month or so for quite a small initial contamination to become a serious nuisance in an unguarded family.

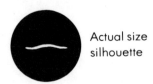

Actual size
silhouette

HELPING YOURSELF

If no-one in your family has symptoms and you have never seen worms in their faeces or around their bottoms, relax. Your defences are pretty good already!

Get everyone to scrub their finger-nails with a good nail-brush (bristles still straight and springy) very first thing every morning, along with thorough washing of their hands and faces. This is the keystone of worm prevention. If you never swallow any eggs from your own worms they die out within six weeks, and any chance INFECTION from outside your family will get nowhere. Everyone will have to keep their finger-nails manageably short, however, for this to work perfectly.

If any of your children suck their thumbs or fingers and worms are about, get them to wear two pairs of pants at night (or one pair plus pyjamas) and launder these daily. Change all bed-linen as soon as you discover an outbreak, and be careful not to billow it about in your haste to get the job done. Keep the dirty linen in a closed bin-liner or separate clothes basket until you can get it all washed.

A whole clove of garlic with its outside skins removed as if for cooking, and moistened with oil, makes an excellent suppository to reduce heavy infestation. Be careful not to bruise the garlic, and to oil it well, or it will make the skin around your anus feel uncomfortably hot; but many worms will be shed with your next bowel action. Two or three cloves of raw garlic, chopped and swallowed quickly with water when fasting, reinforce and prolong this effect. Fresh horse-radish is a less readily available alternative.

It is hard for children to cope with hot-flavoured herbal remedies, so try these others instead. Raw rose-hips have barbs on them which ensnare threadworms quite effectively. Break the hip pods and mix them with jam or peanut butter so that you can swallow them whole. Grated raw carrot is also effective, and no hardship at all for most children. Sage tea (1 teaspoon of herb to $\frac{1}{2}$ pint of water) is a useful complement to either of these.

Powerful one-shot remedies are available from your doctor, but need to be repeated after two weeks to catch newly hatched adult worms. They are not a satisfactory method of long-term control.

*Roundworms** are much larger, the shape and size of earth-worms. They are also far less common, have a more complicated life cycle and can produce significant disease in your lungs as well as your intestine. All the above measures apply, but consulting your doctor is worth while to be sure the infestation clears completely.

WHAT HAPPENS

*Candida albicans** is a yeast which inhabits your COLON from a very early age. In health it usually remains in its *cellular** form, which makes GAS but is otherwise harmless. However if your health breaks down or your DIET deteriorates it can overgrow and spread from your anus onto the surrounding skin. This produces an angry pink damp scaly rash with a fairly sharp edge, with or without crops of red spots. It can be quite ITCHY and sore and is common on babies where their nappies prevent good ventilation.

Unfortunately for women, thrush is very much at home in your vagina and can easily spread there from your bowel. It causes a milky or clotted white VAGINAL DISCHARGE which can itch so badly as to constitute a medical emergency. You can get it in your MOUTH, which usually means it is in your stomach too. BREAST FED babies probably get it in the first place from your nipples.

It thrives wherever there is alkaline moisture, which should not often occur when you are healthy. Most of the *bacteria** that inhabit your skin and colon produce acids which stop thrush flourishing, though there are always a few small colonies around. But the conditions which produce COLITIS, CONSTIPATION and GAS also favour thrush; foremost among them is a meaty diet with sugar and starch but little vegetable fibre.

Women are especially susceptible to thrush because STEROID hormones favour it and dampen your resistance. Pill CONTRACEPTION and PREGNANCY make you particularly vulnerable; you and your partner can pass it to and fro between you, accidentally short-circuiting courses of treatment given to only one of you. DIABETES is sometimes uncovered because thrush has taken advantage of the plentiful sugar its victim provides. But a much commoner cause is repeated or prolonged ANTIBIOTIC treatment, frequently given for ACNE as well as other INFECTIONS.

Milky discharges comprise thrush in its yeast form, which would be fairly easy to deal with. It is the *mycelium** – a network of roots and stems resembling a creeping weed – which is most troublesome. Yeast cells are able to transform into mycelium whenever your health weakens or they are prosperous enough. In mycelial form they are capable of invading your skin, mouth and throat, gullet and upper stomach. Spores from this mycelium can pass unscathed through the acid bath in your lower stomach too, invading your small intestine and reinforcing the colonies already in your colon. Not only can its rootlets penetrate your internal skins, threading their way past your natural defences; but partially digested proteins can travel along them and evade your immune scrutiny. Consequently these fragments do not behave as orderly parts of you, and once in your CIRCULATION can have widespread and devastating effects on your whole body. Its attempts to cope with them can exhaust your IMMUNE system, and produce severe ALLERGIES to a wide range of substances. Once it has the better of you in this way, thrush can take a great deal of time and effort to dislodge.

HELPING YOURSELF

To get rid of stubborn and troublesome thrush you will need to follow a cleansing DIET with plentiful fresh green vegetables and fruit but free of meat, fish, hard cheese, sugar and refined floury food; it would be best to avoid bread altogether to begin with. Start each meal with some raw fresh vegetable or fruit, and add live yoghurt RECIPE to it. Use garlic frequently in salads, and swallow two or three chopped fresh garlic cloves with lots of water at bed-time – if your partner has one with you, neither of you will notice.

Take a SUPPLEMENT of Biotin (50–250 microgm three times daily with food), and a yeast-free B Complex Strong (eg Nature's Own). Extra Iron and Vitamin C sometimes helps in particularly stubborn infections. If your illness has been long and exhausting, supplement your IMMUNITY also.

One or two tablets ($\frac{1}{8}$–$\frac{1}{4}$ level teaspoon powder) Nystatin taken four times daily one hour before your next meal will gradually and harmlessly reduce your thrush population by destroying the part of it in your intestine. This destroys it all eventually, in the way repeated mowing destroys nettles in your lawn. But this may easily take six months, or up to a year if your case is particularly stubborn. Rinse colouring off the tablets and crush them in water to enhance their effectiveness. This remedy is only available on a doctor's prescription, and he may not yet believe yeasts can cause your problems; but you lose nothing by asking him.

Alternatively consult a *Homoeopathic** practitioner, who can offer specific treatment with a potency of Candida Albicans.

When masses of thrush begin to die off you may temporarily be quite ill with 'FLU symptoms as your body struggles to detoxify their remains. Persevere with your cleansing programme, using home-made lemon barley water and cider-vinegar-honey RECIPES to help you. Take courage from this sign that your immune system is getting itself together again, and putting you in order.

'Acidophilus' cultures are expensive and tend to deteriorate; some manufacturers decline to produce them because they cannot guarantee their viability when consumed. Manage without. Remember that any live culture will multiply in favourable circumstances, given time. Therefore repeated daily use of ordinary live yoghurt cultures is in the long run more reliable, and inexpensive.

WHAT HAPPENS

Tiredness is your APPETITE for rest. It arises because you are able to spend energy faster than you can accumulate it, and need a gauge to tell you how fully charged your 'battery' is – not any particular organ, but a whole-body '*colour*'* function. When you feel light-hearted and ready for anything, your battery is well topped up: when you need a great effort of will to cope with STRESS or get going on anything, it is run down.

Like all 'colour' functions it is concerned not only with the amount of your energy reserves but also with their various kinds and qualities. If you exert yourself too intensively in one mode without a corresponding effort in all the others, you tire sooner and in a peculiarly unpleasant way – perhaps with HEADACHE, BACKACHE or an APPETITE or craving you cannot quite define. On the other hand, if the kind of resources available to you are inappropriate for making these deficits good, you cannot properly *re-create*' yourself. But you will try. You may over-eat to appease a yearning you cannot gratify directly or vent your frustrated aggression through sport or log-splitting.

Your automatic NERVOUS system controls this complex ebb and flow, and signals its state to you as some form of tiredness. But, just as you can over-ride the autopilot and take conscious control of your BREATHING, you can out-vote your tiredness and draw deeper on reserves. Their capacity is vast and can cover you through months of perpetual tiredness if need be, but all you spend must eventually be repaid. Otherwise your natural buoyancy and curiosity gives way to irritability, impatience and intolerance of frustration.

You can get into the habit of managing with a half empty battery, but the signs are inescapable if you look for them. First thing in the morning when you should be at your best, you are at your least motivated and need an effort of will to get up and going. Many times daily you do what you feel you should, in defiance of what you would really like to do. A lie-in makes you feel worse rather than better, and at the beginning of a holiday you are like a bear with a sore head. Anything that puts you off your stride – a dental anaesthetic, for example – may set you reeling for days, unable to pull yourself together. All these are signs of your weary instincts reasserting themselves whenever you show the least sign of paying them attention.

If you do not, the process which ran your reserves down this far will exhaust them further. You will gradually become very inefficient, forgetful, NERVOUS, DEPRESSED or diseased in any other way you are susceptible. Eventual breakdown into STRESS disease is almost certain. This may take a benign form, like coming to and finding yourself alone at a cluttered breakfast table, hours after you would normally have cleared it and gone to work yourself. But it may be devastating, like a CORONARY or *stroke*.*

You cannot even hold your own, unfortunately. Chronic depletion of your reserves ages you prematurely; you pay off the debt in lost years. But you need only convert a small net daily loss into a gain to put matters right. After that, RECOVERY is just a matter of time – though quite a bit of it.

Sit down with your partner or confidant and work out where you are going wrong. You may be giving too much, or in too narrow a band of variety; you may be receiving too little good-quality food, or rest, or personal gratification. *Recreation** depends on getting the balance restored, with a small surplus of receipts each day.

Commence the Diet for health, SUPPLEMENTED as for STRESS. Spend enough time on eating each meal to chew it well and relax into good digestion, and eat most of your energy food at breakfast and mid-day. Establish a regular meal routine, and stick to it.

Check yourself for COLDNESS and HYPOGLYCAEMIA.

Stop relying on stimulants such as coffee, strong tea, SMOKING and ALCOHOL. Substitute herbs like camomile, lime (linden), elderflower; roasted grain coffee substitutes; Honey Cider Vinegar and Egg Nog RECIPES.

You need an hour extra rest daily for a minimum of several months. The best time is after your mid-day meal, otherwise when you arrive home. Get your children minded, go to bed properly, and set the alarm. At first you may not sleep, guilty about being there at all. Within two days the alarm will arouse you from deep sleep, to feel groggy for the next hour. But the evening then feels pleasant, and you will sleep better at night as well.

Your reserves cover a wide range of quality, and need to be spent in balance. A narrow '*mono*'tonous job is therefore much more wearing than a varied and '*colour*'ful occupation, particularly one where you can match your mood to what you do. If you are obliged to work monotonously, you need to re-create a balance in your 'colour' signature by spending your leisure on effort of the opposite kind – EXERCISE for office work, something restful after labouring. You know you have it right from the refreshment and ease it gives you in return for the effort you put in. You need about an hour daily and a day each week to re-create yourself from a typical full-time job.

Once you feel all your self-preservative instincts appropriately again and respond to them accordingly, you are on the mend – even though you feel dreadfuly tired and could sleep anywhere. Your reserves will accumulate over three to six months, refreshing your youth.

Never afterwards be tempted to ignore those warning signs again, and take them seriously in your children.

WHAT HAPPENS

If you are underweight, it is not for lack of opportunity to eat. Even if you only managed to offset the OVERWEIGHT tendency enough to keep slim, people would envy your will-power; that you can defy the trend altogether and stay unnaturally thin indicates something much more powerful at work in your nature. So do not expect a simple solution to your problem.

If you were *anorexic** you would not be reading this, but you may wish to help someone who is. She may once have been overweight, and slimmed hard and successfully. But she still thinks she is fat, and is avoiding food to make herself slimmer. She runs on her NERVES, feeling full of energy and really high. She has no insight into what is happening, and cannot accept that she is burning herself out and will be entirely spent within a few months if she carries on this way. From the biological point of view she has lost the ability to conserve herself and is spending her capital.

If you have always been underweight, your growth may have been subtly delayed as a fetus, at the stage when the cells of your metabolic organs were multiplying. If they failed to reach adequate numbers in the time available, the power rating or capacity of those organs is permanently reduced, limiting your growth and stamina to less than your original potential.

The commonest reason for being chronically underweight arises from the way you habitually react to STRESS. Most people are eventually subdued by it, their nervous systems unbalanced into a submissive mood highly conducive to digestion; this helps to explain how they tend to over-eat.

But difficulties in life do not dishearten or slow you down in this way. On the contrary, they arouse you to work harder at solving them. That puts your nervous system in a more anxious, active mood – geared up as if to run away from or fight your assailant in a more primitive world.

This mood is quite incompatible with digestion, so while it lasts you are disinclined to eat. Meanwhile you fret and bustle about, finding things to do, spending much more energy than other people. If you play a court or field game as EXERCISE you seem to your opponents or team-mates to be everywhere at once; yet they may compete with you successfully by standing still and making you do all the moving – and make all the mistakes. You succeed, in sport as in life, by great arousal and alertness, staying carefully in control. As long as you act purposefully and get some respite occasionally you will get more done than others, and succeed better generally; but you may wish you could trade your worrying temperament for their care-free nature.

Prolonged challenges give you a difficult and dangerous time. You never feel free to relax and enjoy yourself, and may go on until you eventually collapse exhausted. Quite a number of students get into difficulties of this kind, faced for the first time with a sustained challenge to cope with on their own. Some young women who become anorexic probably start this way. In both these cases, exceptional circumstances expose a weakness in your otherwise successful and perfectly viable temperament.

HELPING YOURSELF

If you are caring for an *anorexic** young woman, you will already have discovered how futile it is to try persuading her to eat, or convincing her of the danger of her position. Her problem is a serious failure of personal IMMUNITY which would otherwise conserve her resources through her APPETITES and keep her whole.

The key may be those appetites themselves, which have been deranged by nutritional deficiency originating from her previous DIET, made much worse when she began to slim aggressively. One common deficiency is easy to put right. If she needs them she will not notice hidden doses of zinc SUPPLEMENT solution, even though they may taste bitter and conspicuous to you. But she may require a wide range of other minerals, essential fatty acids and vitamins before she will come to her senses. Until then just let your loving care show; persuasion and worry are usually ineffective. If hospital admission and forced feeding are eventually recommended by your doctor, press him to refer you to a centre with particular experience of the condition. But you will probably have to accept his advice in any case, if her danger is extreme.

If you have always been underweight and it seems likely that your *metabolic** organs are undergrown, there is nothing you can do now to change that. But you can cherish fully what you have. Eat well, using the DIET for weight control. Avoid stimulants such as coffee, and never abuse your liver with ALCOHOL. Be careful about PREGNANCY; good FAMILY PLANNING is essential, well beforehand.

If after all you are temperamentally inclined to run on nervous energy and enjoy that, you simply need to be aware of your position. It has great strengths, and is much healthier than submissiveness and complacency in the face of challenge. But it has its weaknesses. You risk burning yourself out and are a prime candidate for alcoholism. So relax deliberately each evening in some other way, and never let your SLEEP pattern get out of hand. Discipline yourself to eat well, and allow enough time to relax over your meals. You do not need stimulant drinks, so avoid them.

Not only will PREGNANCY be a difficult time for you; it may prove quite difficult to conceive in the first place. Once fully mature, your system only settles into pregnancy when your mood is prosperously at ease. You have probably postponed your FAMILY until you are established in life, by which time this protective mechanism is fully operational. Technical investigations will not help you and may increase your anxiety. Instead, act quite out of character for at least a year before going near a gynaecologist. Recognize your nature and the secure establishment you have achieved by it, and set about enjoying their fruits for a while. You may need to give up work, and learn to rest, relax and *re-create** yourself. Get involved with your nieces and nephews and other people's babies. Take your talent for love-making as seriously as you used to take your work. Your *'colour'** will strengthen and come into balance, enabling your *'mono'** fertility to work.

VAGINAL DISCHARGE

Your vagina has to work quite hard to keep healthy and an INFLAMMATORY discharge is evidence of your efforts. It is a *cul-de-sac* rather like your CONJUNCTIVA, ideal shelter for any *microbe** that can reach it. Its entrance lies very close to your *anus,** so that microbes from your COLON have every opportunity to gain access. Once there, they get ample nourishment from the secretions that lubricate it. To make matters more difficult for you, you cannot consolidate your defences: any arrangement you can make is unsettled each month by your PERIODIC blood flow and must be re-established afterwards virtually from the beginning.

What you cannot expect to achieve is total eradication of the microbes that bother you. They are not INFECTIONS from outside, but accustomed inhabitants of your bowel and skin. They have a life of their own, and work out amongst themselves an ecological balance based on the room and resources you are prepared to give them. In health you participate in this debate, and ensure for yourself that the balance achieved will not be at your expense. On this basis it is perfectly possible for all of you to get along very well.

However you need to make alliances to ensure this. Some of the *bacteria** that are inclined to colonize your vagina are quite harmless and inoffensive, whereas FUNGAL INFECTIONS such as THRUSH can be a serious nuisance. Fortunately these two microbes are directly antagonistic to each other, both in your vagina and your COLON where a large reservoir of either can build up. So in health you ally yourself to the bacteria, and let them control the fungi for you.

Under any kind of STRESS, particularly in DIABETES and PREGNANCY, this arrangement breaks down. Even in good health, preventative ANTIBIOTIC treatment can kill off your bacterial allies indiscriminately, opening you up to fungal nuisance. If that is not effectively dealt with, in your bowel as well if necessary, the fungus may transform into a *mycelium** which is much harder to eradicate. Consequently a small minority of women get vaginal THRUSH repeatedly at frequent intervals, yet respond superficially to treatment each time.

Accidental consumption of small doses of antibiotics, present in any flesh-based food you regularly consume, may account for more subtle changes in the variety of bacteria that thrive within you. Some of these can become troublesome a bit too easily. They are resistant to ordinary antibiotics, and some are able to thrive in the absence of air; you can recognize these from the offensive BODY ODOUR they usually cause.

It is well worth consulting a doctor about any stubborn vaginal discharge that is heavy enough to make you wear protection, is accompanied by PAIN or BODY ODOUR or ITCHES severely. If tests reveal no GONORRHOEA,* TRICHOMONAS or other recognizable bacterial INFECTION that your doctor is able to treat effectively, you had better adopt the following measures on your own account.

HELPING YOURSELF

During and after the longest course of anti-fungal treatment your doctor is prepared to give you, reinforce your colonies of acid-forming bacteria by eating two or three cartons daily of live yoghurt made at home according to the RECIPE. You know then that the *Lactobacillus Aerogenes* bacteria, that make yoghurt, are alive and well when you swallow it. Commercial yoghurt has been kept for a variable time, during which the culture stagnates and some bacteria die. And many grocery assistants are not aware of the difference between live and pasteurized yoghurts and give misleading advice. *Natural* yoghurt may still be pasteurized, which kills the germs you need to eat alive.

Support this with a healthy DIET based on fresh raw vegetables and fruit, with whole-grain cereals, a little fresh sea fish if you desire it and a few free-range eggs. Avoid meat in case residues of antibiotics or *steroid** growth promoters should favour THRUSH. Take absolutely no sugar or refined flour, on which fungi thrive.

Avoid the CONTRACEPTIVE pill if you can. You and your partner may otherwise find yourselves needing repeated antifungal medication for many months before coming out on top.

If you use external protection, towards the end of each PERIOD insert a small sponge tampon soaked in live yoghurt high in your vagina overnight. If you use internals, poke the first centimetre out of the introducer and soak it in live yoghurt before you insert it; do this whenever you can, night or day. This gives the lactobacilli a head start over other microbes that may attempt to recolonize your vagina after your menstrual flow has ceased.

Acidophilus cultures are fine in principle, but very expensive and unreliable in practice. Few survive transit and storage consistently, and many that are tested have already died out. Do not be fooled by 'concentrated' cultures – any vigorous colony quickly multiplies to become concentrated, given the chance. You are better off taking fresh home-made yoghurt regularly.

An Iron SUPPLEMENT sometimes helps women with a really stubborn THRUSH problem to solve it finally – one tablet daily is usually enough.

A daily vinegar bath can finally tip things your way. Try douches of Cider Vinegar (two tbsp per litre warm water) or warm *Sitz** baths containing a cupful of Cider Vinegar.

VARICOSE VEINS

WHAT HAPPENS

Blood from your legs has to climb about a metre back to your heart to keep in CIRCULATION. Were gravity the only force involved, it could not be done without intolerable pressure in your FEET. So the journey is designed in stages, between valves that work like the lock gates on a canal. Your leg muscles pump your blood uphill while you move about in the ordinary way; when they relax the valves keep the blood at the height it has gained, waiting to be pumped up the next stage by different muscles. Only in your *abdomen*,* above the top-most valve, do the ordinary pressure rules come back into operation.

The pressure of water in a canal cannot burst lock gates because they rest on rigid walls. Your veins are elastic, so the valves in them are much more easily overcome. Their gates work well as long as they meet easily across the vein's diameter; if it swells fractionally too far, they fail completely. The pressure they let through stretches even more the vein below, so that the next valve down is challenged in its turn. This domino effect can operate whenever the pressure in your abdomen keeps high enough to overstretch the top valve in your legs, and only has a chance to recover when you switch gravity off by lying down.

Your main leg veins are buried deep inside your muscles, where they are pumped most effectively. The smaller low-pressure veins on the inside surface of your legs drain into these unseen deeper ones at intervals, through short connections protected by yet more valves. When these fail the surface veins swell and stretch under pressure into the ugly contortions called varicose veins.

These are unsightly and uncomfortable, but that is only the beginning of your problems. Blood flows through your swollen veins more slowly at the best of times, and stops altogether when the back-pressure from above is at its worst. This stagnation hinders the refreshment of your muscles, which begin to ache. The worst combination of circumstances occurs when you stand around for any length of time; your muscles are POSTURING enough to need a good blood flow, but not pumping sufficiently hard to provide it. A brisk walk usually relieves the congestion and back-pressure well enough to overcome this.

The nuisance to your skin is less acute, but more destructive in the long run. It may ITCH for years before chronic starvation of air and blood eventually cause varicose ECZEMA. If this is not nursed back to health you risk breakdown or *ulceration** in areas whose circulation is no longer sufficient to support the necessary turnover of skin *cells.**

Straining because of CONSTIPATION usually underlies this chain of events, as well as PILES. The weight of a full congested COLON or pregnant womb hinders your chances of recovery between pressure bouts. *Steroids** from PREGNANCY, medication or CONTRACEPTIVE pills make veins baggy and vulnerable. So do the heavy burdens of *waste acids** in your blood after rich meat meals. Standing about in very warm clothing, straining to lift but walking little, is the worst occupation. Rowing and weight-lifting are the sports to avoid.

HELPING YOURSELF

Avoid prolonged hot baths unless you are prepared to finish by splashing your legs generously with cold water. To shower is preferable, finishing on cold for 30 seconds, attending especially to the insides of your legs. You will see the veins contract visibly with this treatment. Do this before going to bed. You can repeat the cold spray whenever your legs feel tired, tight, heavy or swollen.

Block up the foot of your bed 10–15cm (4–6"). This dramatically reduces the night-time pressure of blood in your veins and gives them a chance to contract to a normal size.

Keep your DIET healthy and simple, seldom indulging in rich meaty food.

SUPPLEMENT this with Rutin 50–100mg after three meals daily with Vitamin C 500–1000mg and Vitamin E 200IU each time.

Witch Hazel (Hamamelis) ointment 5–10% or undiluted Cider Vinegar is often very comforting, especially if varicose veins leak or bruise.

Firm support from appropriate stockings is appropriate to both sexes; your doctor can prescribe them, but at a higher prescription charge.

EXERCISE regularly, especially walking, swimming or cycling. If you sit for long put your feet well up, at least level with your hips. Avoid crossing your legs.

Notice how you lift, and how easily your bowel empties. Correct any hint of straining by correcting your POSTURE or dealing with CONSTIPATION, respectively.

If you use the CONTRACEPTIVE pill, consider changing your method.

In PREGNANCY, start precautions against varicose veins early.

VIRUS INFECTIONS

Viruses are among the smallest living things on earth. Some of them are remarkably sophisticated even so, but none carries the apparatus necessary to reproduce itself – only the blueprint for the job. Consequently it is obliged to multiply itself by taking over the reproductive apparatus of an appropriate *cell*.* This constitutes INFECTION, so far as the victim is concerned. What is worse, viruses destroy the cells they use in this way, so that many of the disorders associated with viruses are dangerous to life. Influenza, polio and smallpox are the best known historical examples, but the Human Immuno-tropic Virus of AIDS has all our attention at the moment.

The most commonly encountered viruses have a preference for one of two routes of entry to your body: your BREATHING passages or your intestines. In either case they then fall into two further classes according to whether they remain around the point of entry or tend to spread from there throughout your body. The common COLD is a localized respiratory illness, whereas MEASLES, MUMPS, influenza and CHICKENPOX are generalized ones. *Gastro-enteritis** is typical of local intestinal diseases, whereas polio and 'gastric 'FLU'' spread from the same place to have general effects. This simple classification gives no inkling of the huge diversity within the virus kingdom but it will probably cover your experience. AIDS constitutes an important exception.

People vary a good deal in their resistance to virus attack. The key to this is strong and perfectly formed skin at the points of entry, since viruses which cannot get into the cells of that skin are easy prey for your defensive secretions. And until they penetrate cells, viruses cannot multiply.

Once your resistance is overcome, each virus particle that successfully penetrates a cell takes over its apparatus to make replicas of itself. This is only possible for one virus at a time, as a substance called interferon is also produced which prevents the entry of any other virus.

After a period of *incubation** varying from a few days to several weeks, the cell bursts to release many thousands of virus particles, which then each seek a new cell to infect. It does not take long for the destruction to become widespread, a trend prevented only by mobilization of your IMMUNE proces-ses. Your general defences maintain a stiff resistance while specific *anti-bodies** are prepared. Their arrival in quantity marks the turning point in your disease, sometimes accompanied by a rash – evidence presumably of the reaction which occurs when antibody and virus combine.

Symptoms then rapidly clear, but TIREDNESS and lack of stamina persist while your effort is diverted into replacing the destroyed cells. They are inconspicuous and thinly spread by comparison with SURGICAL wounds, but cost you just as much effort to repair. Until healed they are weak points in your outer defences which can easily let in other INFECTIONS; deterioration in your condition just when you were expecting to RECOVER often means that a *bacterial** complication has set in. Even if you succeed in warding this off, the increased effort of doing so drains your resources further.

HELPING YOURSELF

Ventilate rooms well in good weather. Avoid tobacco SMOKE.

During the autumn and winter when people COUGH a good deal, avoid crowding together in confined spaces. Shop at quieter times, preferably on breezy days. Infections are much more easily spread from person to person on foggy damp days with no wind.

BREATHE through your nose whenever possible (you cannot when EXERCISING hard). This makes excellent use of the organ specialized for filtration, air conditioning and self-defence, and keeps the passages clean.

Dress according to the temperature. Chilling your neck in cold weather can reduce the power of your local defensive lymph GLANDS and let a SORE THROAT begin.

Fresh live raw salads bolster resistance better than preserved, frozen or reheated food. So have some raw carrot, fresh leaves or sproutings RECIPE daily, especially through the winter (from February to May).

SUPPLEMENTS of Vitamin C help your white blood cells defend you. Take a tiny pinch of crystals in a breakfast juice daily, more frequently when under pressure.

Garlic is a powerful natural antiseptic. Keep a Garlic Lozenge RECIPE in your cheek for an hour at a time on days when your throat feels vulnerable. The reek is minimized if you avoid chewing or bruising it.

Live within your energetic means. Otherwise well defended people are much more prone to INFECTION when they over-work. Moving house is an especially difficult time.

WARTS: Verrucae

WHAT HAPPENS

All warts originate as a VIRUS colony settling on your skin from the outside. Like illegal immigrants arriving by sea on a lonely beach, they do not automatically come to the notice of your police force; they are able to thrive there for months or years because they do not attempt to penetrate inland. After about two years a colony tends to die, and the wart either recedes gradually to nothing or degenerates into a shell that can be picked cleanly out of its socket, which then heals over. But until that decay begins the wart is *contagious*, which means that it can be spread by surface contact; so you may discover a younger seedling wart on any piece of nearby skin. Even so they are not usually very INFECTIOUS; the few people who end up covered with them seem to be especially susceptible, and need to boost their general IMMUNITY.

Warts have a special liking for the skin of your hands and feet that is ridged with finger-prints, and can be easily distinguished from other kinds of lump because they disturb the print pattern locally. This is quite clear under a magnifying lens, and warns you that a wart you thought was cured has re-grown. But verrucae, and some warts on hard-worked hands, can get buried under great piles of *corny** skin which obscure their origin; you need to trim off the insensitive skin with a razor to see the tell-tale cauliflower pattern. Bear in mind if you do this that exposing the active wart makes spread more likely; very crusty warts are otherwise slow to spread. The term verruca is simply Latin for wart, but has come to be reserved for warts on your feet. They arise in the same way as warts anywhere else on your body, but then behave a little differently because of the special properties of the skin on the soles of your feet.

When they occur elsewhere on your body, warts may take a different form. Crops of small flat crazy paving stones on your genital skin multiply fast and are very contagious and sore, but also respond quickly to treatment. You will probably need to attend a hospital Special Treatment clinic for venereal diseases to get them adequately dealt with. The kinds of wart that stand out on stalks from your eyelids and elsewhere are a nuisance and tend to recur after treatment, but do not seem to multiply.

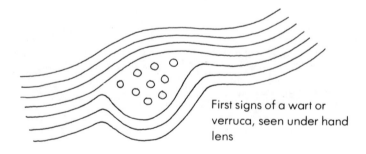

First signs of a wart or verruca, seen under hand lens

Warts are less troublesome on tough, cool, well-ventilated FEET. The DIET for health helps to proof your skin against them.

When you discover a wart, keep it covered with adhesive tape – a dressing is unnecessary. That will prevent spread in dry conditions.

Cover warts on your feet with rubber socks in pools and showers; chemists usually supply them. Most swimming pool authorities now admit you if you cover your verruca properly; it is a pity to miss out on swimming for something so harmless.

Homoeopathic treatment often deals well with warts, but you may need the help of a homoeopathic practitioner to select the right remedy. You can safely try one of these three possibilities first, if you prefer:

> For *a crop of large warts* try Thuja 30, one dose four hourly for three doses. Wait a few days for an effect; no further dose is needed while the warts are waning, but you can repeat it if they do not. *Many small warts* anywhere, especially on your face and eyelids, may require Causticum 12 instead, taken three times daily. Men with *genital warts** should try Antimony Tartrate 12 or Sepia 6, three times daily.

Local treatment of warts on tender skin is tricky, and best done with medical help; but you could safely try using Thuja Ointment first.

If you tackle large crusty warts on your hands and feet, nag away gently for weeks for the best result. Aggressive measures can arouse a wart as if you had only pruned it; a rosette of new seedlings then sprouts around the scar of the old.

A Caustic Pencil (Toughened Silver Nitrate) is very effective, but use it almost dry; the dampness of skin licked meanly or slightly clammy is quite enough. Rub the pencil tip on the damp wart for a minute, and cover it when dry. The surface blackens, parches and separates cleanly in a few days. Treat it three times a week, unless it gets sore or cracks. When you think it has all gone rest for a week, and watch to see if the fingerprint heals undisturbed; resume treatment if tell-tale bubbles appear instead.

If you have a warty growth dangling on a long stalk, you can safely destroy this by positioning a noose of strong thread around its base as near to your skin as possible, and pulling it tight. Any PAIN this causes is quick to settle. After a few days the dead lump falls off, when you should treat its stump once with a Caustic Pencil, as in the previous paragraph. If it recurs, you can repeat the process when it again reaches a manageable size. You are likely to win in the end.

WATER

Life originated in water, and cannot manage without it. When animals began to take greater advantage of sunlight and the air by living on dry land, they had to carry their water with them. The composition of your body liquid still resembles the saltiness of the sea.

Your first home was a bag of water at your mother's body heat, and at birth three-quarters of your body was water too. You have dried out a little since then, but water still comprises about three-fifths of the weight of an average adult. That works out at around forty-one litres or nine gallons.

Three litres of this CIRCULATES in your blood vessels, exchanging freely with another nine litres distributed through your tissues but remaining outside them. This twelve litres of fluid is your portable sea, contained by your skin as an aquarium for your true substance to bathe in. Your real body, the *cells** descended from your mother's fertilized egg, still live very much like sea creatures.

Two litres of water trickle into this reservoir each day, and the same spills out as urine, sweat and other moist excretions. This turnover brings in your food and mineral necessities and flushes out your wastes. Its composition is carefully controlled by your kidneys and primal adaptive system, so that your body cells are kept in absolutely constant conditions.

These cells contain the remaining thirty litres of fluid, but its composition is quite different. Like all sea creatures they work hard to keep out salt, scavenging instead the other minerals on which their life depends. This charges them ELECTRICALLY, which maintains their vital energy.

Chemical pollution of the soil with agricultural chemicals and the fallout from industrial smoke runs off into streams and eventually soaks down into the underground water-courses that feed springs. Both nitrate fertilizers and more complex organic chemical pesticides get into the water supply in this way. The nitrates stimulate growth of vegetation in ditches and streams, which may choke itself to death or be killed by pesticides washed out of the soil by a shower of rain. This vegetation decays into small organic *molecules** like methane (marsh gas), which then combine with the chlorine (and sometimes fluoride) added at the waterworks to produce volatile chlorinated hydrocarbons, similar to the carbon tetrachloride used to clean stains off clothing. These, and residues of the original chemicals, are too expensive to remove from drinking water at present without huge increases in water rates. The water supplies in many parts of the United Kingdom are at times heavily contaminated in this way.

This unwelcome range of additions to your food and water inevitably contaminates your body, unbalancing your mineral economy and spoiling your electrical vitality. But you can use your natural intimacy with water to correct these disturbances. Bathing increases appreciably your excretion, which is made more efficient by careful selection of what you drink.

HELPING YOURSELF

A prolonged warm bath is very relaxing, but not the most efficient way to cleanse your body. If the water comes from a hot copper tank you will in addition have time to absorb more copper than is good for you.

Bathe more briefly in hot water to make you perspire freely, then finish with a cold splash or shower. Sweating through wide open skin pores enhances your excretion. The cold phase then closes the pores, extruding the last of the sweat which would otherwise have dried out to clog and irritate them. It also has a bracing, tonic effect on the whole of you.

Bathing in the sea or fresh water ponds is very refreshing and healthy, hampered only a little by the pollution they usually contain. Indoor swimming pools are spoiled by the chlorine used to control cross-INFECTION between so many people at close quarters. If you are obviously irritated by chlorine use an open air pool instead, or any pool disinfected by an alternative process. Your local government office should have the information you need.

The mineral quality of spring water varies considerably. If you wish to drink fresh water as an alternative to stimulant beverages, try one of the bottled varieties. Buxton, Highland Spring, Malvern and Perrier are good sources that use glass bottles, which are superior to plastic but more expensive. Malvern is now generally bottled in plastic, but can still be obtained in glass by special pleading with the manufacturers. Of the other sources bottled in plastic, Volvic is among the least expensive and the best. Try to avoid sources that contain natural fluoride – you get plenty from other sources if you need any at all.

Avoid cooking in aluminium pans, especially if your water supply is fluoridated and when cooking acid fruits. Very considerable amounts of aluminium dissolve in the cooking water in these circumstances, and are liable to be absorbed and get deposited in your brain *tissues*.* Some people have troublesome *abdominal* PAINS while digesting food contaminated in this way.

Filtration greatly improves the taste and composition of your mains water supply. The range of domestic equipment available at reasonable prices is quickly improving and well worth considering. The least expensive is the 'Brita' jug with a hopper that works on the same principle as a filter coffee jug; the filter candles require renewal every month or so. The 'Mayrei' is next most economical, but fits onto your tap spout and comes off under pressure; if you wire it on, you are obliged to filter washing water as well. There are several systems that overcome this by providing a separate tap for filtered drinking water, but these require plumping into your kitchen main and are therefore more expensive initially. Some of these systems are able to remove fluoride. These filters differ widely in the absorbent systems they employ. The most promising system available avoids these however, and depends instead on the principle of reverse osmosis; its only draw-back is to remove nutrient minerals as avidly as the poisonous ones. It is available from Fileder Systems Ltd (ADDRESS).

WEANING

Weaning is an event whose meaning has been blurred and practically rubbed out by modern infant feeding practice. Worse than that, it has become a negative – the withdrawal or termination of BREAST FEEDING. Some women do it arbitrarily at a certain age, perhaps when they wish to resume their careers. But it more often happens by accident, when you are advised to stop during a minor illness or difficulty. This is the blind leading the partially sighted – no doctor, and few health visitors, understand nutrition or motherood well enough to over-ride wholesome maternal instincts in the way they often do.

To appreciate the full significance of weaning you need to consider the state of affairs in principle, before infant milk formulae and baby foods were invented. A baby is equipped to obtain all his nourishment at mother's breast throughout his infancy. This situation is very simple: his food resembles the bloodstream from which he fed before he was born, and is clearly recognizable as distinct from all the alien creatures met since his birth – *microbes*,* plants, and animal proteins – which compete with him for space to live their lives, and yet must eventually nourish him too. For the moment he is not required to face that conundrum, but has two quite separate functions to perfect – digestion and IMMUNITY to encroachment by other *organisms.**

As the months of his infancy go by, progress is easy to see. Within about six weeks he can take feeding in his stride, and settles into an efficient and reliable routine. Progressive changes in the character of his faeces indicate his increasing digestive skill. The combined benefits of protection conveyed in his milk, and the gathering momentum of his self-defence, keep him disease free. Meanwhile he learns to chew, gains control of his hands and FEET, and makes more and more subtle use of his senses to explore the people and home around him. Step by step he is striding along several paths at once towards the end of his infancy.

You know the moment is approaching when his digestion becomes so efficient as to leave very little residue. Quite a few healthy babies seem CONSTIPATED for a few weeks during their fifth month, yet do not ail for it; at most they pass a little jelly material every day or two. This perfect poise may continue a few weeks, but cannot last – he is about to outgrow what milk can give him.

Then comes one of life's great 'Aha!' discoveries. He suddenly realizes several important things at once; whichever penny drops first sets off an avalanche. He can sit up, use his hands to get objects into his mouth and is accustomed to your behaviour at mealtimes. He begins to hunger for something more than your milk can give him, and has the skill to digest it. He is confident that he can defend himself against anything hostile. Suddenly it occurs to him to taste what you are eating, and he tells you so.

That is weaning – worth waiting for, and celebrating. Your permanence dawns on him soon after, and he is free of infancy for good.

HELPING YOURSELVES AS PARENTS

BREAST FEEDING is the most vivid lesson in the simplicity of living you are ever likely to get. But its clarity is easily obscured, especially by well-intentioned but foolish advice based on gross underestimates of what you and your body are capable of. Plan for it during your PREGNANCY, believe in it, and have the nerve to work it out instinctively, using only your common sense. Let your baby tell you what he wants; rely on his wisdom, not on books – neither yours nor those of your advisers!

Do not allow anyone to give your baby anything else at all, right from birth. This is more difficult at first if he is very premature or tiny, when you need to express your wishes and work them out with your doctors and nurses. But there is never any reason to give any other food or drink as a matter of routine. Many families have reared several children without ever buying a baby's feeding bottle!

If your baby digests his food so perfectly as to excrete nothing solid for a week or two in his fifth month or so, do not panic. CONSTIPATION is quite different; he is obviously straining and uncomfortable at times, quite unlike the contentment of this natural state. On the other hand, do not worry if this phase seems not to happen. It may be obscured by overlapping trends which do not mean he is any less healthy.

When you are accustomed to reading your baby's moods, it is not difficult to spot when he first wants to taste something solid; do not keep on offering things before then, 'just to be sure'. You should not hurry his weaning any more than you should hurry his birth.

When the moment comes, mash something suitable from your plate and offer him a *very small* amount on a spoon. It is the *'colour'** he needs, not the quantity. He will repeatedly savour and marvel at a lot of new things before hungering for them. Do not stuff him to prove a point of your own. You can save him from the habit many adults have, of eating lots just to get full.

Weaning is positive – *to* solid food, not *from* your breast. Assume he will go on feeding from you just as before, probably for another six months if you will let him. Meanwhile he will gradually want more and more of the foods he gets a liking for. So long as large undigested lumps do not appear in his faeces, you can let the quantity grow at his pace. Give things that are poorly digested a week's rest, and then be sparing with them.

There is no use or advantage in manufactured baby foods, and one serious snag to all of them – they have lost all the 'colour' they ever possessed. Your milk is live and full of 'colour', and to lose it is a serious set-back for your baby. So wean him to your own healthy DIET of fresh foods, prepared from the best live produce you can get. It is terribly sad to see a loving mother breast feed proudly for six months, then fall back on 'baby foods' in the false belief that they are superior. They are not even particularly convenient: nothing can be easier than feeding him from your own plate.

WHAT HAPPENS

'Health for All by the Year 2000!' is a slogan adopted a few years ago by the World Health Organization. Few doctors in Europe believe this can be done. They know the volume of disease and misery presented to them and suppose it to be only a fraction of the sum of human suffering. They go on to argue that if this is true in the developed world, how much more it must be so elsewhere!

This reasoning is grounded in a fundamental misconception, that health is some perfect or ideal *'mono'** state of body, mind and spirit. Were this so, it would indeed be scarcer than the rarest of diseases. On the contrary, health rather than sickness is the rule for most people, throughout most of your body, for practically your entire life span – even in 'mono' terms. It is unimaginable otherwise that you could succeed in being born.

To argue otherwise would be like agonizing over road accidents without appreciating how tiny a proportion of all journeys involve one. There is a remarkable degree of order in drivers' behaviour on the road: most people drive carefully almost all the time. The secret of this remarkable accomplishment is not difficult to see. Your safety on the road depends not on your destination, on your knowledge of the Highway Code or on the car you drive (assuming it is in working order). It depends entirely on how you are driving it, every instant of the journey, every inch of the way.

Health is well portrayed in this analogy. It is not any destination in life but a way of travelling through it. It stems from a *'colour'** APPETITE for harmony and ease that you share with all things living. This hunger drives all that happens in your body and everything you do. It holds the simplest *molecule** and *microsome** in place yet enables your entire person to function as one simple whole, itself in turn a comfortable part of larger wholes – your family, your school, your community.

Once you have seen this for yourself, a great many puzzles become clear. You realize that technology, far from promoting your health, tends to undermine it. Material development has accustomed you to act through machines and adopt a mechanical or economic outlook on life in which your individual health lies hidden and dormant. You are not even encouraged to trust it as an organizing force any more, but urged to rely instead on 'mono' screening tests and MEDICAL CHECK-UPS which merely search intermittently for signs that your 'colour' wholeness has already broken down. This seems good to the doctors and technologists who design services like these; they have the most invested in this outlook. In reality it is far too costly to be practical for all, and achieves nothing real. Above all, by questioning your integrity yet doing nothing to promote it, this approach actually undermines your health as well as your happiness.

Health is not available at all this way, in twelve years or twelve thousand. But you can have it today, by a simple 'colour' transformation in your outlook on life. Real health is readily and freely available to all, right now.

HELPING YOURSELF

Read Templegarth Trust's BOOKLET (ADDRESS) or Mansfield's BOOK to explore the nature of health further. You cannot deduce it logically, but you can get near. The main thing is to see it clearly for yourself; it does not matter whether or not you can explain it to anyone else.

Having got the general idea, set about exploring it in practice – there is no other way. Your health is a matter of your own experience, not of scientific proof.

Start where you are now, by acting from resources you already command; it gets you nowhere to be wistful for what you do not have. Healthy action is self-reinforcing, so your situation will automatically improve. But the work may initially be hard – it does get easier, as things come into order.

Start with your body. Correct your DIET, cut down your ALCOHOL and SMOKING, get good SLEEP and deal with chronic TIREDNESS. Work hard to reduce TENSION and overcome DEPRESSION, which could stop you in your tracks. Look at your other ailments, many of which are topics in this book. You need your body to become an efficient vehicle for what you want to do.

Your personal relationships will probably by then be already thriving better, on healthy body-work. To improve them further, listen carefully to what people say and how they say it. Pay attention to them, and to what you say and do towards them. You do not need to think out any kind of plan – simply get the communications right.

Notice what this has done for your emotional life. Once you have clear and honest communication with the people around you, there is much less reason to accumulate emotional rubbish. Your self-respect comes into balance because others are also listening to you; everybody holds one another in high regard.

If you are already adapted to unemployment your time is your own, to extend your income by growing food and developing crafts, services and human-scale technologies, as you think fit. Unemployment is not so much a handicap as an opportunity.

A job that serves your own purposes poorly is more difficult, especially if you are used to, and dependent on, a high wage or salary. Work towards changing it, but take your time.

Living this way is real and wholesome, each day complete in itself. There is no need to set targets and fret when you miss them. Savour and enjoy every moment of the process of living for its own sake, and trust the direction and destination of your life to look after themselves.

Index and Glossary

Apis mel Homoeopathic

Appendix/itis/Grumbling Appendix *Inflammation in/pain of the short
narrow cul-de-sac of intestine,
resembling the finger of a glove,
attached where the intestine joins to
the bowel.* COLITIS; CONSTIPATION;
THREADWORM

Arnica Homoeopathic

Arsen alb Homoeopathic

Arterial disease ANGINA;
ARTERIOSCLEROSIS†

Arthritis BACKACHE

Ascorbic acid Vitamin C; SUPPLEMENTS

Atheroma ARTERIOSCLEROSIS†

Athlete's Foot FEET; FUNGUS DISEASES†

Atopic ⎰
Atopy ⎱ ASTHMA; ALLERGY;† HAY FEVER

Bach Flower Remedy Chapter Four;†
ADDRESS; BEDWETTING; EARACHE;
SHINGLES; SMOKING

Bacteria *Microbes (singular bacterium)
unlike plants or animals, able to
multiply independently, usually
susceptible to destruction by
ANTIBIOTICS.* ANTIBIOTICS; BOILS;
COLITIS; CONJUNCTIVITIS; CYSTITIS;
EARACHE; FOOD POISONING; FUNGUS
INFECTION; NAPPY RASH; NITS; PERTUSSIS:
SORE THROAT; TEETH; THRUSH; VAGINAL
DISCHARGE

Bad breath BODY ODOUR†

Baldness HAIR LOSS†

Basal temperature COLDNESS;† MEDICAL
CHECKUP

Béchamp, Prof. Antoine INFECTION;†
MUMPS

Bee BITES

Behaviour, bad HYPERACTIVITY

Belladonna Homoeopathic

Bidor Anthroposophic

Bifidus *A bacterium that favours
digestion.* NAPPY RASH

Bile ALCOHOL; COLITIS; GALL STONES†

'Biodynamic' *Grown according to 'organic'
principles on a farm managed as a
whole, self-sufficient organism; as
advocated by Rudolph Steiner.*
Anthroposophy; DIET (Nutrition); FOOD
POISONING

Biofeedback *Indicating unconscious or
'colour' events in your body by 'mono'
means, so that you can learn to control
them consciously.* NERVES†

Biotin SUPPLEMENTS†

Bircher-Benner, Dr M. DIET (Nutrition)†

Blackcurrant seed oil SUPPLEMENTS†

Blackhead ACNE;† OVERWEIGHT

Blisters ECZEMA

Blood Cell ANAEMIA; BLEEDING; Lymph
GLANDS; IMMUNITY

Blood Sugar DIABETES; HYPOGLYCAEMIA

Bones, soft OSTEOPOROSIS†

Borage seed oil SUPPLEMENTS†

Bowel *The large intestine or COLON, which
functions mainly as a cauldron in
which nutrients and moisture are
salvaged, aided by some bacterial
fermentation, to leave useless faeces
which are then expelled*

Bowel, irritable COLITIS†

Breakdown STRESS†

Breath-holding *A common reaction to
anger and frustation in the toddler age-
group. May result in collapse and a
brief fit.* EPILEPSY

Bronchiectasis PERTUSSIS†

Broncho-pneumonia BRONCHITIS†

Bruise SPRAINS

Bryonia Homoeopathic

Bunion FEET†

Burial DYING

Calciferol Vitamin D; SUPPLEMENTS†

Candida (albicans) BOILS; FUNGUS
INFECTION; NAPPY RASH; SUPPLEMENTS;
THRUSH†

Cantharis Homoeopathic

Cap CONTRACEPTION†

Capsule SPRAINS†

Carbohydrates *Foods like starch and
sugars that can be digested to simple
sugars like glucose that can be
absorbed into the CIRCULATION.*
DIABETES

Carbo veg Homoeopathic

Carbuncle *A BOIL with many
interconnected compartments*

Caries TEETH†

Cartilage *Flexible gristly material which
lines the surfaces of bones inside joints
to aid their lubrication and
nourishment.* SPRAINS

Causticum Homoeopathic

Cells *The smallest independent building-
block of the body, with the same basic
design but many variations according
to tissue.* BREAST PROBLEMS; CHICKEN

POX; COLDS; DANDRUFF; IMMUNIZATION;
MULTIPLE SCLEROSIS; PROSTATE
PROBLEMS; RADIATION; RECOVERY;
RHEUMATISM; SORE THROAT; SPRAINS;
THRUSH; VIRUS INFECTIONS; WATER

Red blood cells ANAEMIA; ANGINA

White blood cells AIDS; COLDS;†
IMMUNITY

Cerebrospinal fluid CONCUSSION†

Cervical smear *A microscopic examination
of cells in mucus scraped from the neck
of the womb, to detect pre-*CANCEROUS
*changes at a very early and treatable
stage.* MEDICAL CHECK-UP

Chamomilla Homoeopathic

Change, the c. (of life) MENOPAUSE†

Chartered Physiotherapist Chapter Four;†
ARTHRITIS; BACKACHE; JOINTS; PAIN

Cherry plum Bach flower remedy

Chestnut bud Bach flower remedy

Chilblain CIRCULATION†

Chill *A feeling that you cannot get warm,
perhaps with muscle pains and shivers.*
'FLU

Chiropractor Chapter Four;† BACKACHE;
JOINTS; POSTURE & MOVEMENT

Cholesterol *A fatty substance present in
certain foods and made in the blood
from sugars, especially when these are
eaten in excess.* COLDNESS; CORONARY;
GALL STONES

Choline Vitamin B group; SUPPLEMENTS†

Chronic *Protracted, because healing effort
is insufficient or frustrated*

Chronic bronchitis BRONCHITIS†

Cirrhosis ALCOHOL†

Clinical Ecologist Chapter Four;†
INFLAMMATION

Clinical Psychologist Chapter Four;†
SMOKING; STRESS

Cocculus indicus Homoeopathic

Coffea cruda Homoeopathic

Cold sores CHICKEN POX†

Cold urticaria CIRCULATION†

Colic *A pain that comes in short sharp
pangs lasting up to a minute or two,
separated by rests of similar length.
Usually arises from the opposed
involuntary contraction of intestinal,
urinary or uterine muscle.*
CONSTIPATION; PAIN; THREADWORM

Coliforms BOILS; COLITIS; GAS; NAPPY RASH

Colloidal *Stable mixture of a solid in
water to form a jelly-like semi-solid
substance.* CATARACT

Colon COLITIS;† ANTIBIOTICS

'Colour' Chapter One;† ACNE; AIDS;
ALLERGY; ANGINA; APPETITE; ASTHMA;
BACKACHE; BREAST FEEDING; BREATHING;
CANCER; CIRCULATION; COLDS;
CONCUSSION; CORONARY; COT DEATH;
DEPRESSION; DIET (Nutrition); DYING;
FAMILY PLANNING; FUNGUS INFECTION;
HEADACHE; HYPERACTIVITY; IMMUNITY;
INFECTION; ITCHING; MENOPAUSE;
MISCARRIAGE;† MOUTH ULCER; MULTIPLE
SCLEROSIS; NERVES; PAIN; POSTURE &
MOVEMENT; PREMENSTRUAL TENSION;
RADIATION; RECOVERY; RETIREMENT,
AGEING; SCHIZOPHRENIA, PSYCHOSIS;
SLEEPLESSNESS; SUPPLEMENTS; SURGERY;
TEENAGE MEDICAL PROBLEMS; TEETH;
TENSION; TIREDNESS; UNDERWEIGHT;
WEANING

Community Counsellor Chapter Four;†
Psychiatrist

Concepsus *The products of conception.*
MISCARRIAGE†

Conception *Creation of a fertile egg and
the very beginning of* PREGNANCY.
FAMILY PLANNING†

Congenital *Inherited, or acquired before
birth.* SURGERY

Contagious *Capable of transmission by
touch.* WARTS†

Contrast bathing CIRCULATION;†
INFLAMMATION

Convalescence ELECTRICITY DISEASE;
RECOVERY†

Convulsion EPILEPSY;† FEVER

Corns ECZEMA; WARTS

Cough Drops Anthroposophic

Counselling Chapter Four;† HEADACHE;
SMOKING

Cramp CIRCULATION; MIGRAINE;
RHEUMATISM

Cranial osteopath Osteopath; CONCUSSION

Cremation DYING

Dance/drama ADDRESS; IMMUNITY;
POSTURE & MOVEMENT

Death Chapter Three;† DYING

Delirium *Acute and severe confusion and
excitement of the mind.* CHICKEN POX;
FEVER

Dermatitis ECZEMA†

Diaphragm ANGINA; BREATHING;† PILES;
RECOVERY

Diarrhoea COLITIS; FOOD POISONING;
SICKNESS & DIARRHOEA

Dieting OVERWEIGHT
Difficult child HYPERACTIVITY
Digestion *Process of rendering down food into fragments small enough to be absorbed from the intestine.* INDIGESTION
Diphtheria IMMUNIZATION
Disc, slipped BACKACHE†
Dislocation JOINTS;† SPRAINS
Disseminated Sclerosis MULTIPLE SCLEROSIS†
Diverticular disease COLITIS; CONSTIPATION†
Diverticulitis COLITIS; CONSTIPATION†
Dolomite Mineral SUPPLEMENT†
Double pneumonia BRONCHITIS
DS MULTIPLE SCLEROSIS
Ductless gland see gland, ductless below
Dyspepsia INDIGESTION†

Elbow JOINTS†
Electro-magnetic radiations ELECTRICITY DISEASE;† HYPERACTIVITY
Eleutherococcus senticosis Siberian Ginseng, SUPPLEMENTS†
Emphysema BRONCHITIS†
Encephalitis *Inflammation of the brain.* CHICKEN POX;† HEADACHE; MEASLES; MUMPS
Endometriosis PERIOD PROBLEMS†
Engorgement BREAST PROBLEMS†
Enuresis BED-WETTING†
Enzyme *The basic machine tool of metabolism, made of protein and designed to carry on a specific chemical reaction very efficiently and very fast. Thousands of different types exist in human cells and body fluids.* INDIGESTION; PROSTATE PROBLEMS
Epidemic *Major outbreak.* INFECTION; MEASLES
Essential fatty acid DANDRUFF; SUPPLEMENTS
Eurhythmy Anthroposophic; POSTURE & MOVEMENT; Chapter Four†
Eye BLEEDING; CATARACT; CONJUNCTIVITIS

Faeces *Waste material in or emptied from the bowel*
Fascia SPRAINS†
Fat ARTERIOSCLEROSIS;† DANDRUFF
Fatigue TIREDNESS;† MULTIPLE SCLEROSIS
Fatty Acids, essential ARTERIOSCLEROSIS;† DANDRUFF; SUPPLEMENTS

Fetus *Baby in the course of development before birth*
Fever, glandular Glandular fever
Fissure *A crack in the lining of the anus.* BLEEDING; CONSTIPATION
Fitness *Readiness for efficient and sustained effort, indicated in 'mono' by the maximum rate at which oxygen can be consumed.* EXERCISE
Fits EPILEPSY;† FEVER
Flat feet FEET†
Flatulence *GAS in the bowel*
Floater *Small particles in or parts of the eye which interfere with its functions sufficiently to be visible.* CATARACT
Fluoride TEETH
Folic acid Vitamin B group; SUPPLEMENTS†
Foot bath HEADACHE
Fragador Anthroposophic
Free radical CATARACT; INJURY; RADIATION;† RECOVERY; SUPPLEMENTS

Galea HAIR LOSS†
Gastritis *Inflammation of the stomach.* INDIGESTION
Gastroenteritis ANTIBIOTICS; VIRUS INFECTIONS
Gene *A unit of the chemical code of inheritance; conveying a single characteristic.* RADIATION
Genital herpes CHICKEN POX†
Genital warts WARTS
Gentian Bach flower remedy
Germ *Microbe, but usually confined to mean bacterium;* ANTIBIOTICS; BODY ODOUR; INFECTION
German Measles IMMUNIZATION
Gingivitis TEETH†
Gland, ductless *An organ or tissue that produces a hormone and secretes it directly into the CIRCULATION*
Gland, lymph Lymph GLANDS
Gland, swollen Lymph GLANDS
Glandular fever 'FLU; Lymph GLANDS;† NITS
Gonorrhoea VAGINAL DISCHARGE
Gorse Bach flower remedy
Graphites Homoeopathic
Growth, a growth *A new lump of tissue that is getting larger, but is not necessarily CANCER*
Gut *The complete intestinal tube, from mouth to anus*
Gymnastics POSTURE & MOVEMENT

Habituation *Acclimatization to repeated exposure to a chemical, by intensifying its metabolism to a harmless end-product.* ANTIBIOTICS†

Haemoglobin *The red oxygen-carrying pigment of red blood cells.* CIRCULATION

Haemolytic Streptococci *Streptococcal bacteria that produce a toxic chemical capable of breaking up red blood cells and causing a variety of prolonged illnesses.* SORE THROAT

Haemorrhoids PILES†

Hallucination SCHIZOPHRENIA†

Hand ARTHRITIS†

Hardening of arteries ARTERIOSCLEROSIS†

Head injury CONCUSSION

Healer Chapter Four;† INJURY; SCHIZOPHRENIA, PSYCHOSIS

Healing crisis INFLAMMATION

Health Chapter One;† WELLBEING

Heart ARTERIOSCLEROSIS; CIRCULATION; CORONARY;† CYSTITIS

Heartburn INDIGESTION†

Herbs Chapter Four;† INJURY

Hernia SURGERY†

Herpes CHICKENPOX†

Hips ARTHRITIS; FEET; JOINTS;† SPRAINS; TEENAGE MEDICAL PROBLEMS

Histamine ALCOHOL; ITCHING; SCHIZOPHRENIA, PSYCHOSIS

HIV AIDS;† INFECTION

Hogweed BITES

Homoeopathy Chapter Four;† ACNE; ADDRESSES; ASTHMA; BITES; BLOOD PRESSURE; BOILS; BRONCHITIS; BURNS; CATARRH; CHICKEN POX; COLDS; CONCUSSION; EARACHE; ECZEMA; EPILEPSY; FOOD POISONING; GAS; HAY FEVER; INDIGESTION; INFLAMMATION; INJURY; MEASLES; NITS; PAIN; PERIOD PROBLEMS; PERTUSSIS; PSORIASIS; SPRAINS; SURGERY; WARTS

Hormone *Chemical messenger, produced by an internal ductless gland to regulate a bodily function.* CONTRACEPTION; OSTEOPOROSIS; PERIOD PROBLEMS; PROSTATE PROBLEMS; steroids

Hydroxocobalamin Vitamin B_{12}; SUPPLEMENTS

Hypersensitivity ALLERGY†

Hypertension BLOOD PRESSURE†

Hypnotherapy Chapter Four;† NERVES;† PAIN

Hysterectomy *Surgical removal of the uterus.* MENOPAUSE†

Ignatia Homoeopathic

Immunosuppressive *A drug intended to damp down IMMUNE reaction.* HAIR LOSS

Impaction *Interlocking of two jagged ends of a broken bone, eliminating movement and concealing the fracture.* JOINTS†

INCUBATION *Hidden development prior to outbreak.* CHICKEN POX; MEASLES; MUMPS; VIRUS INFECTIONS

Infludo Anthroposophic

Influenza (Immunization) 'FLU; IMMUNIZATION

Inositol SUPPLEMENTS†

Insect repellent BITES

Insulin *The chief hormone concerned with sugar metabolism.* DIABETES;† HYPOGLYCAEMIA

Intermittent claudication ANGINA†

Intestine *Synonymous with gut, but usually refers to the part between the stomach and the bowel*

Intolerant, Intolerance ALLERGY;† HAY FEVER; PSORIASIS

Ionizer BRONCHITIS; COUGHING; ELECTRICITY DISEASE;† SICKNESS & DIARRHOEA

Ipecacuana Homoeopathic

Irritable bowel COLITIS;† TENSION

IUCD CONTRACEPTION*

Jaundice ITCHING†

Jelly fish BITES

Kinesiology Chapter Four;† MIGRAINE; TEETH

Knees ARTHRITIS; FEET; JOINTS;† SPRAINS; TEENAGE MEDICAL PROBLEMS

Lactation *Milk-making.* BREAST PROBLEMS

Lactobacillus *A digestive bacterium found in yoghurt.* THRUSH†

Lecithin SUPPLEMENTS†

Lens CATARACT

Leukaemia *A CANCER of blood cells.* RADIATION†

Life, change of MENOPAUSE†

Ligaments *Sinews holding bones together.* BACKACHE; BREAST PROBLEMS; FEET; SPRAINS

Liver *The body's principal* organ *of metabolism.* GALL STONES; OVERWEIGHT

Lobar pneumonia BONCHITIS†

Louse NITS†

Lumps, breast BREAST PROBLEMS

Lymphatic Lymph GLANDS;† NOISES IN YOUR HEAD

Lymphocytes *White blood cells made in lymph* GLANDS, *recording and conveying* IMMUNITY

McCarrison, Sir R. DIET (Nutrition)

Malignant, malignancy *A* CANCEROUS *growth*

Massage Chapter Four;† INJURY

Mastitis *Inflammation of the breast.* MUMPS

Mastoiditis *Abscess in the middle ear, forcing its way into deeper cavities; a serious cause of severe* EARACHE

Medical herbalist Chapter Four;† EPILEPSY; MENOPAUSE; PERIOD PROBLEMS

Meditation BLOOD PRESSURE; HEADACHE; NERVES†

Membrane *Lining skin.* MULTIPLE SCLEROSIS

Menière's Syndrome NOISES IN YOUR HEAD†

Meningitis *Inflammation of the wrappings of the brain.* HEADACHE; IMMUNIZATION; PERTUSSIS

Merc sol Homoeopathic

Metabolism *The 'mono' business of the body, taking the form of chemical reactions controlled by enzymes.* ACNE; ALCOHOL; COLDNESS;† DEPRESSION; EXERCISE; FEVER; 'FLU; GALL STONES; INJURY; MIGRAINE; OVERWEIGHT; RADIATION; RHEUMATISM

Microbe *Any micro-organism – bacterium,* FUNGUS, *or virus.* ACNE; ANTIBIOTICS; APPETITE; BOILS; BREATHING; CANCER; CONJUNCTIVITIS; ECZEMA; FOOD POISONING; Lymph GLANDS; IMMUNIZATION; INFECTION; NAPPY RASH; PERTUSSIS; PSORIASIS; SORE THROAT: VAGINAL DISCHARGE; WEANING

Microsome *The basic component of independent life identified by Béchamp as the microzyma, capable of transforming into a microbe, aggregating with others to form a cell or surviving dormant for immense spans of time.* INFECTION; WELLBEING

Microwaves ELECTRICITY DISEASE;† FAMILY PLANNING; MULTIPLE SCLEROSIS

Minerals SUPPLEMENTS†

Mixed Pollen Homoeopathic

Molecule *The basic particle of a stable chemical substance.* RADIATION; WELLBEING

'Mono' Chapter One;†AIDS; ANGINA; APPETITE; ASTHMA; BACKACHE; BREAST FEEDING; CANCER; CIRCULATION; COLDS; CORONARY; COT DEATH; DIET; DIET (Nutrition); DYING; ELECTRICITY DISEASE; EXERCISE; FAMILY PLANNING; HEADACHE; HYPERACTIVITY; IMMUNITY; ITCHING; MENOPAUSE; MOUTH ULCER; MULTIPLE SCLEROSIS; NERVES; OSTEOPOROSIS; PAIN; POSTURE & MOVEMENT (see BACKACHE); PREMENSTRUAL TENSION; RETIREMENT, AGEING; RHEUMATISM; SCHIZOPHRENIA, PSYCHOSIS; SLEEPLESSNESS; TEENAGE MEDICAL PROBLEMS; TIREDNESS; UNDERWEIGHT; WELLBEING

Morbillinum Homoeopathic

Moschus Homoeopathic

Movement POSTURE

MS MULTIPLE SCLEROSIS

Mucus *Clear* CATARRH.

Mustard Bach flower remedy

Mycelium ANTIBIOTICS; FUNGUS INFECTION;† INFECTION; THRUSH; VAGINAL DISCHARGE

Nat mur Homoeopathic

Naturopath Chapter Four;† APPETITE; INFLAMMATION; SUPPLEMENTS

Nausea *A feeling that you want to vomit.* SICKNESS & DIARRHOEA

Neck HEADACHE; JOINTS;† TENSION

Negative Ions *Microscopic particles charged with negative electricity.* ELECTRICITY DISEASE

Nettle BITES

Neuralgia *A* PAIN *arising in a malfunctioning nerve.* SHINGLES†

Neurotic, Neurosis SCHIZOPHRENIA,†

Niacin Vitamin B_3; SUPPLEMENTS†

Nose ALLERGY; BLEEDING; COLDS

Nutrient *Basic component of nutrition, ready for metabolism*

Nutrition DIET†

Nutritional Medicine Chapter Four†

Nutritionist *Graduate of a course in nutritional science.* APPETITE

Nux vomica Homoeopathic

Oestrogen *Woman-hormone. Steroid;* MENOPAUSE

Oral contraceptive   CONTRACEPTION†

Organ   *Any multicellular part of an organism with a distinct structure and function, exercised on behalf of the whole organism.* ACNE

'Organic'   *Grown without recourse to chemical sprays in naturally cultivated soil, fertilized only with composts.* APPETITE; DEPRESSION; DIET (Nutrition); FOOD POISONING; NOISES IN YOUR HEAD; PERIOD PROBLEMS; RETIREMENT, AGEING; SUPPLEMENTS; TEENAGE MEDICAL PROBLEMS

Organism   *A living whole creature, fending for itself as part of Nature.* Chapters One & Two; WEANING

Osteoarthritis   ARTHRITIS;† FEET

Osteochondritis   TEENAGE MEDICAL PROBLEMS†

Osteopath   Chapter Four;† ARTHRITIS; ASTHMA; BACKACHE; JOINTS; MULTIPLE SCLEROSIS; PAIN; PERIOD PROBLEMS; POSTURE & MOVEMENT

Ovary   *The female sex organ, producing eggs and steroid hormones.* MENOPAUSE; MUMPS

Ovulation   *Production of an egg by an ovary.* BREAST PROBLEMS; COLDNESS; FAMILY PLANNING; PERIOD PROBLEMS

Oxygen   *The atmospheric gas in which animals burn food metabolically to release usable energy.* COLDNESS

Palpitation   *Heartbeats violent enough to draw your attention to them.* STRESS

Pancreas   *A digestive organ and* ductless gland, *best known for making the hormone insulin.* DIABETES; HYPOGLYCAEMIA; MUMPS

Pangamic Acid   Vitamin B$_{15}$; SUPPLEMENTS†

Pantothenic Acid   Vitamin B$_5$; SUPPLEMENTS†

Paranoia   *Unreasonable feeling of being persecuted.* SCHIZOPHRENIA†

Parotidinum   Homoeopathic

PAS   *Primal Adaptive System,* Chapter One;† AIDS; RECOVERY; TENSION

Pasteur, Louis   INFECTION

Peptic ulcer   INDIGESTION;† BLEEDING

Peritonitis   *Inflammation of the inside lining of the abdomen.* CONSTIPATION; PAIN

Pertudoron   Anthroposophic

Pertussin   Homoeopathic

Petroleum   Homoeopathic

Phagocyte   *Cell that consumes and destroys waste material or microbes, making them harmless.* IMMUNITY

Pharynx   *The chamber behind the throat where the nasal cavity joins it.* COUGHING

Physiotherapy   Chapter Four;† MULTIPLE SCLEROSIS; and see Chartered Physiotherapist

Pill, the   CONTRACEPTION

Pink eye   CONJUNCTIVITIS†

Pinworms   THREADWORMS†

Placenta   *Organ by which the fetus is attached to his mother's womb.* FAMILY PLANNING

Plaque   TEETH†

Plasma cells   *White blood cells actively making* IMMUNE *antibody.*

Platelets   BLEEDING†

Pneumonia   PERTUSSIS; SURGERY

Podiatrist   Chapter Four;† BACKACHE

Poisoning   FOOD POISONING

Post-natal depression   DEPRESSION

Pre-conception   FAMILY PLANNING

Premenstrual tenderness   BREAST PROBLEMS

Pressure   BLOOD PRESSURE; TENSION

Priessnitz pack   ECZEMA;† ITCHING;† PAIN; SLEEPLESSNESS

Primal adaptive system   Chapter One;† BREATHING; CANCER; CONCUSSION; CONTRACEPTION; COT DEATH; DEPRESSION; NERVES; PERIOD PROBLEMS; PREMENSTRUAL TENSION; STRESS

Primrose, Evening   SUPPLEMENT† of essential fatty acid

Pruritus   ITCHING†

Psychiatrist   Chapter Four;† *A medically qualified doctor who specializes in the diagnosis and treatment of mental illness.*

Psychosis   SCHIZOPHRENIA†

Pubescence   *Onset of puberty, the physical component of adolescence.* BREAST PROBLEMS

Pulsatilla   Homoeopathic

Pulse pressure   *Difference between the highest and lowest levels of aortic* BLOOD PRESSURE *during a single pulse beat. At rest this is a measure of the rigidity, and therefore ageing, of the walls of the arteries.* MEDICAL CHECK-UP†

Pyridoxine   Vitamin B$_6$; SUPPLEMENTS†

Pyroluria   *Congenital inability to break down the waste metabolic product* cryptopyrole and thereby save zinc and pyridoxine; cryptopyrole is wasted through the urine instead. SCHIZOPHRENIA

Quinsy SORE THROAT†

Rabies INJURY
Recreation *Re-creation and rebalancing of spent 'colour' vitality.* BLOOD PRESSURE; EPILEPSY; FAMILY PLANNING; NERVES; RETIREMENT, AGEING; SLEEPLESSNESS; STRESS; TEENAGE MEDICAL PROBLEMS; TIREDNESS;† UNDERWEIGHT
Reflexology Chapter Four;† FAINTING
Relaxation Chapter Four;† BLOOD PRESSURE; NERVES;† SMOKING; TENSION
Relaxation for Living ADDRESS; HEADACHE; INDIGESTION
Rescue Remedy Bach Remedies, Chapter Four;† BURNS; CONCUSSION; FOOD POISONING; SPRAINS
Rest TIREDNESS
Rheumatoid Arthritis ARTHRITIS; RHEUMATISM
Rhinitis ALLERGY;† ASTHMA; CATARRH
Riboflavin Vitamin B$_2$; SUPPLEMENTS†
Ribs JOINTS†
Riding POSTURE & MOVEMENT
Ringworm FUNGUS INFECTION
Roseola ACNE†
Roundworms THREADWORM
Rubella IMMUNIZATION
Rutin SUPPLEMENTS†

Saccharine disease *A term coined by Surgeon Cdr Cleave RN to cover all those seemingly separate disorders that frequently occur together in one individual, and have as a common cause overconsumption of sugar.* ARTERIOSCLEROSIS; CORONARY; DIABETES; GALL STONES; OVERWEIGHT; PILES; peptic ULCER
Sailing POSTURE & MOVEMENT
Scabies *Infestation of the skin by a burrowing mite.* ITCHING
Scald BURN† *caused by a hot liquid or vapour.*
Scurf DANDRUFF†
Scurvy *The disorder arising from gross deficiency of Vitamin C.* DANDRUFF
Sebaceous (gland) ⎱ ACNE; BODY ODOUR;
Sebum ⎰ DANDRUFF;†
Seborrhoeic dermatitis ⎰ EARWAX; ECZEMA†

Seizure EPILEPSY†
Selenium Essential trace mineral; SUPPLEMENT†
Selye, Prof Hans BOOKS; STRESS
Septic spot BOILS
Sepia Homoeopathic
Shock *Collapsed condition of the body arising from mental or physical blow.* BITES; FAINTING; INJURY
Shoulder JOINTS†
Siberian Ginseng SUPPLEMENTS†
Sickness 'FLU
SIDS *Sudden Infant Death Syndrome.* COT DEATH†
Silica Homoeopathic
Sinew SPRAINS†
Singing BREATHING
Sinuses *Caves in the head bones.* TEETH
Sinusitis *Inflammation of the sinus(es).* ASTHMA; CATARRH; MIGRAINE;† PAIN
Sitz bath CYSTITIS;† PERIOD PROBLEMS; VAGINAL DISCHARGE
Slipped disc BACKACHE
Solar plexus BREATHING†
Special diet DIETS for special purposes
Speech therapist *Graduate of a recognized course in elocution and voice production.* BREATHING
Spine BACKACHE;† FEET; POSTURE
Spore FUNGUS INFECTION
Spot ACNE; BOIL
Sputum *Mucus or CATARRH produced by COUGHING.*
Staph BOILS
Star of Bethlehem Bach flower remedy
Steiner, Rudolph Anthroposophy, Chapter Four†
Sterilization *Surgical stoppage of ability to have further children without interfering with other sexual functions.* MENOPAUSE
Steroid ACNE; BLEEDING; CONTRACEPTION;† DANDRUFF; ECZEMA; INFLAMMATION; MENOPAUSE; MOUTH ULCER; MUMPS; OSTEOPOROSIS; PERIOD PROBLEMS; PILES; VAGINAL DISCHARGE
Stimulant *Substance that excites or arouses.* RHEUMATISM
Sting BITE
Stomach CATARRH;† GAS; INDIGESTION
Strain STRESS†
Strep(tococcus) *Type of bacterium.*
Stress disease STRESS†
Stroke ARTERIOSCLEROSIS; BLOOD PRESSURE; DIABETES; MENOPAUSE

Subarachnoid haemorrhage BLEEDING *from an artery near the base of the brain, a surgical emergency.* BLOOD PRESSURE

Sudden infant death COT DEATH

Sugar see carbohydrate; saccharine disease

Sugar diabetes DIABETES†

Sugar, low HYPOGLYCAEMIA†

Suicide DYING

Sulphur Homoeopathic

Survival Chapter Two;† STRESS

Tamus Homoeopathic

Temporal lobe epilepsy EPILEPSY†

Tenderness *Painfulness to pressure.* RHEUMATISM

Testis *Male organ of reproduction.* MUMPS

Tetanus IMMUNIZATION; INJURY

T-helper lymphocyte AIDS†

Thiamine Vitamin B₁; SUPPLEMENTS†

Thuja Homoeopathic

Thymus IMMUNITY†

Tinnitus NOISES IN YOUR HEAD†

Tissue *A characteristic arrangement of cells and supportive structures, specialized for a particular functional purpose within an organ or part of the body.* ASTHMA; CANCER; CIRCULATION; 'FLU; PAIN; SURGERY; WATER

Tocopherol Vitamin E; SUPPLEMENTS†

Tone POSTURE; TENSION

Tonsillitis *Inflammation of the tonsil(s).*

Tonsils and Adenoids SORE THROAT

Trachea *Wind-pipe*

Traditional Chinese Medicine Chapter Four;† ADDRESS; ASTHMA; BACKACHE; BLOOD PRESSURE; CIRCULATION; EPILEPSY; FAINTING; IMMUNITY; MENOPAUSE; PAIN

Trichomonas VAGINAL DISCHARGE

Trimethylamine BODY ODOUR†

Tryptophan, L-tryptophan SUPPLEMENTS†

Tuberculosis COLDNESS; IMMUNITY; IMMUNIZATION

Tumour *Growth, not necessarily* CANCER

Ulcer
Ulceration
  } *A hole through a skin or membrane.* BURNS;† INDIGESTION;† MOUTH ULCER; VARICOSE VEINS

Umbilical cord *Pipeline connecting fetus to placenta.* FAMILY PLANNING

Urinary *To do with kidneys, bladder, and all connecting pipework.*

Urticaria ITCHING†

Uterus *Female organ in which the fetus grows; otherwise the source of* MENSTRUATION

Vaccination IMMUNIZATION†

Varicella CHICKENPOX†

Vasectomy *Male sterilization.* PROSTATE PROBLEMS

Vegan *One who chooses to eat food exclusively from plants.* DIET

Verruca FEET; WART†

Vertigo *False sensation that the world is spinning round you.* NOISES IN YOUR HEAD

Vine Bach flower remedy

Virus *A class of primitive microbe that depends for reproduction on using the cellular apparatus of another organism.*

Visualization *Technique for concentrating one's* IMMUNE *resources upon a specific problem by imagining the scene.* ANGINA;† PAIN

Vitamin *Originally 'vital amine', a class of nutrient essential to human survival.* SUPPLEMENTS†

Vocal cords COUGHING†

Vomiting FEVER; FOOD POISONING

Walnut Bach flower remedy

Wasp BITES

Waste acids BREAST PROBLEMS; CYSTITIS; 'FLU; MIGRAINE;† RECOVERY; RETIREMENT, AGEING; RHEUMATISM

Whooping cough PERTUSSIS†

Wild Oat Bach flower remedy

Wind-pipe COUGHING†

Windsurfing POSTURE & MOVEMENT

Womb Uterus

Worm THREADWORMS†

Wound *Local damage to some part of the body.* BLEEDING; Lymph GLANDS; SPRAINS

Wrist See SPRAINS

Yoga Chapter Four;† ARTHRITIS; BACKACHE; BLOOD PRESSURE; BREATHING; IMMUNITY; MULTIPLE SCLEROSIS; NERVES;† PAIN; RETIREMENT, AGEING; SMOKING

Zinc *Essential trace metal.* SUPPLEMENTS†

Zoster SHINGLES†